Milady's
SKIN CARE
AND
COSMETIC
INGREDIENTS
DICTIONARY

Third Edition

Natalia Michalun
and
M. Varinia Michalun

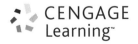

CENGAGE
Learning™

Australia • Brazil • Japan • Korea • Mexico • Singapore • Spain • United Kingdom

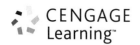
CENGAGE
Learning™

Milady's Skin Care & Cosmetic Ingredients Dictionary, Third Edition
Natalia Michalun and M. Varinia Michalun

President, Milady: Dawn Gerrain

Publisher: Erin O'Connor

Acquisitions Editor: Martine Edwards

Senior Product Manager: Philip Mandl

Editorial Assistant: Elizabeth Edwards

Director of Beauty Industry Relations: Sandra Bruce

Senior Marketing Manager: Gerard McAvey

Production Director: Wendy Troeger

Senior Art Director: Joy Kocsis

For product information and technology assistance, contact us at **Professional & Career Group Customer Support, 1-800-648-7450**

For permission to use material from this text or product, submit all requests online at **cengage.com/permissions.** Further permissions questions can be e-mailed to **permissionrequest@cengage.com.**

Library of Congress Control Number: 2009923921

ISBN-13: 978-1-4354-8020-9

ISBN-10: 1-4354-8020-1

Milady
5 Maxwell Drive
Clifton Park, NY 12065-2919
USA

Cengage Learning products are represented in Canada by Nelson Education, Ltd.

For your lifelong learning solutions, visit **milady.cengage.com**

Visit our corporate website at **cengage.com.**

Printed in the U.S.A.
3 4 5 11

CONTENTS

FOREWORD

This book is already in its third edition, which represents a significant passage of time since it was initially written. However, the same elements that motivated us to write the first dictionary remain true today. Cosmetic ingredients continue to be a mystery to most consumers and to many professionals in the skin care area. This is becoming even more daunting now, given the pace at which new ingredients and concepts are making their appearance into the market—not to mention the quantity. Cosmetic consumers continue to wish to understand products' confusing names, government regulations, and cosmetic-industry naming and labeling practices. However, consumers and professionals are increasingly more savvy in their evaluation of skin care products and are paying more attention to ingredients. People want to know (and justifiably so) what to expect of the products they are using. If no one can give them a satisfactory answer, they are more often seeking ways to find out for themselves. This book intends to provide the reader with the tools necessary to achieve this understanding.

We have always believed that the value of ingredients lies in their interaction with the skin or with one another to make a formulation effective. Thus, to better understand product performance, this book contains a short section on skin care physiology and theory. Please note that this is a dictionary and not a skin care book. The skin care section is presented as an aid for overall understanding and should not overshadow the book's main purpose.

If this dictionary were to be read from cover to cover, some information would seem repetitive, especially in the initial chapters. This repetition has been purposely created, as we believe that readers will search for specific information or definitions, and we want them to find detailed information under each heading.

Finally, Chapter 4, the definition of terms, almost always represents how an item relates to the formulation and to the skin. It does not provide a technical definition of the item, as we consider this a separate issue.

For this edition, we have used many U.S. and European sources of information. We are grateful to all of them, but there are far too many to mention individually. We wish to express our very special appreciation to Mr. Joe DiNardo, who, as always, and with infinite patience, helped us to understand the newest ingredients and the nuances of formulations. Our four reviewers have been invaluable and we want to express our most sincere appreciation for their efforts. They have done an incredibly careful job of reading every page and making useful comments and notes that often required us to refine some concepts and/or review our entries to make them more precise and clear. This edition is much better for it. Finally our appreciation goes to Martine Edwards and Philip Mandl of Cengage Learning, whom we thank for their gracious understanding of the personal factors that postponed, for several months, the completion of this edition.

We hope this book provides the answers to the many skin care cosmetic ingredient questions that estheticians and cosmetic consumers share.

Dedication
To the estheticians who,
with great dedication and sincerity,
work to help their clients have and maintain
healthy, more beautiful skin.

PART I
The Skin

Introduction

Cosmetic products without the human skin have no purpose. Their value, efficacy, function, virtue, and problems are valid only within the framework of the skin they are supposed to beautify and enhance. To give cosmetics, especially skin care products, any value, it is important to understand how the products work on the skin, what function or functions they perform, what problems they solve, and how the skin may react to them. Without this understanding, the use of skin care cosmetics remains a mystery, for some translated into "hope in a jar," and for others the "miracle solution" to a multitude of skin problems. The first step to solving the mystery of skin care product performance is by asking two basic questions: What are cosmetics? And what can they be expected to do?

Rigorously defined, cosmetic products are those that remain on the surface of the skin. More loosely defined, skin care cosmetics are those that penetrate the top layer of the skin but do not reach the skin dermis and are not absorbed by the blood capillaries. Products that penetrate the dermal layer and are absorbed by the capillary system are classified as pharmaceuticals and are subject to Food and Drug Administration (FDA) safety requirements. In the strictest sense of the FDA's interpretation, cosmetic products are formulated for the beautification of the skin and should make no claim of performing in a drug-related fashion.

The original definition of cosmetics was established in 1938, when the skin was believed to be almost impermeable. While this is still the legally applicable definition, there is now a vastly improved understanding of the skin's physiology, its chemical components, and the relationship between skin structure, skin chemistry, and cosmetic ingredients. There is no longer doubt about the capacity of a large number of ingredients to penetrate the skin and provide a level of benefit. While this rapidly advancing comprehension has benefited skin problems such as acne and hyperpigmentation, the primary beneficiary has been the antiaging category. It has also balanced the emphasis in skin care among ingredients and ingredient combinations that not only "correct" but also "prevent" skin problems and damage from occurring. It is now recognized that one of the "prevention" keys are antioxidants. They are particularly important as a means to minimize cellular damage caused by free radicals, and hence help to prevent skin aging. Therefore, antioxidants are now incorporated into a wide range of products, from moisturizers to eye creams to sun and post-sun products.

New knowledge has led to the development of new, "high-tech" cosmetics and the cosmeceutical category—a term fusing "cosmetic" with "pharmaceutical." Some manufacturers specialize in cosmeceuticals, and the leaders in this category are often found in the United States. They tend to patent specific ingredient technologies, and frequently complete molecules, as well as trademark their names, using these as themes running throughout a brand. This results in the leading cosmeceutical companies often developing, incorporating, and using their own set of specialty ingredients.

The speed of development in cosmetic technology may continue to accelerate with results that are currently difficult to predict. Nanotechnology is an example. Leading cosmetic companies are investing heavily in nanotechnology research. It may be the next "big thing" in cosmetics, however, its future is still uncertain.

While there is a proliferation of "high-technology" ingredients and an expansion of new cosmetic categories, such as cosmeceuticals, this is being complemented by a simultaneous increase in the scientific understanding of botanicals. As researchers identify with greater precision the individual chemical constituents of botanicals, more specifically targeted and sophisticated natural ingredients are being incorporated into cosmetics. Carotenoids, for example, are now recognized for their vast number of individual components, each performing specific functions. Cosmetic chemists are also emphasizing the use of individual flavonoids, peptides, polyphenols, and phytoestrogens. In addition, cosmetic chemists are combining natural ingredients with synthetic ones, providing a larger set of ingredients with which to formulate. The result is that products formulated with natural ingredients represent one of the fastest-growing cosmetic market segments.

Consumer interest in natural and/or organic cosmetics is growing together with confusing marketing terminology. Natural and organic cosmetics fall into poorly defined and unregulated categories, where an array of different terms are used to present product benefit. Consumers can be easily confused by the nuances of such terms as "natural," "derived from natural materials," "extracts from natural plants," "organic," and "percentage of organic content within the total content of botanical materials." At times, statements are presented in ways that seem to indicate that consumers should seek products that are only 100 percent natural if they want cosmetic purity or something that is "best." In reality, "natural products" all contain a certain percentage of synthetically manufactured ingredients.

In an attempt at differentiation, statements such as "preservative-free" are made. However, this is not possible since the addition of preservatives in a cosmetic is a regulatory requirement for product safety and health reasons. "Paraben-free" may be the case, but this does not mean the product is preservative-free, as the formulation may contain another preservative system that does not have the same long research history of safety as parabens.

There have been significant changes in cosmetic formulations since 2000. Dermatological and chemical researchers have increased their understanding of skin physiology, the chemical components of the skin, and how these interact with chemicals applied to the skin in the form of cosmetics. The cosmeceutical concept has expanded and become even more sophisticated and effective. Botanically based products are experiencing a renaissance and renewed credibility as formulations become increasingly sophisticated in their technologies and results. Sunscreens are including more UVA protection and PABA has been practically eliminated from all sunscreen formulations. Animal-based ingredients are now replaced with plant-based or synthetically manufactured equivalents. Antioxidants are strongly emphasized as a means to prevent skin damage and skin aging. Nanotechnology is coming to the forefront of research and development with unknown limits. No one can promise a solution to all skin problems, nor can they promise "eternal youth." However, the cosmetic industry is continuously working toward vast improvements in the appearance and health of the skin, while making "aging slowly and gracefully" an attainable and pleasing reality.

Cosmetic products and the chemistry behind them can be extraordinarily valuable to the skin. Since a product's ultimate purpose is to benefit the skin, in order to properly evaluate the positive actions or potential problems of cosmetic products and their ingredients, it is crucial to have an understanding of how the skin works, how and why a product may or may not penetrate it, and what care individual skin types and conditions may require. It is, therefore, impossible to meaningfully discuss product ingredients without correlating product performance to skin function.

Throughout the following chapters, a large number of the skin's chemical components and other technical terms will be introduced. They are purposely presented and/or discussed to familiarize the reader with the new terminology used by cosmetic chemists, which is also being incorporated into new product formulations. For definitions of some of these terms, see Chapter 4.

Skin Physiology

The skin is a complex, multipurpose organ, one that attracts much attention and scientific study. Science is constantly unraveling the intricacies of skin physiology, of the chemical substances present in the skin, and of their interaction. This knowledge, in turn, increases the understanding of the process of skin disease and skin aging. Scientists are identifying the skin's individual chemical compounds and the chemical and physiological reactions that accelerate aging. With the aging process better understood, laboratories are developing and incorporating new ingredients into cosmetic products that can reduce or decelerate aging and other skin problems, as well as counteract and/or correct them. A large number of new cosmetic ingredients have been incorporated into cosmetic products in the last 10 years and this is expected to continue at a fast pace. Many of these ingredients are intended to delay the aging process, rejuvenate the skin, improve skin problems, and even reduce the risk of skin cancer. An increased understanding of skin physiology allows for more targeted and effective skin care cosmetic formulations.

THE SKIN'S FUNCTIONS

As the body's largest organ, the skin performs a series of key functions resulting from multiple chemical and physical reactions that take place within it. The skin is a barrier, protecting the body from the elements, injury, and oxidation. It helps maintain a constant body temperature by helping the body adapt to different ambient temperatures and atmospheric conditions through the regulation of moisture loss. It gathers sensory information and plays an active role in the immune system, protecting from disease. In order to play all of these functions—protective, metabolic, sensory, and immunological—the skin must maintain its own auto-repairing capacities and functional integrity.

Cosmetic products are very important to the skin's protective function. Sunscreens protect against UV radiation and, therefore, against premature skin aging and skin cancer. Creams and lotions with a bactericidal effect reduce and/or control excessive proliferation of bacteria on the skin, a problem particularly associated with oily skin, and one of the main causes of acne development. And, by forming an invisible barrier on the skin's surface, specific moisturizing ingredients can help reduce the skin's moisture loss that results in dehydration. The skin also protects internal organs from exposure to oxygen. Without the skin, the body's organs would rapidly oxidize, much like a peeled banana or apple does when its interior is left exposed to air.

Through the secretion of sweat and sebum, the skin performs an excretory function, eliminating a number of harmful substances resulting from the metabolic activities of the intestine and the liver. The skin also secretes hormones and enzymes. When the skin's chemistry and chemical composition are not compatible with a particular product's ingredient(s), the result is overall product sensitivity and even allergic reactions.

The large number of nerve endings in the skin makes it sensitive to touch. As a result, the skin is a sensory organ and the point of receptivity for cold, heat, and pain.

The skin plays an immunological role, primarily through the Langerhans cells, which carry antigens from the skin to the lymphatic system. Excessive UV radiation either destroys or inhibits the performance of Langerhans cells, increasing the risk of skin cancer.

The skin tends to be discussed and treated as an entity unto itself, so this close relationship between the skin and the body is often overlooked or forgotten. Although it protects the body in a variety of ways, the skin and its condition are governed by a number of internal body functions. For example, skin oiliness arises from oil gland hyperactivity. Pigmentation problems are due to the tyrosinase enzyme, and are regulated by hormonal functions. Given this relationship between the skin and the body, for the skin to look its best, there is a need for overall health through proper nutrition, exercise, and rest. This connection also highlights the potential problems that ingredients penetrating deep into the dermis may cause if they are systemically absorbed by the capillary system.

When the skin performs in perfect harmony, the result is a beautiful, glowing, healthy complexion. If the skin is not in harmony because of deterioration due to age, sun damage, bacterial infection, hyperkeratinization, or simply loss of natural moisture, cosmetic products are meant to assist in restoring its balance and beauty. They must do so, however, by working in conjunction with the skin's very complex structure.

THE SKIN'S COMPONENTS AND STRUCTURE

The skin has a very intricate microanatomical structure. In addition to thousands of skin cells, within one square inch of skin, varying from 0.04 inches (1 mm) to 0.16 inches (4 mm) in thickness, there are some 650 sweat glands, 65 hair follicles, 19 yards of capillaries, 78 yards of nerves, thousands of nerve endings, Merkel cells for sensory perception, and Langerhans cells for immunological protection. The skin also contains melanocyte cells responsible for producing the melanin that gives the skin its color and pigmentation spots, or freckles. For a solid visual understanding, draw a one-inch square and attempt to make 650 dots representing the sweat pores in the square. Then take a spool of thread, measure 19 yards, and place it within the square. If you are having a hard time with 650 dots and 19 yards of thread, imagine trying to add 1,300 nerve endings and 78 yards of nerves! All of this is found in one square inch of skin, about as thick as a few stacked sheets of paper.

The skin is home to a variety of glands. These glands are important not only because of their intrinsic functions but also because they represent a route of entry into the skin for certain chemical compounds. Their main function is to synthesize substances that can cool the body, protect the skin, increase skin suppleness, or eliminate impurities such as mineral elements or cholesterol. Among these glands are the sebaceous glands and two sweat glands: the eccrine and apocrine glands.

Sebaceous glands, also known as oil glands, are attached to the same duct that contains the hair follicle. They are responsible for oil secretion in the skin, and are held within little sacs. The ducts of the oil glands open into the upper portion of the hair follicle. Usually, there is only one oil gland per follicle, but in some locations there may be more, resulting in greater oil (sebum) secretion in that area. Oil glands are found in almost all parts of the body. The face and back contain the highest number per square inch of skin, whereas the palms of the hands and soles of the feet contain none. The sebum secreted by the oil glands lubricates the skin and helps prevent the evaporation of moisture. It also possesses antifungal properties. Excessive oil secretion is associated with the development of acne, while insufficient oil secretion is associated with skin dryness.

Sweat glands are abundant throughout the skin. Eccrine glands are the most numerous. Their secreting duct opens as a pore directly onto the skin surface. Very abundant on the soles of the feet and the palms of the hands, they secrete a transparent fluid composed mainly of water, lactic acid, urea, toxins, and even bacteria-fighting substances. The primary function of this secretion is to cool the body and to maintain thermal equilibrium with the environment. The apocrine sweat glands are situated in the axillae, the eyelids, the pubic area, and the genitals. They are inactive until puberty and are stimulated by the emotions and stress. The apocrine sweat glands' excretion is very limited; it does not occur directly onto the skin's surface, but rather into the upper part of the phylosebaceous orifice, and from there to the skin surface. The perspiration from apocrine sweat glands can smell unpleasant due to a chemical reaction between the excretion, oxygen, and the enzymes produced by the microflora of the hair follicle.

It is important to note that dirt, impurities, and the asphyxiation, or clogs, seen in the pores occur in the hair follicle. They are the result of a mixture produced by oil and the keratinized and corneocyte cells present in the follicle. Cleansing the skin means eliminating impurities from these pores. Perspiration is not a cleanser. It may help clean the tiny opening of the sweat pores, but perspiration will not cleanse the hair follicle pore—the pore through which oil is secreted. This is a regular misconception by those who feel that saunas or perspiration cleanse the skin.

The surface of the skin is acidic. Its pH, also known as its protective mantle, is formed by a number of components. On the stratum corneum, these include naturally secreted sebum and perspiration (which contains lactic acid), as well as chemical reactions that occur in the epidermis, generating several relatively strong water-soluble acids. At the stratum corneum, the skin's pH level ranges from 4.4 to 5.6, depending on the individual and the place on the body from which the reading is taken. It also appears to vary by individual and race. As one moves past the stratum corneum through the epidermis and into the dermis, the pH level increases and becomes neutral (pH 7.0) at the dermis. This process is not completely understood.

The skin's acidity helps maintain the strength and cohesiveness of the skin, helps ward off infection by preventing the growth of bacteria, and allows for easier and more normal exfoliation of surface dead cells. One of the principal reasons why soaps—especially harsh soaps or cleansers with high pH values—are detrimental to the skin is because the skin needs an acidic environment to function properly. Thus, after the use of certain skin care cleansers, the use of a balancing lotion is needed. When cleansers have a neutral or alkaline pH, the skin's acidic level needs to be restored. Left alone, the skin will regain its acidic value in about 20 minutes or more depending on the level of acidic imbalance created.

Sensations, such as cold, heat, pressure, vibration, and stretching (both of skin and tendons), result from a stream of nerve impulses detected and transmitted to the brain by encapsulated nerve endings.

All of these components and actions are found within the basic building block of skin tissue, treated and discussed as three layers.

THE SKIN'S LAYERS

The skin is a highly specialized and complex set of tissues divided into three layers: the epidermis, the dermis, and the hypodermis, also known as the subcutaneous layer (see Figure 1.1).

There are several different types of cells in the skin, the most important of which are keratinocytes, melanocytes, fibroblasts, immunocompetent cells (Langerhans cells), migrating mononuclear cells, and mastocytes. In addition to these various cell types, the skin also contains connective tissues that are rich in extra cellular matrix (ECM), the components of which are primarily responsible for the flexibility of the skin—its suppleness and elasticity.

Other physiologically important functions such as hydration, temperature regulation, and the regulation of the skin's permeability depend on specific cells and the chemical composition of the ECM. These regulatory functions are closely linked to the interaction between the cells and the chemicals in the skin through special receptors located on the cell's membrane. These receptors can be thought of as antennae that help cells communicate with each other and with their environment. They are also able to bind with various chemical components that pass between cells. Among these chemical substances are certain cosmetic ingredients (such as retinol) that interact with cells and perform their therapeutic function only through cellular

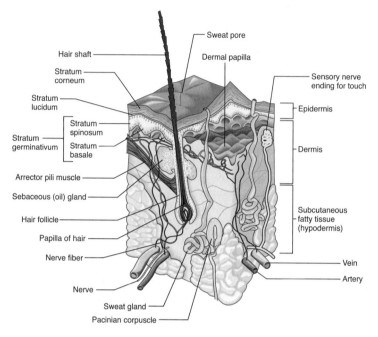

Figure 1.1 *The Layers of the Skin*

receptors. Some of these receptors fulfill important physiological functions. When receptors do not function properly, the skin's physiological performance may be impaired, accelerating damage or deterioration, such as aging. While work with receptors is a concept studied in greater depth in medicine and pharmaceuticals, in cosmetics the role of receptors for retinol effectiveness is well established.

The epidermis is the part of the skin visible to the naked eye. It is a very thin layer: its thickness varies from 0.63 inches (1.6 mm) on the soles of the feet to 0.002 inches (0.04 mm) on the eyelids. The epidermis contains a variety of cells, including keratinocytes which are engaged in a constant process of reproduction to replace exfoliated cells; Langerhans cells for immunological protection; melanocytes for skin color; and Merck cells that are involved in the function of touch. This is the layer of skin to which products are applied, and the one with which an individual (and cosmetics) comes most in contact when cleansing, exfoliating, healing, or hydrating.

The second skin layer, or dermis, lies below the epidermis and is connected to it by the basement membrane. The dermis represents the most important part of the skin. It is made of connective tissues, collagen, elastin, hair follicles, sebaceous glands, sweat (eccrine) glands, blood vessels, and nerves that transmit sensations of pain, itch, and temperature. There are also specialized nerve cells that transmit the sensations of touch and pressure.

The third skin layer, the hypodermis, is the deepest of the three layers. Consisting primarily of connective and fatty tissues, the hypodermis is much thicker than the dermis. Its measured thickness, however, depends on the part of the body being evaluated and the fat content of the individual. This layer is important for body temperature regulation.

A close examination of each layer, including composition and function, is important for further understanding of the impact a cosmetic product may have on the skin.

The Epidermis

Understanding the epidermis is extremely important for discussing product penetration, the definition of cosmetic versus pharmaceutical action according to FDA regulation, and product efficacy. The epidermis gives the skin its glow, youthfulness, texture, and good looks. It is responsible for the health of the skin, protecting it from moisture loss and the penetration of bacteria. Ultraviolet rays, an acne condition, visible skin disease, cigarette smoke, pollution, and skin cancer all affect this layer.

It is a metabolically active tissue that synthesizes the lipids and contains all the individual components required to form the protective barrier layer. Since the epidermis represents the outermost layer of the skin, it acts as the initial barrier to oxidant assault. The epidermis has a higher protective and antioxidant capacity than the dermis because it houses essential free radical scavengers such as vitamins E and C and superoxide dismutase. This layer also contains large amounts of glycosaminoglycans and ceramides.

The epidermis is further divided into five sublayers of cells, all metabolically very active. From the surface of the skin down to the dermis, these five layers are:

1. Corneum layer
2. Lucidum layer
3. Granulosum layer
4. Spinosum layer
5. Germinative layer

The epidermal cells are formed in the germinative layer and move upward toward the corneum layer. In their upward process, epidermal cells undergo a number of chemical modifications, transforming from soft, protoplasmic cells into flat surface "scales" that constantly rub off.

The epidermis holds a large amount of water. The layer with the highest water content is the germinative layer, holding about 80 percent. Each subsequent layer has less water as a percentage of its total chemical composition, with the corneum layer containing only 10 to 15 percent water. Water is held in the cell's cytoplasmic gel and in the intercellular channels (spaces between the cells). The younger the body, the more water there is in the skin. The skin's capacity to retain water decreases with age, making the skin more vulnerable to dehydration and wrinkles.

The epidermis is also the first barrier against immunological aggressors, thanks to the Langerhans cells. These dendritic cells are formed in the bone marrow and migrate to the skin's dermal and epidermal layers. Once they complete their migration, Langerhans cells typically are found in the lower layers of the epidermis, comprising about 5 percent of the total epidermal cell population. These cells engulf foreign bodies, carrying the invaders to the lymphatic system to be processed and eliminated. Langerhans cells are sensitive to ultraviolet radiation, and are easily damaged by UV rays. Even minor UV exposure will damage the Langerhans cells enough to reduce the skin's immune capacities. With age, these cells also decrease in number. This is one reason why the potential rate of skin disease increases with age.

In a young person, it takes approximately 28 days for a cell to travel from the germinative to the corneum layer. With age, the speed of this process is greatly reduced. It is estimated that after the age of 50, it takes about 37 days to complete the same process. Put in terms of skin aging, this indicates that stimulating skin functions, either manually through facial massage or through cosmetic product activity, would improve cellular metabolism. The 28- and 37-day time span is also important when it comes to skin sensitivity and the misuse of facial scrubs. If it takes 28 days or more for a cell to reach the surface of the skin, then we are naturally exfoliating one layer of dead cells a day. Depending on the harshness of the material, the use of scrubs may remove more layers of surface dead cells than appropriate, potentially increasing skin sensitivity. Furthermore, the misuse of scrubs may exacerbate oil gland activity, thereby increasing oil production, the opposite of what the user generally wishes to achieve.

Epidermal layers. Understanding the epidermal layers allows us to comprehend some of the problems of dehydration, sensitivity, aging, and pigmentation, which in turn helps associate product and ingredient effectiveness with skin requirements. The cells of the four epidermal layers from the germinative to the lucidum layer are referred to as keratinocytes and are the predominant cell species found in the epidermis. The primary function of the epidermis is to manufacture the uppermost layer, the corneum layer. An improperly functioning keratinocyte formation system cannot generate a cosmetically acceptable corneum layer. Therefore, an important factor for beautiful skin appears to be the appropriate metabolism of keratinocytes in order to generate a healthy corneum layer. This is important in order to protect against moisture loss and the penetration of bacteria and microbes.

The germinative layer, also referred to as the basal layer, is where the cells reproduce by mitosis: one cell divides into two, creating two cells identical to one another and to the original parent cell. After subdivision, one cell remains in the basal layer and the other is pushed upward toward the mucosum layer. In young skin, the germinative layer is the thickest layer of the epidermis. Here, the cells are large and supple, and contain a high percentage of water.

As the cells move upward, they begin to fill with a granular substance called keratin (hence the term *keratinocyte*). The keratinocytes lose water, become flatter, and their nucleus begins to degenerate. They secrete a "cement" made up of lipids, cholesterol, free saturated fatty acids, and ceramides into the intercellular spaces, increasing cohesion between the cells and thereby contributing to making the epidermis an effective barrier.

In their last state of migration, the cells reach the corneum layer (also referred to as the stratum corneum). This layer is considered so important and critical to product penetration, skin hydration, and the reduction of skin sensitivity that it is often studied separately from the other epidermal layers. The corneum layer is what we see as our skin. In healthy, young skin, it is made of 18 to 23 layers of flattened, dry cells (corneocytes) firmly cemented together. The actual number of layers depends on a variety of factors, including oil secretion and the skin's own desquamation system. The stratum corneum is thicker on the palms of the hands and soles of the feet. Scientists divide the stratum corneum into two distinct layers: the compact layer, where the corneocytes are linked one to another and have the role of a barrier, and the outer sloughing layer. In this second layer, the breakdown of cellular union provokes desquamation, allowing for the continuous elimination of corneocytes. Here, as the corneocytes gradually detach, numerous spaces are formed between the cells where the bacteria living on the skin find refuge and thrive, feeding on the remaining corneocytes. These bacteria are adapted to the acid environment of the stratum corneum. Other bacteria, known as transients, may be present on the surface of the skin, but the pH conditions are not favorable for them and they do not develop.

The natural cellular sloughing process is enzymatically controlled. Specific enzymes dissolve the bonds holding the corneocytes together, enabling them to slough off. If this process is not functioning properly, too many dead cells will accumulate on the skin surface. Oily skin may look thick and rough, and aging skin may look thin and fragile. However, both tend to have a thick stratum corneum. The corneum layer retains only about 10 to 15 percent of its original moisture. Its principal activities are to prevent excessive dehydration of the skin tissues and foreign matter from penetrating the skin. The cells are held together and surrounded by lipids and ceramides, as well as glycoproteins, desmosomes, peptide breakdown products, sebaceous products, and active enzymes. The intercellular lipids play a crucial role in the skin's water-retention properties by acting as a barrier, trapping water, and preventing excessive water loss. Ceramides account for up to 40 percent of the total intercellular lipids and also play a vital role in the skin's water-retaining capacity.

The corneum layer includes a natural moisturizing factor (NMF) made of hydrosoluable (able to dissolve in water) and hygroscopic (able to retain water) substances that regulate the corneum's selective permeability. The NMF is composed of about 40 percent free amino acids, some 12 percent PCA, 12 percent lactose, 7 percent urea, and approximately 30 percent of a large variety of other materials. Exposure to harsh detergents and climatic conditions can result in decreased NMF levels, rendering the skin fragile and dry.

The thickness of the corneum layer, the appropriate arrangement of its surface cells, and the strength of the cellular cement greatly determine a product or ingredient's ability to penetrate. A well-formed stratum corneum tends to be thin and compact, with an orderly cellular structure, or basket-weave, and strong barrier function. This is normal in young, healthy skin. When the corneum layer is thick and its cells are arranged in a scaled, uneven pattern, the natural barrier action of the skin is reduced, allowing for faster substance penetration. This is one reason why products may have a burning sensation on skin that is very dry and scaly. When the skin is excessively moist, sensitivity also may occur because the "barrier" has been softened, resulting in increased ease of product penetration. For aging or damaged skin, ingredients such as alpha hydroxyacids (AHAs) tend to restructure an abnormal stratum corneum, giving it a healthier and normal basket-weave structure.

Skin pigment or melanin is formed at the deepest layer of the epidermis by the melanocyte cells. This pigment is later transferred to the keratinocytes, giving the skin its color. Excessive melanin production is induced either by UV light exposure (e.g., sunbathing, tanning beds) or hormonal imbalances. In the first case, the melanocytes produce additional melanin to protect the skin from free radical damage. Once excessive UV light exposure is interrupted, the process of exfoliation and cellular upward movement allow the skin to slowly eliminate its excessively pigmented cells and recover its normal color. For example, a few months after summer vacation, the skin recovers its normal color. In the second case, the melanocyte tendency will be to continue to produce melanin at a new higher rate, regardless of changes in hormonal balance, making it very difficult to improve hyperpigmentation.

Immunological protection is provided in the epidermis by the Langerhans cells. Their function is to detect foreign bodies that have penetrated the epidermis, capture them, and carry them to lymphocytes in the lymphatic system. An immune response is then triggered, neutralizing and finally eliminating the foreign element.

Touch is sensed by the Merkel cells that are situated between the keratinocytes.

These three specialized epidermal cells, the melanocytes, the Langerhans cells, and the Merkel cells, account for 13 to 20 percent of total epidermal cells.

The complexity of the epidermal layer is astonishing, especially when considering its thinness. In addition to the different cells present, their individual functions, and their relationship to one another, there is the activity of cellular receptors and their communications and physiological and chemical interactions. All of these elements need to maintain a proper equilibrium in order to ensure the appropriate metabolism and functioning of keratinocytes and the corneum layer. Without such balance, the beauty and the health of the skin are impaired. Thus, the care of the skin and the avoidance of unnecessary harshness becomes most relevant if skin health and beauty is the desired goal.

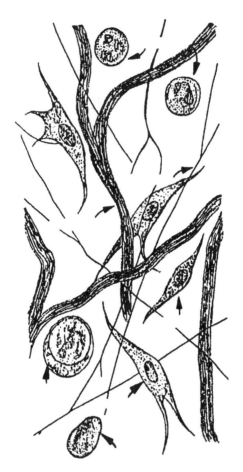

Figure 1.2 *Dermal Fibers* (*courtesy of Geo. A. Hormel and Co.*)

The Dermis

The dermis is the second layer of the skin. It is 10 to 40 times thicker than the epidermis (see Figure 1.1). Within the dermis are the appendages of the skin, the hair follicles, sebaceous glands, two sweat glands (eccrine and apocrine glands), plus a complex capillary and nerve network. It is made of 80 percent moisture, elastin tissues that supply elastic properties, and collagen fibers that provide a structural framework (see Figure 1.2). Collagen represents about 70 percent of the dermal proteins and provides resistance, resilience, and traction. About 20 different types of collagen fibers have been identified. Optimum wound healing is achieved when the repair process begins with the production of very thin collagen and continues with collagen of increasing thickness. Keloids are formed when wound healing begins with thicker forms of collagen. In addition to collagen and elastin, the dermis has a variety of other fibers, grouped together as structural glycoproteins, and a set of chemicals grouped under the term glycosaminoglycans. These are responsible for hydration, suppleness, and water retention. They also regulate permeability, provide resistance to pressure, and are responsible for the orientation of proteins.

By means of its vast network of capillaries and blood vessels, the dermis provides energy and nutrition to the epidermis, and plays a critical role in healing and thermoregulation. It is responsible for the supporting framework and elasticity of the skin, which also depends on a well-balanced water content in the dermis and other skin layers. To facilitate this essential hydration, the dermis acts as a water storage site. It also protects the body from mechanical injury and plays an important role in sensory perception and as an internal regulator.

Langerhans cells, responsible for immunoprotection, are also present in the dermis.

The dermis consists of a thick connective membrane crisscrossed by blood vessels, lymphatic vessels, nerve fibers, and many sensory nerve endings. Collagen and elastin protein fibers, the two main components of the dermis, act as a structural support system for the nerve fibers, hair follicles, blood vessels, and oil and sweat glands located in this layer, and also provide the skin with strength and elasticity.

Collagen is the dermis' principal component and is basically a chain of amino acids including alanine, arginine, lysine, glycine, proline, and hydroxyproline. Its production begins with the elaboration of procollagen which later undergoes a series of modifications and is transformed into regular collagen. Procollagen is very hygroscopic and binds many times its weight in water. A decreasing procollagen content over time may be related to the increased dryness and lack of elasticity associated with mature skin. In undamaged or normal skin, different types of elastin fibers account for 2 to 4 percent of the dermis. They form an interconnected structure that provides skin elasticity and resilience. Under a microscope, elastin looks like short, overlapping fibers that form an irregular network within the dermis, primarily concentrated in the layer's lower segments. The importance of elastin is disproportionate to the relatively small quantity found in the dermis. Filling the space between collagen and elastin are glycoproteins, forming something akin to a protective mantle. Among these glycoproteins are glycosaminoglycans and fibronectin. Glycosaminoglycans are a mixture of a large number of chemicals that are responsible for the arrangement of proteins in the skin and for regulating its permeability, as well as for hydration, suppleness, water retention, and the proper environment for the development of dermal cells. Glycosaminoglycans are a fundamental dermal material that provide support, lubrication, and the proper environment for the development of dermal cells. They also have a great water-binding capacity and are, therefore, crucial for the healthy turgor (normal distention), water content, and elasticity of the skin. Although they are sometimes referred to as mucopolysaccharides, they are not exactly the same. Mucopolysaccharides are a component of glycosaminoglycans. With age, the skin's glycosaminoglycan content diminishes, thus decreasing the skin's capacity to retain water and increasing the propensity for skin dryness.

The proper functioning of the dermal layer, as well as its water content, accounts for the skin's smoothness and elasticity. A properly functioning dermis is key for a youthful appearance and beautiful skin.

The Hypodermis

The hypodermis, the skin's third and last layer, connects the skin with the muscle tissues. This layer is highly elastic and has fat cells acting as "shock absorbers," thereby supporting delicate structures such as blood vessels and nerve endings. The hypodermis may be regarded as the extension of the strong fibrous and elastic bundles forming the dermis.

The skin, with its many tiny components and multilayered structure, is astonishingly complex. For the skin to be healthy and beautiful, balance and the proper working of all interrelated elements is essential. As more light is shed on how the skin works, cosmetic chemists have new elements to consider when exploring improvements in the functioning of different skin mechanisms and the formulation of appropriate skin care products.

The cosmetic chemists' concerns include:

- Preventing or reducing skin damage at the dermal and epidermal layer. This, in addition to correction, has become a strong focal point for product development and ingredient selection.

- Increasing skin hydration in order to ensure proper skin function. This also involves preserving and strengthening the epidermal barrier function.
- Helping the skin maintain its chemical balance to ensure proper function.
- Targeting ingredients for optimum performance in the layers where they are supposed to perform a specific function.

Augmenting the challenge to the cosmetic chemist is that this must be done within the established guidelines that define cosmetics and product penetration.

As more is known about the skin and its complexity, its chemical composition, and how it functions and why, there are greater opportunities to identify ingredients or compounds that can provide significant benefit to the skin. This includes maintaining the beauty and health of the skin, and delaying the damage caused by the passage of time—assuming, of course, that these ingredients reach their targeted destination within the skin unchanged. This is yet another challenge for the cosmetic chemist.

Product Penetration

Today, most cosmetic consumers are aware of and focus on a product's active ingredients and their ability to penetrate into the skin. However, the concept of penetration is not that simple; it is more accurate to think in terms of "ingredient delivery" to a target site within the skin. This includes target sites on the skin surface—the stratum corneum—as not all ingredients ought to penetrate.

In order to establish product effectiveness, it is important to consider the total formulation of a product, not just its active ingredients. Active ingredients need to be delivered to their target site, even if the target site is the surface of the stratum corneum. Therefore, delivery agents or delivery vehicles that facilitate penetration, such as liposomes, also need to be considered. Encapsulated retinol, for example, penetrates with less irritation than does free retinol. In addition, cosmetics contain many other ingredients, including emulsifiers, thickening and gelling agents, stabilizers, and preservatives. Each performs a function that helps make a complete product. In order not to hinder or neutralize activity, these also need to perform their own function while being compatible with the active ingredients.

There is no doubt that ingredients penetrate. There are, however, numerous issues that arise from this understanding—including how deep they can or should penetrate, both in order to be effective at their target site and/or to remain within the realm of cosmetics rather than pharmaceuticals. Another important issue is how to maintain the integrity of the active ingredients throughout their journey to a target site. One question cosmetic chemists pose is what percentage of the active ingredient actually reaches its target site.

Hyperpigmentation and the use of tyrosine/melanin inhibitors are a good example of how difficult and yet critical the concept of penetration is for product efficacy. The designated active ingredient needs to cross the stratum corneum's lipid barrier, traverse the cellular structure of the epidermis, penetrate the melanocyte, and then reach the melanosomes there—all the while maintaining its chemical and structural integrity in order to provoke the chemical reaction that can inhibit the transformation of tyrosine into melanine. This is no small challenge. At the other end of the spectrum are sunscreen chemicals. These need to remain on the skin's surface in order to be truly effective.

Thus, product effectiveness is not only a function of the active ingredients. It is a function of the whole formulation, as the formulation's full range of ingredients work in synergy to ensure that the active component reaches the target site without hindering its ability to act.

To understand product effectiveness, the traditional questions are still valid: How do products penetrate? Is penetration important for cosmetic product efficacy? Is product penetration crucial for actual cosmetic treatment of specific skin types and conditions?

We can begin to answer these questions by clearly understanding the defined parameters of product penetration, including the whys, hows, and factors that could affect it.

WHAT IS PRODUCT PENETRATION?

By definition, product penetration is the movement of substances or chemicals through the skin. While the stratum corneum provides a barrier to penetration, the skin is now recognized as a semipermeable membrane. Microorganisms cannot penetrate an intact skin, but chemicals can. The skin selectively allows molecular passage in and out. In spite of this, a significant amount of topically applied chemicals in the form of cosmetics and lotions are absorbed by the skin (possibly as much as 60 percent). Most agents that penetrate the skin need to pass through the intercellular lipid matrix, because these lipids form an almost continuous barrier in the stratum corneum. This barrier may vary considerably depending on individual age, the anatomical site considered, and even the season. In skin disorders, including dry and very dry skin, this barrier—and thus the permeability of the stratum corneum—is compromised and products can penetrate more easily.

For many consumers, product efficacy appears to be a function of product penetration. In reality, product efficacy is determined by a large variety of factors, including the active ingredients incorporated, the quantity of the actives used, the vehicles selected to help transport these actives to their target sites, the amount of actives that actually reaches the target site, and the actives' capacity to remain there long enough to function optimally and impart the desired benefit. The most efficient use of an active ingredient requires attaining an effective concentration at the target site and minimizing concentrations where the active is either unproductive or potentially harmful.

An important issue for cosmetic formulators is to ensure that ingredients will not penetrate into the dermis and be carried from there into the bloodstream through the capillary system. This would be product absorption through the skin into the circulatory system, and falls within the realm of pharmaceuticals.

The concept of ingredient delivery to a targeted site must also distinguish between dermal delivery and transdermal delivery. In the first case, the site of activity is the stratum corneum, viable epidermis, and/or dermis. In the second, the site of action is beyond the dermis, with the normal target being the circulatory system. Traditionally, cosmetic delivery refers only to surface epidermal delivery. Transdermal delivery is strictly a pharmacological area. This results in a clear parameter of understanding: cosmetic ingredients need to be delivered *to* the skin rather than *through* the skin. Therefore, one of the key issues surrounding cosmetic product penetration is the avoidance of transdermal delivery and the maintenance of the active principle within a specific skin layer. Presently, scientists are investigating two methods to accomplish this. One is to ensure that the active principle reaches its target and remains active there. The other is to be certain it becomes inactive if or once it moves beyond the desired site. Cosmetic chemists are often faced with a series of related questions: How much remains as residue on the skin? How much arrives at the target site? How much might be traveling further through the skin, reaching the circulatory system? And what is the optimal balance or ratio of these possibilities?

It is also important to remember that when evaluating a product's efficacy, basing conclusions on penetration potential alone can be misleading. For example, skin lighteners must penetrate the epidermis and reach the basal layer in order to inhibit the tyrosinase enzyme responsible for melanin production. However, bleachers may also remain on the surface of the stratum corneum to bleach out accumulated pigment. In both cases they may be efficacious but their penetration potential differs. UV absorbers are a good example of products that need to remain on the skin surface to be truly beneficial. If they penetrate, they become less effective because they have moved beyond the site of action. At the opposite end of the spectrum from sunscreens are antioxidants and molecules with antiaging properties. These tend to exert most of their benefit once they are in the epidermis or even the dermis, and, therefore, their efficacy is highly dependent on targeted penetration. Moisturizers can work in different ways. Those that work by occlusion should remain on the skin surface; others, such as humectants, ought to penetrate into the superficial layers and help retain water there. Thus, the need for and efficacy of product penetration ought to be in direct correlation to ingredient function.

WHY PRODUCTS PENETRATE

Products penetrate via two main channels: the extra cellular and the intercellular. In topical treatments the absorption organ is the skin, yet within the skin there are numerous different target sites. Among these are the philosebaceous pore and the sweat ducts, the stratum corneum, the viable epidermis, and the epidermal–dermal junction. More often than not the same active substances will act on several of these target sites. The rate of penetration depends on molecular size, the delivery vehicle, and the skin's state of integrity and health.

It is clear that the skin's ability to serve as a barrier is largely dependent on an intact corneum layer. Removal or alteration of this layer by scraping or scaling (due to dryness), the application of products like Retin-A™ or alpha hydroxyacids, skin dryness, or skin diseases such as eczema and psoriasis may increase product penetration.

Movement through the corneum layer depends on the molecular size of each ingredient and its tendency to metabolically interact with the skin's chemistry and with cellular receptors. If movement through the corneum layer is slow, a significant concentration of the product will develop. This results in a reservoir-like situation where the corneum layer holds that which has penetrated and supplies the underlying tissues with a particular compound over a period of time after application. The corneum layer can, therefore, function in a dual capacity—as a barrier and as a reservoir—storing compounds for hours after application on the skin.

Illness can change the rate of topical absorption. For example, diabetes is known to change the structure of the epidermal–dermal junction and the capillary function, increasing the skin's absorption capabilities in chronic diabetics. In addition, chemical penetration varies on different parts of the body. On the face and scalp, for example, absorption is often 5 to 10 times higher than elsewhere.

HOW PRODUCTS PENETRATE

The corneum layer, with its strongly and tightly bound cells, is the greatest obstacle to product penetration. The second barrier is the epidermal–dermal junction, or basement membrane. If one skin function is to serve as a barrier, protecting the body from penetration by foreign matter, how is it that chemicals or cosmetic ingredients can penetrate? Structurally, the skin absorbs. This absorption takes place through the philosebaceous pores, the ducts of the sweat glands, the intercellular channels that bind cells together, and the cellular system itself.

In reality, a large percentage of topically applied products never penetrate the corneum layer due to one or more of the following reasons:

- molecular size (too large)
- retention or binding on the surface by other ingredients present in the product
- evaporation (if volatile)
- adhesion to surface corneum cells and then loss by exfoliation

What does manage to penetrate can:

- permeate through the epidermal cells and cellular cement
- form a reservoir by binding in the corneum layer (or in the subcutaneous fat), from which it may be released very slowly
- be metabolized by the skin's own process
- penetrate into the dermis and remain there
- penetrate into the dermis and be absorbed into microcirculation by the capillaries (this is an absorption method used in the pharmaceutical field; nicotine and estrogen patches are examples)

Although the whys and hows of product penetration have been established, it is also important to look at what can affect this action.

Factors Affecting Product Penetration

The corneum layer's health is a major factor affecting the rate and extent of skin absorption. Another is skin hydration. One of the most common methods to increase penetration is through occlusion (trapping liquid or gas, in this case in the corneum layer) in order to prevent surface evaporation of water, which further increases corneum layer hydration. This is the concept behind the use of masks in skin care.

Environments with relative humidity greater than 80 percent may also result in significant skin hydration. It must be noted, however, that while the skin has great water-absorption capabilities, it does not have equally great water-retention capabilities. As the corneum layer softens due to excessive hydration (as during prolonged baths), its barrier function is weakened, allowing for increased moisture loss and dehydration.

One main path for chemical penetration of the corneum layer is through the lipid-containing intercellular spaces. Therefore, the stratum corneum's lipid composition affects permeation. Given the miscibility (ability to mix) of oil with oil, chemicals dissolved in oil-based carriers will permeate more easily through the epidermal layers than those dissolved in water. However, lipophilic (oil-based) chemicals have a harder time continuing down the path of penetration because the lower epidermal layers have a higher water content than the stratum corneum and, therefore, are lipophobic. As we all know, oil and water do not mix very easily, if at all. The carriers in which ingredients are dissolved or mixed for convenient application and control of ingredient concentration play a major role in determining the rate of penetration. In some instances, chemical absorption may be limited by the carrier used rather than by the barrier function of the skin layers. For example, in products where the active principles need to remain on the surface of the skin (such as UV absorbers and protective moisturizers), oil-based formulations provide optimal results. On the other hand, overcoming the challenge of passing hydrophilic (water-based) actives through the lipid-based intercellular spaces of the stratum corneum requires either a number of various cosmetic reactions that can increase the stratum corneum's moisture content, or delivery technologies, such as liposomes.

The fact that products penetrate is now so thoroughly accepted that the current concern is the speed and depth at which ingredients travel. Multiple techniques have been developed to achieve controlled product penetration. These include the use of vehicles (liposomes), natural encapsulating materials, and other systems.

With each delivery system, the objective is to send an active to its target site and keep it there so it can provide maximum benefit while avoiding any negative reactions such as irritation, dermal absorption, or other undesirable effects.

PRODUCT TESTING

A variety of testing methods are used to determine the function of an active ingredient in the skin and where the active ingredient is located once introduced topically. These tests can be in vitro and in vivo, often using extensive and complex computer programs. For in vitro testing, skin is cultured in glass containers where cells reproduce 20 times or more. Skin samples are also obtained from patients undergoing plastic surgery or some other type of surgery where a segment of skin is eliminated. Work in vitro presents great advantages in terms of time, cost, and ethical considerations when toxicity is a potential problem.

Products tested in vivo are tested on animals and human beings. In vivo studies provide the most direct, relevant, and conclusive information, especially when a product's systemic effect is being questioned—i.e., how the product may affect the body as a whole. The methods used in in vivo testing depend on what scientists are trying to prove. For example, in order to establish the moisturization level and repair benefits of a product or ingredient for dry skin, scientists use volunteers who are instructed to treat the skin with standard soap products for several days without using supplemental moisturizers. After a period of time, measurements are taken to determine skin dryness. Researchers then proceed to give a moisturizing product to some of the volunteers and a placebo product to the others. At periodic intervals, skin hydration is measured among all testing subjects in order to determine the rate of hydration over time. In the case of sunscreen testing, the aim is to keep the active ingredients on the upper layers of the stratum corneum to achieve their effectiveness and prevent toxicity issues. Tape-stripping techniques are mostly used in this case, plus blood and urine samples. In these tests, some organic sunscreens have been found in blood plasma and urine. This has not been the case with mineral-based sunscreens.

In the case of products that remain on the skin's surface or in the corneum layer, researchers apply the product on the skin and then remove the skin by stripping with adhesive tape or by scratching. The rate of product penetration and cellular change at different levels of penetration is then studied, usually through complex computer models.

For products believed to penetrate into the dermal layers, their systemic effect is also evaluated with sophisticated computer models that allow researchers to see not only how deep the product penetrated but also what changes it caused in the cellular structure. The compounds under consideration are marked and their penetration is followed into the skin and the blood, urine, and other body fluids. However, the amounts penetrating the skin are frequently quite small and require extremely sensitive equipment to detect their presence in the body.

Given what is known about how the skin functions, products (or more accurately, specific ingredients contained therein) can, under the right conditions, penetrate, generally through absorption. Penetration, however, may not be all important for product efficacy. In certain cases, it may actually be undesirable or counterproductive.

Great progress is being made in cosmetic chemistry and in understanding how the skin works. With this knowledge, new product technologies are available that facilitate product penetration to the exact point of maximum efficacy with minimum side effects.

Skin Types and Skin Conditions

The correct identification of skin types and conditions is key for successfully selecting effective cosmetic products. Although there are as many subtle variations to skin types and conditions as there are human beings, certain prevalent characteristics allow skin types to be grouped into three classifications and skin conditions into another six. In most cases, individuals have a combination of skin types plus one or more skin conditions. Products are generally formulated to address specific situations.

This chapter is designed to help relate skin requirements to the cosmetic ingredients most beneficial to an individual's skin. It is also useful for identifying why a given product may or may not provide expected results, and for identifying potential negative reactions.

SKIN TYPES

Skin types are hereditary and are the result of oil gland functioning. Skin types can be classified into three categories: normal, oily, and dry. In most cases, individuals have a combination of skin types such as an oily T-zone (around the eyes, nose, and chin) and normal cheeks. Of course, these skin types occur in varying degrees, such as very oily or very dry, slightly oily or slightly dry.

The notion that one person's skin can be oily and dry is more commonly a confusion in concept than a reality. For example, when people describe their skin as having been oily and all of a sudden being dry, they are referring to an oily skin type that is losing moisture because of overdrying. This is usually caused by excessive use of astringents, soaps, and/or scrubs in an attempt to reduce the amount of oil secretion. While the skin is an oily type, this dryness should be considered a skin condition and be properly referred to as dehydration, a lack of water moisture rather than oil.

In general, there seems to be such an obsession with oiliness that people forget about moisture. It is quite common to hear, "I don't need a moisturizer, my skin is oily." It is important to remember that the skin has oil from the oil glands and water from the intercellular channels, and that both are important for its beauty and for retarding the aging process.

Normal Skin

Normal skin has perfect hydration, muscle tone, and resilience produced by moisture and the adipose tissues. There is strong biological activity at the basal layer, blood circulation is active, and the metabolism is balanced. Normal skin looks soft, moist, plump, and dewy, and has a healthy glow and color. The corneum layer shows a fine texture, and there are no visible wrinkles, fine lines, or open pores.

The best example of normal skin is that of children, from birth usually until puberty. Oil glands functioning at a normal rate of secretion are also seen in mature individuals who once had oily skin. With age, the rate of oil gland secretion slows down and becomes normal. However, the normal skin found in this second case varies from the normal skin of youth insofar as there is no strong biological activity at the basal layer and, in most cases, suppleness and color have deteriorated.

Aging due to the passage of time, sun exposure—and other external elements such as harsh climate, dehydration, and poor care—is the primary factor that causes the deterioration of normal skin. Other factors include insufficient water intake and an inadequate diet. Tea, coffee, and sodas do not make up for water because the body processes them differently. Food devoid of vitamins, enzymes, and amino acids does not provide the cells with the nourishment necessary for cellular reproduction and growth. Improper skin care, such as lack of cleansing, is quite prevalent in children and teenagers due to the lack of skin care awareness. The use of harsh soaps and scrubs, climate, and environment contribute to the deterioration of normal skin. Sun exposure and exposure to the elements without protection dries, dehydrates, and ages the skin.

Normal skin requires proper morning and evening cleansing and protection from oxidation caused by free radicals. The consistent use of protective moisturizers during the day to prevent moisture loss and hydrating creams at night is essential. It is important that these moisturizers contain antioxidants such as vitamins E and C, idebenone, or coenzyme Q 10. An occasional exfoliation is also beneficial. Sun protection is extremely important, even for children. Children should not be allowed on the beach without a proper sunscreen or in the snow without a good protective cream, including SPF protection. For normal skin the key is damage prevention.

Oily Skin

Oily skin is a hereditary condition that develops due to overactive sebaceous glands. This activity is controlled by the androgen, or masculine, hormone. Oily skin can be recognized by its shiny, thick, and firm appearance. Pores look enlarged, usually due to oil entrapped in the philosebaceous follicle. Enlarged pores become aggravated with a dehydrated skin condition. An oily complexion tends to look dirty and uncared for—with occasional blemishes on the chin or the forehead area—and feels oily to the touch.

Hot and humid climates tend to exacerbate oil gland secretion, making the skin more oily. Oily skin problems can be aggravated by the misuse of skin care products and the tendency to dry the skin either through the use of harsh soaps or the excessive use of astringents or scrubs. Overstimulation of skin functions through scrubbing or stimulating massage should be avoided.

Oily skin can be classified into two subcategories: oily (*without* water deficiency) and oily dehydrated (*with* water deficiency). In the first case, the skin has proper hydration; while it feels and looks oily, it does not have the sensation of "dryness." In the second subcategory, the skin lacks moisture. All the characteristics of oily skin are present but the individual tends to complain of "dry skin." Often those with oily skin tend to use drying, dehydrating ingredients in an effort to feel "less oily." The end result is skin that feels flaky, rough, and scaly. The usual thought when this type of condition develops is to "self-diagnose" as a dry skin type and purchase products rich in oils. As the skin already has enough oil, these products only aggravate the oily condition and result in blemishes, blackheads, etc. It is not unusual for individuals with oily skin to conclude that they do not need a moisturizer because they have oily skin. Thus, it is important to distinguish that oiliness comes from the oil glands, and moisture from the intercellular channels.

Care of oily skin requires thorough yet gentle cleansing morning and evening. Daytime protective moisturizers will help the skin maintain its suppleness and moisture. Night creams, gels, or lotions should help regulate oil gland secretion. It is essential to keep oily skin clean and hydrated with appropriate cleansing and care. Exfoliators, such as AHAs or BHAs, or the weekly use of enzyme peels is highly recommended to help improve the look and texture of oily skin by reducing hyperkeratosis. When properly cared for, this is the preferred skin type since the wrinkle process is delayed.

Active substances, including botanicals that may help regulate or reduce oil gland secretions, are highly beneficial. Suitable actives could include, but are not limited to, royal jelly and vitamin F. Among the appropriate botanicals are rosemary; lemon oil and lemon balm for their antiseptic and depurative action; all citrus, which are antibacterial, antiseptic, and astringent; rose hip for its antiseptic properties and ability to regulate oil gland secretion; sage, which is antiseptic and antibacterial; yarrow, which has astringent and antiseptic properties; and mint and thyme, which act as solvents on the fats and have additional action on the sebaceous glands.

Dry Skin

Dry skin develops as a result of under-active sebaceous glands. Dry skin, while hereditary like oily skin, is also a result of aging. As all body activities slow down with time, oil gland activity slows as well. Dry skin tends to be dehydrated. It can feel scaly, rough, and itchy. It rarely has comedones, and when it does, they tend to be on the nose area. The lack of oil in dry skin reduces its ability to retain moisture, since oil in the skin acts as a natural barrier against moisture loss. Dry skin is characterized as very fine, overly delicate, and thin. Insufficient oil secretion deprives the skin of enough "glue" to retain cells in the corneum layer. As a result, dry skin has fewer cells in the corneum layer than does oily skin. In dry skin, pores are almost invisible. The skin also tends to wrinkle easily and is often filled with tiny superficial lines.

Dry skin problems are aggravated by exposure to the sun, wind, and heat. Improper skin care, especially the lack of protection against moisture loss, further exacerbates this problem. Care for dry skin should include the use of products that will stimulate skin functions, activate oil gland secretion, and provide deep hydration. Moisturizers that can form a "sealing" film on the skin surface will prevent or reduce moisture loss. These should include high molecular weight ingredients, such as collagen, hyaluronic acid, and natural silicones (e.g., dimethicone). Other moisturizing ingredients are also essential to activate the skin's natural water-retention ability and to place additional moisture into the skin. These ingredients include glycolic and lactic acids, glycerin, urea, ceramides, and cholesterol. Such multifunction moisturizers are essential for dry skin. Nourishing creams that can stimulate oil gland secretion and skin functions are highly recommended. As with every skin type, the use of products with antioxidant ingredients is essential to delay cellular damage. The use of nourishing, hydrating masks is also advisable for dry skin.

Appropriate ingredients for dry skin can include, but are not limited to, vitamin E (tocopherol), PCA, ginseng, dandelion extract, avocado oil, macadamia nut oil, hyaluronic acid, ceramides, and mucopolysaccharides. Specifically beneficial botanicals can include St. John's wort, effective for improving circulation; aloe vera, for its deeply hydrating capacities; sage, which is stimulating and invigorating; and orange flower extract, which is calming and soothing.

Combination Skin

Combination skin tends to have either normal cheeks and an oily T-zone, or dry cheeks and a normal T-zone. The skin cannot be dry and oily at the same time. The skin does not tend to be that extreme within such a small space. Usually when the skin is classified as dry and oily, it is oily or oily and normal-dehydrated.

SKIN CONDITIONS

Skin conditions develop over time and apply to all three skin types (with the exception of acne, which is not usually found together with dry skin), leading to the many combinations that make everyone's skin unique. The most common skin conditions are dehydration, couperose, sensitivity, pigmentation, aging, acne vulgaris, and rosacea. Skin conditions develop for a variety of reasons, including a low water content in the skin; the excessive production of corneum cells; a poor skin metabolism; free radical damage; unbalanced or excessive melanin production; improper daily skin care; excessive sun exposure and use of tanning beds; and a lack of protection from the environment, including the sun.

Dehydration

Dehydration—a lack of sufficient moisture in the cellular system and intercellular channels—is one of the most common skin conditions. Dehydration is caused by the compromised permeability of the lipid barrier; cracks in the skin due to a decrease in the suppleness, softness, and flexibility of the stratum corneum; a reduction in size of the flattened corneocytes and the stratum corneum; and a lower capacity by the skin to retain moisture, which is usually as a result of lower glycosaminoglycans levels due to skin aging.

Dehydration is aggravated by atmospheric conditions that include too much sun and wind as well as not using sunscreens and/or daytime protective moisturizers. It is also aggravated such factors as using inappropriate skin care products; cleansing with harsh soaps and water; drinking tea, coffee, soda, or diuretics; and not drinking enough water.

Dehydrated skin looks dry, scaly, and flaky. It feels tight. When gently pulled, the skin "crinkles" in a way that is similar to pulling a corner of very thin tissue paper. Sometimes the skin appears as if it had an additional thin layer of skin placed on top. This is particularly evident on the nose and forehead.

Dehydration is one of the most difficult skin conditions to diagnose. It is usually confused with dryness, which is technically a lack of oil. Unfortunately, dehydration and dryness have many similarities. Both dry and oily skin types may be dehydrated. Dry skin can be dehydrated because thin skin has difficulty retaining inner moisture. Oily skin becomes dehydrated through the use of harsh soaps and the excessive use of astringents. When oily skin becomes dehydrated, the surface layers of cells harden up and block oil secretion. The result is an entrapment of the oils under the corneum layer. This is particularly detrimental in the case of someone with acne because it also results in the entrapment of the infection. To end the confusion between dehydration and dryness, the best approach is to first diagnose the skin type and then the skin condition.

Care for dehydrated skin requires the use of moisturizers containing ingredients that will protect the skin from moisture loss as well as restore internal skin hydration. Moisturizing ingredients that can help the skin retain inner moisture by reducing transepidermal water loss are generally high molecular weight ingredients, for example collagen and hyaluronic acid. In addition, to help increase the skin's inner moisture, the use of AHAs can activate the water-retention capability of glycosaminoglycans, and could be complemented with ingredients that add moisture to the skin, such as glycerin, urea, and propylene glycol. In order to restore or improve the skin's lipid barrier (and thereby reduce transepidermal water loss), ingredients such ceramides, cholesterol, and fatty acids are essential. Aloe is an outstanding botanical ingredient for dehydrated skin. In addition to moisturizers with these ingredients, proper care can include the application of hydrating masks on a weekly or biweekly basis, depending on the level of dehydration.

Couperose

Couperose is a temporary or chronic redness appearing on the face. It shows up as small, dilated, winding, bright red blood vessels on the cheeks, around the nose, and sometimes on the chin.

Couperose occurs primarily as a result of poor elasticity in the capillary wall. When there is a sudden rush of blood because of blushing, excessive heat, or other stimuli, the capillaries expand, making room for the increase of blood. When the amount of blood recedes, the capillaries contract to their normal size. If the capillary wall is not sufficiently elastic, it will expand but not contract again to its original shape or size. The result is a distended capillary that will hold blood cells within its structure, thus giving the appearance of diffuse or local redness.

Couperose is aggravated by atmospheric conditions such as hot or cold climates, by the use of excessively cold or hot water, nervous disorders, digestive disorders, saunas, exercise that causes the face to turn very red, drinking alcohol and very hot liquids, eating spicy foods, blushing, and excessive sun exposure. Individuals with couperose that are also using Retin-A™ should consult with a physician, as this product may aggravate the condition as well.

Care should be taken that skin with this condition is not exposed to excessively hot or cold water. Night creams or lotions that help strengthen the capillary walls are helpful. Products with soothing, vasoconstrictive ingredients are also beneficial. Botanical ingredients of benefit for couperose include plantain; grape; horse chestnut; St. John's wort, for anti-inflammatory activity; and acacia, for its soothing capacities.

Sensitivity

Generally speaking, the term sensitive skin is used when the skin readily experiences adverse reactions or unwanted changes in response to external factors, such as cosmetic or pharmaceutical products or regular toiletries.

Skin sensitivity can be experienced as inflammation, redness, tightness, itching, burning, spots, flaking, scaly patches, bumps, etc. It is important to distinguish between reactive skin and sensitive skin. Reactive skin can experience any of the abovementioned occurrences, but it will do so inconsistently; in other words, it will not react to the same product or ingredient in the same way each and every time it is used. In fact, it may react once and never again. Skin that is considered clinically (i.e., truly) sensitive will respond predictably (in the same fashion) each time a specific ingredient or product is applied. The general consumer perception of skin sensitivity is high. Surveys show that in some countries, over 60 percent of women report they have sensitive skin. However, from a scientific standpoint, it is estimated that no more than 20 percent of the population may have sensitive skin and of this, only 2 to 5 percent can be attributed to cosmetic ingredients.

The skin reacts sensitively when the stratum corneum is damaged and products can penetrate directly into the deeper layers of the epidermis and/or dermis. In addition, the skin's own chemical components, its bacterial flora, and/or its antigens—substances that stimulate an immune response—may react with a product's chemical components and cause a sensitivity reaction. Because the chemical composition of each person's skin varies, this might be sufficient for one person to react sensitively to an ingredient while another may not. Factors such as climate and ambient pollution levels, also combine with the skin's own chemistry. This can produce a chemical reaction and chemical by-products that then react with the ingredients in a cosmetic product, leading to a sensitivity reaction by the skin.

Sensitive skin is highly complex and difficult to resolve. Possible reasons for why skin may be sensitive include a sensitive nervous system in the skin that has an enhanced response to otherwise minor skin stimulations; a strong immune responsiveness consisting of high antibody response; and a defective barrier function that permits rapid penetration of ingredients into the epidermis and dermis, and that rapidly activates sensory response.

Ingredients that can most often cause sensitivity are fragrances, preservatives, and some chemical sunscreens. It is important to note that an ingredient may not be sensitizing as a rule, but that a given individual's skin may be sensitive to that particular chemical. An ingredient itself is deemed sensitizing if most individuals react to it with sensitivity. When a reaction occurs in isolated cases, it is considered that the individual is sensitive, not that the ingredient is sensitizing. Ultimately, sensitivity reactions are very complex and depend on the individual who experiences them.

It is most logical that people with sensitive skin use very gentle and delicate cosmetics. From a formulatory standpoint, cosmetic chemists are constantly assessing new antiallergenic, anti-inflammatory, and anti-irritation ingredients. Interestingly, these tend to be botanical derivatives. Popular among them are chamomile, licorice root extract, aloe vera, geranium, coltsfoot, and St. John's wort.

Pigmentation

Pigmentation is a normal process in the cellular activity within the skin. Hyperpigmentation results from an uneven distribution of melanin over the skin surface, either due to pigment accumulation, as in the case of age spots and lentigo, or because of uneven melanin production by the melanocytes, as in the case of melasma.

The melanocyte cell is located in the basal layer of the epidermis. From there it projects a series of dendrites (tentacles), each surrounding approximately 36 keratinocytes. Within the melanocytes are the melanosomes that produce melanine. When appropriate new keratinocytes surround a dendritic portion of the melanocyte, there is a chemical process by which the melanosomes are able to pass into the keratinocytes. Once in the keratinocyte, the melanosome loses its membrane and releases the melanin. This gives the keratinocytes—and thus the skin—its natural color. Melanine is produced by the tyrosine protein, which is activated by the tyrosinase enzyme in an oxidative environment (i.e., due to free radicals). Thus, exposure to UV light and the consequent free radical formation incentives an increase in melanin production. The reaction is also hormonally controlled, which explains why melasma can be a result of pregnancy and the use of contraceptives. Prolonged periods of intense stress are also believed to cause melasma in susceptible individuals.

The rate of melanin production varies from person to person and from race to race, being greater in darker-skinned individuals. Melanin acts as a filter, protecting the skin and body against the harmful effects of the sun's radiation. Surface irritation, often caused by sun exposure, triggers increased melanin production, augmenting the amount of pigment in the skin. Therefore, a suntan is basically the body's protective response against internal skin damage from free radicals.

Lentigo, commonly known as age spots, occurs when there is an uneven accumulation of melanin deposits in the epidermal surface layers. In the case of melasma, or local hyperpigmentation, the pigmentation results when the melanocytes produce a greater amount of melanin in a given area of the skin, and/or when the melanin is not properly absorbed by the keratinic cells. Melasma occurs as a result of hormonal imbalances caused by pregnancy, the use of birth control pills, menopause, or nervous disorders. Dark spots can also be the result of surface irritation of the skin as those caused by acne conditions.

The best treatment for pigmentation is based on bleaching agents and ingredients that can help regulate melanocyte activity. Bleaching and skin lightening agents, both botanical and synthetically manufactured, can include all citruses, idebenone, kojic acid, lemon oil, linden, and yarrow. Hydroquinone, a very effective bleaching ingredient, has been removed from the cosmetic ingredient category in a number of countries due to potential melanocyte-damaging effect. Some bleaching agents should only be applied at night, as some of the ingredients tend to react with sunlight and further aggravate the problem.

Key ingredients that regulate melanin production include antioxidants, as these can reduce the free radicals that stimulate melanocyte activity. Such ingredients include alpha lipoic acid, green tea, idebenone, super oxide dismutase, and vitamins E and C. In addition, anti-inflammatory and soothing ingredients are essential in order to reduce potential skin irritation, which also aggravates melanin production. Exfoliating ingredients such as glycolic acid or salicylic acid will help eliminate surface accumulated pigmentation. It is important to avoid provoking strong skin irritation with exfoliating ingredients, as this could aggravate the pigmentation problem.

In all cases, when attempting to correct hyperpigmentation— one of the most challenging skin conditions—it is essential to use a sunscreen with a high SPF at *all times* during the day, regardless of whether it is sunny or cloudy, summer or winter. Direct sun exposure in the summer should be avoided, as UV light increases the process of oxidation responsible for pigmentation. The use of tanning beds should be avoided, of course.

Failure to use a sunscreen could neutralize whatever result the treating product may give.

Aging

Skin aging is a complex, biological process affecting various layers of the skin—most significantly the dermis—and includes a modification of genetic material. Among the events that occur in the aging process are a deficiency in the nutritional components within the different tissues, cellular destruction through excessive sun exposure, the effect of free radicals on the cellular membrane, a deterioration in the genetic programming of the DNA, and a decrease in cellular proliferation. The impact on skin tissue is a loss of elasticity, a reduced ability to regulate water, and a less efficient replication or renewal process. The consequences are skin atrophy and a general process of degeneration. Aging skin is characterized by a thick stratum corneum with a thin epidermis and dermis. It suffers an accentuation of lines and wrinkles as a result of increased dryness and of dehydration caused by skin thinning and reduced oil gland activity. The complexion looks withered, and assumes an "old ivory" shade as melanin production diminishes. Aging skin can be recognized by its poor elasticity, lack of normal firmness, and sagging due to the loosening of collagen and elastin in the dermis. Aging is accompanied by a slowing down of cell proliferation. Skin thickness decreases with age. On average, the skin loses about 6 percent of its thickness every 10 years. This means that someone who is 100 years old will have lost approximately 60 percent of their initial skin volume. This impacts both the epidermis and dermis.

Skin aging can be grouped into two categories. The first is intrinsic or chronological aging, which results from the passage of time, and is the slow irreversible process of tissue degeneration. Intrinsic aging is linked to the transformation of connective tissue and the decrease of cellular regeneration. The second category is extrinsic aging. It is often referred to as photoaging since it is primarily due to sun (UV) exposure, which damages or destroys cellular reproductive abilities and degenerates collagen. Its clinical characteristics include fine lines and wrinkles, roughness, pigmentation, couperose, actinic keratosis, and skin cancer. Other factors that can cause or accelerate extrinsic aging are exposure to outdoor elements, stress, and lifestyle choices. In addition, skin aging is compounded by health problems, hormonal imbalances, improper care while young, and improper nutrition, which robs the skin of appropriate nourishment for cellular reproduction and growth.

Antiaging treatments emphasize the return to a smoother, more youthful appearance by softening and normalizing the look and feel of sun-damaged or otherwise extrinsically aged skin. With today's skin care technology, however, it is increasingly possible to emphasize the prevention of skin aging as well as the correction or improvement of its visible signs. It is well established that skin aging is mediated by free radical damage, and stems from UV light (followed by cigarette smoke). Thus, the first step in antiaging treatment is to protect the skin from free radical formation and damage by using UV filters and by increasing the skin's antioxidant levels through antioxidant-rich products. Furthermore, if correction is attempted with no prevention, what is corrected at night can be damaged during the day. Highly effective ingredients are available for correction. Among the most sophisticated currently available are idebenone, a powerful antioxidant that reduces collagen destruction and appears to affect intrinsic aging; various forms of vitamin A, especially retinol or retinoic acid, which are recognized as among the best ingredients for stimulating skin functions; glycolic acid, for normalizing skin metabolism; neuropeptides (CL-F5), tiny strings of amino acids that act as messengers to the cells; and pheromones, which serve as chemical messengers that communicate between individual cells and elicit behavioural or neurological responses. Among the beneficial botanical ingredients in antiaging treatment are apricot, for its vitamins A, B, C, and D and antioxidant content; carrot, for its vitamin A and mineral salts; and horseradish, for its ability to improve skin connective tissues, regulate skin functions, increase the skin's defense mechanisms, and prevent and/or counteract wrinkle formation.

When treating aging skin, it is important that the active principles be revitalizing, normalizing, stimulating, and hydrating, as well as protective. No single ingredient or product can accomplish all of these requirements. A complete skin care regime should include daily sunscreen applications for protection; properly hydrating and antioxidant moisturizers; and corrective creams, lotions, gels, or emulsions with active principles that stimulate and revitalize skin function, nourish the skin, neutralize damaging chemicals formed in the skin, and activate intercellular activity and communications. The weekly use of masks can aid in the hydration process, and lead to an improved skin color and texture, together with the softening of fine lines and wrinkles.

Acne Vulgaris

This acne condition is recognized by small infection spots and pustules, either numerous or sparse. Skin with acne vulgaris is oily, and in many cases, it may look improperly cared for, with blackheads, whiteheads, and clogged pores. Acne is not an internal disease surfacing on the skin. Rather, it is the combined result of four elements: the skin's androgen hormones, excessive cellular keratinization and agglomeration in the corneum layer and sebaceous follicle, oil production, and an overpopulation of a bacteria known as the *Propionibacterium acnes* (*P. acnes*). Other types of acne, such as cystic and rosacea, should be referred to a dermatologist, with care given under medical supervision. Some of the many factors said to aggravate acne include excessive oiliness, a failure to thoroughly remove oil and dirt from the skin, hormonal imbalances, hyperkeratinization, food allergies and sensitivities, lack of vitamins (especially vitamin A), and insufficient acidity in the skin. Acne is also aggravated by climatic conditions, especially heat and humidity, which increase bacterial development; the use of astringents and drying cosmetics; improper diet; stress; and picking.

Those with acne should emphasize cleansing at home and by a skin care professional, and skin hydration. The most effective products are those with ingredients that regulate oil gland secretion, hydrate, heal, balance the skin's pH, soothe, reduce inflammation, are antibacterial, and gently exfoliate excessive layers of corneocytes.

Rosacea

Rosacea is an inflammatory, long-lasting skin condition of the face. Although the exact cause of rosacea is still unknown, various theories about its origin have evolved. These include facial blood vessels that dilate too easily, whereby the increased blood near the skin surface makes the skin appear red and flushed; certain bacteria present on otherwise harmless Demodex mites that could prompt an inflammatory response; overproduction of two inflammatory proteins that increase the levels of a third protein that leads to rosacea symptoms; a high level of stratum corneum tryptic enzymes (SCTE), the precursor of a rosacea-causing peptide. None of these possibilities have been proven as a cause.

People with rosacea will experience inappropriate flushing that is not usually associated with sweating and/or persistent facial redness. They commonly have broken blood vessels (telangiectasias or couperose) and experience bouts of inflammation that cause red papules (small bumps) or pustules. However, comedones (blackheads and whiteheads) are not part of rosacea.

Clinically, rosacea may resemble acne vulgaris and is often confused with couperose and/or sensitive skin; however, these are separate conditions requiring different solutions. In contrast to acne, comedones are absent. Acne vulgaris is associated with plugging of the ducts of the oil glands, resulting in blackheads and pimples on the face and sometimes the back, shoulders, or chest. Rosacea seems to be linked to the vascular network of the central facial skin and causes redness, bumps, pustules, and other symptoms that rarely appear anywhere other than on the face.

The presence of rosacea is independent of skin type, as it can affect dry, flaky skin as well as normal or oily skin. The key is to identify the skin type and use the skincare products most suitable for it.

Skin with a rosacea condition may be sensitive and easily irritated. It is important to avoid ingredients and products that burn, sting, or irritate the skin, including those with alcohol, witch hazel, fragrance, menthol, peppermint, eucalyptus oil, clove oil, salicylic acid, scrubs, toners, astringents, and exfoliants. Products containing a sulfur drug or azelaic acid may be medically prescribed as an alternative or adjunct to antibiotic therapy. Rosacea cannot be cured.

Sunscreens or sunblocks that are effective against the full spectrum of UVA and UVB can be especially important for rosacea skin, as this condition may be particularly susceptible to sun damage resulting in rosacea flare-ups. An SPF of 15 or higher is recommended, and physical blocks utilizing zinc oxide or titanium dioxide may be effective if chemical sunscreens cause irritation.

The U.S. National Rosacea Society is the world's largest support organization for rosacea, offering information and educational services to hundreds of thousands of rosacea patients and health professionals each year.

Final Comment

In diagnosing the skin, it is recommended to *first identify skin type*. This will avoid confusing dryness (lack of oil) with dehydration (lack of water). It will also greatly assist in the proper identification of a skin care product with ingredients of most benefit to the skin in question. Proper diagnosis of a skin type and/or condition is key to identifying the correct skin care product with the most valuable therapeutic ingredients.

Definition of Terms

acid—refers to the pH level of a substance ranging from 0 for the most acidic substance to 6.9 for the least acidic. Acids are used in cosmetic formulations for a variety of reasons: to neutralize substances that otherwise would be too alkaline for the skin; as active principles that perform a specific function based on their own particular properties (for example, hyaluronic acid, essential fatty acids, etc.); and as exfoliating and peeling agents (for example, alpha hydroxyacids). Only those acid ingredients with a very low pH will be irritating to the skin. It is important to remember the skin is acidic.

active principle (active ingredient)—an ingredient with "treatment" value. When placed on the skin, it performs a therapeutic or beneficial function for the skin, such as healing, hydrating, soothing, toning, etc.

alcohols—widely used in cosmetics as solvents, carriers, and astringents. When incorporated as active ingredients, it is for antiseptic, antiviral, and bactericidal purposes. Alcohols are organic compounds containing a hydroxyl group (OH) in their molecule. They are recognized by the suffix *-ol,* such as ethanol for ethyl alcohol and isopropanol for isopropyl alcohol. Compounds listed with an *-ol* ending should, therefore, be recognized as alcohols, even if the word "alcohol" does not follow. Alcohols are also present in essential oils. Geraniol, nerol, and linalool are examples.

aldehyde—can be used as a chemical reagent, solvent, fragrance, or, when used as an active ingredient, as a soothing or antiseptic compound. An aldehyde is an organic

45

compound containing a carboxyl group (O and H) in its molecule. This is different from the OH of the alcohols. In an aldehyde, the "O" for oxygen and the "H" for hydrogen are each individually attached to the "C" carbon atom. In the alcohol group, the "OH" is attached as a unit. Aldehydes are generally recognized by the suffix -al, such as citral, geranial, or ethanal for ethyl aldehyde.

$$
\begin{array}{cc}
\text{H} & \\
| & \\
\text{C}\!=\!\text{O} & \text{C}\!-\!\text{OH} \\
\text{aldehyde} & \text{alcohol}
\end{array}
$$

alkali—a pH level measurement: a substance of 7.1 is the least alkaline and a substance of 14 is the most alkaline. Alkalis are used in cosmetics to balance formulas that have an undesired acid level: they raise the pH of formulas with a low acid level that might be irritating to the skin. For example, if a formulation has a pH below 4, an alkali may be added to raise the pH to 4.4 or 5.6, which is closer to the pH value of the skin. At the same time, cosmetics with a high alkaline level will be irritating to the skin.

antioxidant—refers to the ability of an ingredient to slow down, prevent, or block oxidation caused by the damaging effects of free radical activity.

The skin's own antioxidant defense system of enzymatic and nonenzymatic components protects it from free radical damage. However, when the amount of free radicals formed is greater than the capacity of the skin's natural defense system, cellular damage immediately occurs. Thus, as part of a "damage prevention process," antioxidants are being added to cosmetics to increase the natural antioxidant reservoir of the skin. Some of the most common antioxidants used in cosmetics are beta carotene, coenzyme Q10, gluthathione, green tea, idebenone, superoxide dismutase, and vitamins E and C. It is well established that a mixture, or "cocktail," of antioxidants may enhance the photoprotective effects of a formulation. A single antioxidant exposed to free radicals may become a free radical itself, albeit a less active one. When used in conjunction with other antioxidants, there is often a chain reaction that occurs among the various antioxidants, where each "takes a turn" in a process of continual neutralization of a free radical until it is totally neutralized.

Antioxidants are key to age prevention and their daily use in cosmetic products helps reduce UV-induced aging damage. The term antioxidant can also apply to a compound that prevents other compounds from oxidizing or becoming rancid (in the case of fats and oils). Thus, some ingredients with antioxidant properties are also used in preservative systems. *See also* free radicals; free radical scavengers.

aromatherapy—refers to the use of essential oils for therapeutic purposes and perfumery. Its use in skin care ranges from a marketing tool to the fragrancing of cosmetics to the therapeutic value associated with the topical applications of essential oils. The therapeutic value is derived both from topical use as well as more subtle psychological changes that result from scent inhalation. These can include an overall feeling of well-being, mood changes, and even an increase and/or decrease in productivity levels. *See also* botanicals.

astringent—refers to the constriction of tissues. It is considered to improve the appearance of large, open pores. An astringent is also used to reduce the oil content on the skin's surface, and rebalance the skin's acid level after the use of certain cleansers. This is particularly the case with cleansers that have a pH that is higher than the pH of the skin. Excessive use of astringents may result in surface dryness.

atom—the smallest component of an element that still retains the element's properties. An atom is made up of positive and negative charges called protons and electrons, respectively. The protons are in the nucleus of the atom and the electrons are found in layers around the nucleus. Each atom has the same number of electrons and protons. A combination of atoms forms a larger substance called a molecule.

bioavailable (bioactive; bioavailability)—refers to the amount of ingredient(s) absorbed and made available at the action site in the skin, after its application.

botanical—a plant element containing active plant constituents that can elicit certain biological responses when applied on the skin. Botanicals provide a wide range of benefits depending on the specific constituents of the plant. Efficacy is often associated with the concentration level of the active constituents present in the formulation, the skin's capability to absorb these, the effect that other ingredients present in the formulation might have on the active constituent, and the constituent's degree of penetration. Although botanicals were traditionally used by ancient societies as remedies for any number of external and internal disorders, their value was nearly reduced to pure folklore and hearsay when compared to the identified, measured, and tested effectiveness of synthetic ingredients. As research unravels the different molecular components of botanical extracts, it is being established that all botanicals have biologically active molecules. These molecules are responsible for providing the plant's attributed therapeutic properties. For example, bisabolol has been isolated and identified as one of the calming constituents in chamomile, and flavonoids, present in a large variety of plants, are now recognized as powerful antioxidants with anti-inflammatory, antiallergenic, antiviral, antiaging and anticarcinogenic activity.

Botanicals can be incorporated into a product in several forms: as the whole phytocomplex (for example, macerated rose petals or macerated carrots), as extract (for example, licorice root extract); fractions or particular elements of the extract (for example, flavonoids or terpenes); and individual constituents or active chemical components of the extract (for example, glycyrrhetinic acid, naturally occurring in licorice root). The therapeutic activity associated with a botanical can also vary based on the part of the plant used. A plant's fruit extract may have therapeutic values not found in an extract from the plant's leaf, for example. Regardless of the form in which the botanical is incorporated (whole, fraction, or individual constituent), the proper concentration of an active chemical component incorporated into the cosmetic formulations is crucial to determine the benefit provided by that particular plant extract. Merely adding an extract into a cosmetic product does not guarantee treatment benefits. Awareness of botanical performance and the part of the botanical incorporated into the formulation is important in order to differentiate actual benefits from marketing techniques.

Research continues to identify the actives present in botanical compounds that give them their therapeutic value. As more becomes known about how the biologically active constituents of botanicals work, the use of botanicals in skin care preparations will continue to rise. Currently, cosmetics based on botanical ingredients represent one of the fastest growing market segments.

Not all botanicals are appropriate for skin care. Depending on the ingredient, the skin type and condition, or amount of product used, some botanicals can cause severe irritation and/or react with other chemical ingredients on the skin, resulting in allergic reactions. As an understanding of botanicals and their therapeutic properties increases, knowledge of their proper use and management in cosmetics will as well.

buffered—refers to a chemical process by which a compound (or compounds) is added to a formulation in order to keep the formulation's pH unchanged regardless of the other ingredients added.

carbomers—a group of high molecular-weight polymers widely used as thickeners, suspending agents, and emulsion stabilizers in a variety of skin care products. The high clarity and unique texture they impart have led the way in the evolution of the gel product form. The benefits associated with carbomers include specific texture and formulation flow control, highly effective oil/water emulsion stabilization, and permanent suspension of insoluble or immiscible ingredients.

carrier (vehicle)—a component of a cosmetic formula that may affect the active ingredient's efficacy, stability, and time release, as well as skin tolerance and final location of the active in the different skin levels. Carriers also determine the ease of product application and depth of penetration.

chemical reaction—refers to the transformation of one or more substances into one or more different substances.

color—can be found listed as FD&C, D&C, and Ext. D&C. FD&C colors are approved for use in food, drugs, and cosmetics. D&C colors may be used only in drugs and cosmetics, including those that come in contact with mucous membranes and those that are ingested. An Ext. D&C listing indicates the use of a color certified for use in drugs and cosmetics that do not come in contact with mucous membranes and that are not ingested. (Note: these definitions should be used only as guidelines, as some FD&C colors are no longer approved for cosmetic use.)

A color listing can be broken down into three parts. For example, with FD&C Red No. 4, the first part indicates under which category of FDA certification the pigment falls, the second gives the color, and the number indicates which red is being used. If listed as FD&C Yellow No. 6 Al Lake, the Al Lake refers to "aluminum lake," and indicates the use of an organic pigment of the lake group, a water-soluble dye absorbed on alumina.

Three types of coloring matter are used in cosmetic products: inorganic, organic, and dyestuffs. Inorganic pigments are insoluble compounds based on metal ions. They tend to have good stability, and are widely used in eye and face makeup. Organic pigments tend to be bright but offer less variety in shades. This type of pigment is further divided into three subsets: lakes (water-soluble dyes absorbed on alumina), toners (organic barium or calcium salts), and true pigments. Although the true pigments are the least popular for use in cosmetics, they are the most stable of the three. The lakes are the least stable, and toners fall in between. Dyestuffs are used primarily in toiletry products such as shampoos and lotions. There are six classes of water-soluble dyestuffs commonly used in cosmetics and whose stability is dependent on chemical structure. These include azo, indigoid, and xanthene. Dyestuffs are also naturally occurring in some plants.

The colors listed on an ingredient label fall under FDA jurisdiction. Currently there are 65 different ingredients that are approved by the FDA for use as color additives in cosmetics. These can range from naturally derived ingredients such as beta-carotene, to minerals such as mica and zinc oxide, to the FD&C, D&C, and ext. D&C previously discussed. Most of these were approved prior to 1988.

comedogenic—describes an ingredient that tends to increase keratinocyte agglomeration in the philosebaceous follicle, thus creating a blockage of the follicle and causing the formation of comedones.

controlled release—describes a gradual and systematic release of an active ingredient into the skin, thereby avoiding the "peaks and valleys" of availability characteristically associated with regular topical applications. It includes encapsulating technologies such as liposomes or polymer entrapment. Encapsulated or entrapped actives can have a more controlled evaporation and greater skin compatibility, cause less irritation, and maximize the amount of time an active ingredient is present on the skin surface or within the epidermis. When required, such a system will reduce potential penetration. These systems can release their content, usually at once, by breakage due to pressure, abrasion, or dissolution of their shell. *See also* encapsulation.

cosmeceutical—a combination of the words *cosmetic* and *pharmaceutical*. This term is applied by the industry and in marketing to both a type of ingredient and a category of cosmetics. There is no legal or official definition of a "cosmeceutical." It is used to describe a range of products that promote attractiveness and affect the structure of the skin. With increased knowledge of skin physiology and chemistry, many more of these types of ingredients are being incorporated into products marketed as cosmetics. These are positioned primarily as "correctors" that influence the biological function of the skin for antiaging, antiwrinkle, and skin rejuvenation purposes. Some of the mechanisms of action attributed to cosmeceutical ingredients include activating cellular receptors (retinoids); enhancing barrier function (most moisturizers); increasing exfoliation (AHAs and BHAs); normalizing cellular repair (copper peptides): inhibiting oxidation (antioxidants); and regulating cellular communication (peptides). As knowledge increases, it is expected that the cosmeceutical category will continue to grow and increase its use of sophisticated ingredients. From the commercial standpoint, the term cosmeceuticals is being used to indicate that a given product may have greater efficacy than whatever can be said under cosmetic claims.

cytokines—a generic name used to describe a group of soluble peptides and proteins that act as regulators modulating the functional activities of individual cells and tissues.

delivery system—a chemical system that delivers the active to the targeted site of action in the skin in order to optimize performance. Delivery systems can affect skin reaction, ingredient penetration, and ingredient efficacy. Unless the active ingredient is delivered to the right place within the skin and at the appropriate concentration, the efficacy of the product can come into question. *See also* Chapter 2, Product Penetration.

emollient—a fatty substance with lubricating action that makes the skin feel softer and more pliable. Emollients also have a hydrating effect by reducing moisture evaporation from the skin surface through water diffusion into the corneum layer and underlying tissues. Although virtually any fatty material can make the skin feel softer, different emollients produce different results and skin feel. There are over 600 emollients, providing a variety of characteristics to a formulation, such as oily, dry, draggy, slippery, penetrating, nonpenetrating, shiny, dull, or any combination the formulator wishes to achieve. The selection of an emollient is a formulator's choice based on desired product performance and the other ingredients present in the formulation.

emulsifier—in a homogenized system, an emulsifier holds the oil-based and water-based ingredients together, helping stabilize the interaction between both phases, and thereby avoiding their separation in the cosmetic formulation.

emulsion—oil and water blended together as one substance, such as a cream or lotion, by use of an emulsifier. When oil is dispersed in water, the emulsion is called an oil-in-water emulsion, abbreviated as o/w. The oily phase of such emulsions can include oils, fats, and waxes. Oil-in-water emulsions provide a number of benefits: they can act as emollients imparting a pleasant skin feel by filling in the crevices between dead cells; or soften and improve the skin's moisture retention properties by leaving a water repellant film. The contrary emulsion form is a water-in-oil or w/o emulsion where water is dispersed into oil. Depending on the ingredients and product purpose, this can facilitate ingredient penetration to a desired target site. When emulsions destabilize, it may be due to any one or combination of such factors as high temperature, water evaporation, microbial contamination, or undesired chemical reactions. Emulsions are the most common delivery system used in cosmetic products because they enable the quick and convenient delivery of a wide variety of ingredients.

encapsulation (microencapsulation)—the process of enveloping microscopic amounts of substance in a thin film of polymer or in a vesicle. Liposomes are an example of encapsulation. Some of the many reasons for the use of encapsulation in cosmetic formulations are controlled release, reduction of irritation, reduction of evaporation, and easier delivery through the lipid barrier. *See also* controlled release.

enzyme—biologically, a highly specific and complex protein present in cosmetic formulations for at least three reasons: as a catalyst, an exfoliant, and an antioxidant. As a catalyst it can accelerate or produce a chemical reaction. Without enzymes, given the temperature and pH usually found in cells, most chemical reactions would not proceed fast enough to maintain the cell's life. Enzymes are specific to the type of reaction they catalyze, and they can increase a reaction rate anywhere from 100 to 1,000 times.

As exfoliants, the most common enzymes are of vegetable origin, such as papain from papaya. They tend to be used for augmenting the activity of naturally occurring enzymes in the skin that are responsible for surface exfoliation of dead cells by breaking intercellular bonds. As antioxidants, enzymes such as superoxide dismutase (SOD) work to convert dangerous and highly reactive oxygen free radicals into a less reactive form. Enzymes have also been used in cosmetics to reduce the preservative content since some of them can protect cosmetic formulations from bacterial attack.

The correct concentration of any enzyme in a product is very important: too little will not be effective and too much might cause adverse reactions or be toxic.

essential fatty acid (EFA)—the basic building blocks of body fats and cellular membranes. If the skin's EFA content declines, so will its elasticity. Meanwhile, transepidermal water loss will increase, together with skin roughness and scaliness. Since cell membranes are largely made of phospholipids, topically applied EFAs may be metabolized in the skin, normalizing the cell lipid layer and improving the water-retention capability of the corneum layer. Examples of EFAs are Omegas 3, 6, and 9.

essential oil—a volatile oily substance produced from plants. Essential oils contain vitamins, hormones, antibiotics, and/or antiseptics. These oils are present as tiny droplets between the plant's cells. They play an important role in the plant's biochemistry, and are also responsible for its fragrance. Essential oils have many established and attributed properties, including antiseptic, antibiotic, soothing, and calming and can also act as preservatives. These oils are extracted by a variety of methods that allow the integrity of the oil to be maintained. Distillation is the most common method used to obtain a plant's essential oil. The yield of essential oils varies between 0.005 percent and 10 percent of the plant, depending on the type of plant. The lower the yield, the more expensive the oil. The quality and chemistry of essential oils may vary according to the part of the plant from which the oil was extracted (root, bark, flowers, leaf), the time of day and/or year in which it was picked, the location where the plant grows (lowlands, highlands), and the methods of cultivation.

esters—products resulting from the combination of organic acids and alcohols. They can be natural or synthetic, liquid or solid, depending on properties of the reacting substances. Insoluble in water, they replace oils and fats to provide a more uniform composition and preservation. They have good skin tolerance and a lubricating and emollient action. Esters are also found in essential oils. Often even small amounts of characteristic esters are crucial for the finer notes in the fragrance of an essential oil.

fatty acid—*see* essential fatty acid.

flavonoids—also known as bioflavonoids. The term refers to a type of plant extract classified as flavonoids, isoflavonoids, and neoflavonoids. There are approximately 3,000 identified flavonoid substances. In addition to an antioxidant effect, flavonoids have also demonstrated anti-inflammatory, antiallergenic, antiviral, antiaging and anticarcinogenic activity. They are used in the treatment of skin aging, as they appear to improve collagen and, to a lesser degree, elasticity, roughness, and skin hydration. In addition, they seem to regulate oil gland secretion.

Flavonoids are widely distributed in plants and fulfill many functions. They provide flowers with their yellow or red/blue pigment and protect the plant from attack by microbes and insects. The beneficial effects of fruit, vegetables, and tea or even red wine have been attributed to their flavonoid components rather than to known nutrients and vitamins. Flavonoids are found in berries, citrus fruits, cocoa, green tea, parsley, red wine, and soybean.

The most important flavonoids are quercetin, which is considered the most active of flavonoids and found in many medicinal plants, and epicatechin, which is found in cocoa. Studies show that these flavonoids, together with those from grape leaf, citrus fruits, and green tea, can penetrate the skin.

fragrance—natural and synthetic compounds are added to a cosmetic formulation to give an aroma, mask chemical odors, and even to achieve subtly communicated messages such as image and market positioning. Studies conducted on consumer perception of product efficacy demonstrated that, using the same product base, consumers gave the product a different performance rating depending on the fragrance used.

Fragrances have also been the source of cosmetic allergies. An FDA study determined that more than 1 percent of all cosmetic allergic contact dermatitis cases were due to fragrances. Observations indicate that in reality, 7 to 18 percent of all individuals may have some form of sensitivity or intolerance to fragrances. Thus, products positioned as hypoallergenic are fragranceless.

On an ingredient label, it is very difficult to determine if the fragrance used is natural or synthetic, a known fragrance, or a proprietary blend. Terminology such as "plant extracts" indicates extracts used for therapeutic purposes and/or fragrancing. There is no definite way of knowing the origin of a fragrance by just looking at the label.

With the increased popularity of aromatherapy, many skin care products depend on already incorporated botanicals for fragrance. Its dual function is appealing: the formulator achieves potential therapeutic value and fragrance without offending a consumer's sense of "green" or creating a fear of increasing skin sensitivity.

free radicals (reactive oxygen species)—electrically charged, highly unstable, and very reactive oxygen atoms or molecules. Free radicals are formed when an oxygen atom loses an electron. The loss of the electron makes the atom or molecule electrically unstable. To regain stability, free radicals tend to capture electrons from other substances in order to neutralize. This reaction can give rise to two different processes: a) the neutralization effect of one free radical can cause the formation of another, causing a chain reaction of free radical formation where innumerable free radical reactions occur within seconds of the initial reaction; or b) it can attach itself to the cellular membrane, allowing the free radical to restabilize, but in the process a new oxidation compound is formed that ends up damaging the cellular membrane, the DNA, and the cellular repair mechanisms, etc. This is why it is important that the skin has a reservoir of antioxidants.

The instability and high reactivity of free radicals is corrected when they either give an electron to another molecule or take one from another molecule. The oxygen molecule, necessary for an organism's survival, is a primary producer of free radicals in the body. Internally, free radicals are produced by metabolic reactions. Externally, they are a result of UV radiation, pesticides, air pollution, drugs, cigarette smoke, stress, and unhealthy lifestyles. The body has its own natural mechanism of protection against free radical-induced damage. This protective ability diminishes with age and when the body is exposed to situations where the quantity of free radicals formed is greater than the body's natural ability to neutralize them. In addition, the production of free radicals over and above that from which the body can protect itself is responsible for numerous undesired problems. Free radicals are considered the number one factor behind skin aging. They damage DNA, cellular membranes, and the connective tissue components of the dermis, particularly collagen, by stimulating collagenase enzyme production. The overall result is cellular damage, alterations in the structure of the cellular membrane, and decreased skin elasticity and pliability. Free radicals also harm the Langerhans cells, diminishing the efficacy of the skin's immune system. In addition, free radicals favor production of secondary chemicals in the skin. These cause negative chemical reactions and cellular damage that further accentuates skin aging. It is important to note that a certain amount of free radicals are necessary for proper skin functioning. It is the excessive amount that causes serious and often irreversible damage.

free radical scavengers (anti-free radicals, antioxidants)— components that counteract the destructive effect of free radical activity. Compounds such as vitamin E (the different tocopherol forms), vitamin C (ascorbic acid form), and the flavonoids are examples of ingredients currently considered free radical scavengers. They can be systemically or topically incorporated to help reduce the free radical effect by decomposing the free radicals into compounds against which the body has defenses.

humectant—used in cosmetic formulations to increase the skin's moisture content. Humectants have the ability to bind moisture and are considered moisturizers.

hydrolysis—a chemical process by which complex proteins are degraded to smaller molecules of lower molecular weight, including into their individual amino acid components. Hydrolysis can be performed by means of acid reactions or enzymatic action. Hydrolyzed proteins, therefore, are proteins of lower molecular weight than their source and have greater skin affinity. Therefore, they are more easily incorporated into cosmetic formulations. Generally, the term hydrolyzed, so commonly found on cosmetic labels, does not identify the amino acids involved or the process or hydrolysis used.

hygroscopic—describes an ingredient that readily absorbs and retains moisture.

hypoallergenic—describes a cosmetic product as one that is not likely to produce allergic reactions. Usually, this term is applied to products that are fragrance-free and have a select type of preservative. The causes and varieties of allergies are so broad and widespread that it is very difficult to state that a product is truly hypoallergenic. Allergenicity is not a matter of the product but rather the sensitivity of the individual.

lipid—refers to fat or fat-like substances (oils, waxes), and encompasses diverse compounds, including triglycerides, phospholipids, and sterols such as cholesterol. Lipids are an important element for the corneum layer's healthy structure and function. They account for a significant volume of the stratum corneum, constituting 6 to 10 percent of the normal corneum layer by weight. They are found primarily in the intercellular spaces. Intercellular lipids provide a barrier to the passage of a variety of substances through the skin.

Lipids incorporated into cosmetics help moisturize the skin by renewing its barrier function, either by replacing lipids that have been removed with washing, by allowing epidermal lipids to remain despite adverse environments, or by renewing the skin's ability to bind moisture. The skin's barrier function against moisture loss is proportional to the lipid content within the corneum layer.

liquid crystal—defined as a substance that flows like a liquid but maintains some of the ordered structure characteristics of crystals. In cosmetics, it applies primarily to compounds that can encapsulate active substances and allow for a time-release pattern. They are considered intermediates between solids and liquids.

masking—refers to an ingredient that can help "hide" any unpleasant odor that may naturally arise from the combination of chemicals that are used to formulate a cosmetic. A masking ingredient may be very different from a fragrance. While a fragrance may impart a pleasant odor, a masking ingredient may simply help neutralize unpleasant ones.

molecule—a substance made from a combination of similar or different atoms held together by chemical bonds. Molecules have their own characteristic set of properties. For example, a water molecule is composed of two hydrogen atoms and one oxygen atom. The size of a molecule is established by its number of atoms and will determine its ability to penetrate the skin layers. The larger a molecule, the less it is able to penetrate the skin. In addition, the larger the molecule, the lower its ability to evaporate and diffuse through the skin. Smaller molecules have a greater volatility (evaporation ability).

nanotechnology—a rapidly developing technology based on extremely small (nano) particles (one nanometer is to a meter like a marble is to the size of the Earth), with multiple applications. At nanoscale, molecules tend to change many of their characteristics. For example, zinc oxide and titanium dioxide change from white to being colorless. The cosmetic industry also classifies nanotechnology into insoluble and soluble nanoparticles, nanoemulsions, and nanodelivery systems.

Insoluble nanoparticles of titanium dioxide and zinc oxide have been used for many years as UV filters in order to provide a broad spectrum of UVA and UVB protection. These two molecules are transparent at nanoscale rather than their characteristic white color, and thus they do not leave a white film on the skin. It has been established that the insoluble nanoparticles, titanium dioxide and zinc oxide, do not penetrate further than the stratum corneum.

Nanotechnology utilizing organic ingredients is now being used in formulating antiaging products with the belief that smaller particles are more rapidly absorbed into the skin and will repair damage more easily and more efficiently. However, at a nano size, organic compounds have deeper penetration capabilities and different toxicity characteristics than the same compound or chemical at its "regular" size. Thus, organic nanoparticles that do penetrate can have the risk of possible secondary reactions, the nature of which is not yet established. Nanoemulsions and nanodelivery systems are being used for the efficient delivery and rapid penetration of active principles through the skin.

Given expressed concerns over the potential unintended effects of nanotechnology, a comprehensive regulatory system is seen as key to ensure the safe implementation of this technology. Both the U.S. FDA and the European Commission are looking into nanomaterials because of uncertainties surrounding the rapid and unknown level of penetration. The FDA and the Scientific Committee for Cosmetic Products of the European Union concluded that titanium dioxide and zinc oxide nanoparticles are safe for use in sunscreens. For other nanoelements, the FDA is seeking feedback from the cosmetic industry to develop the recommendations that its

Nanotechnology Task Force will utilize to establish guidelines for this field.

Capitalizing on the nano concept, some companies are already renaming a variation of this technology as "mega-small" ingredients. Therefore, consumers will need to be aware of the manipulation of nano concepts.

Nanotechnology can either become a revolutionary concept in skin care or it can become a government-regulated area that requires special approval for use. At the time of writing, the newness of the technology and its potential controversy have not been sufficiently developed to foresee its future in cosmetics.

natural cosmetics—strictly speaking, natural cosmetics should refer only to cosmetics made of all natural ingredients. However, this terminology is applied to a variety of concepts that range from products made using mostly organically grown plants to chemically manufactured products that contained some plant extracts.

The term "natural" in cosmetics can be misleading, since everything that comes from nature is considered natural, including plants, minerals, animals, and insects. From this very strict perspective, mineral oil and petrolatum should be considered natural, as they are found in nature.

This classification also covers products formulated with "ingredients of natural origin." These products include those with natural ingredients that have been, or might have been, chemically processed.

In almost all instances, chemical products are present in "natural cosmetics." In almost all instances, except in the case of essential oils, preservatives are added to these products. The more organic compounds a product has, the greater its chance to perish in a short period of time if not properly preserved. A consumer needs just to consider how long an apple or a container of milk lasts even when refrigerated.

While consumers increasingly insist on "natural" and/or "organic" products, it is important to examine manufacturers' claims with a level of skepticism. The term "natural" is not regulated by any government agency and therefore guidelines and standards have not been set as to what can and cannot be considered a "natural cosmetic." It is thus left open to interpretation by manufacturers and consumers. *See also* organic cosmetics.

natural moisturizing factor (NMF)—found in the corneum layer, the NMF is comprised of hygroscopic, water-soluble substances that regulate the layer's selective permeability. The NMF is composed of about 40 percent free amino acids, 12 percent PCA, 12 percent lactose, 7 percent urea, and approximately 30 percent of a large variety of other materials. Exposure to harsh detergents and climatic conditions can result in decreased NMF levels, rendering the skin fragile and dry.

The design of modern moisturizers has depended on selecting various hygroscopic ingredients with properties and effects similar to the NMF and combining them with effective vehicles.

neutralized—when a chemical product has been added to bring the formulation's pH to near 7, or neutral. Partially neutralized is when a chemical product is added to move the compound up or down the pH scale toward 7 or a more neutral value.

occlusive ingredients—used to decrease the level of moisture loss by the skin. Occlusive ingredients tend to be film-formers because of their large molecular size.

oligoelement—refers to trace elements with important catalytic action in enzymatic reactions to ensure normal cell metabolism. These elements include copper, magnesium, selenium, and zinc. Some sources indicate that indiscriminate application of these oligoelements, whether alone or in combination with one another, may be absolutely ineffective and may even harm the skin. Others cite that experimental tests showing that the presence of selected oligoelements in a formulation may improve a protein derivative's affinity to increase moisturization.

organic cosmetics—tend to refer to cosmetics that incorporate either the extracts of organically grown plants or macerations of the organically grown plants themselves. The latter are usually more active than the former, may have a greater tendency to cause sensitivity or allergic reactions, and have a shorter shelf life.

Unlike the case with organic food products, the term "organic" in cosmetics is not government regulated or even defined. The standards have been given by laboratory or manufacturer associations in individual countries and follow no uniform pattern from one country to the next. In Europe, the European Cosmetics Standards Working Group, comprising seven organizations, is working to harmonize organic personal care standards. In 2005, the U.S. Department of Agriculture stated that agricultural products, including personal care products, that have an organic agricultural content may meet the National Organic Program (NOP) standards and be labeled as "100 percent organic," "organic," or "made with organic [ingredients]" pursuant to the NOP regulations. Prior to the use of this statement, companies could receive organic certification for the agriculturally produced ingredients but not for the finished product. However, cosmetics that do not conform to the NOP's organic standards still can use the word "organic" in their products because the word "organic" is an unregulated marketing claim.

Lack of regulation and a consumer perception that "organic" is better has resulted in a significant level of marketing manipulation with respect to the concept of "organic" cosmetics. Under the best self-imposed guidelines, organic cosmetics are made with certified organically grown vegetal materials, do not use genetically modified ingredients, use only selected preservatives (usually a significant amount of natural alcohols and salicylic acid), follow a list of restricted raw materials used for processing, do not use radioactive radiation for disinfection, and do not use synthetic dyes and fragrances. Often, a small amount of chemical ingredients, about 5 percent of formulation total, is allowed.

However, even the best guidelines can be manipulated and lead to misinterpretations. For example, a product can cite a percentage value of organics as if it represented the total value of organic ingredients. More careful reading would indicate that in reality, the percentage listed represents the amount of organic materials in the total quantity of the product's vegetal material. Since the label does not indicate the total percentage of vegetal material present in the formula, the true amount of organic materials cannot be calculated. For example, the product may have 20 percent of vegetal material, and 80 percent of that may be of organic agriculture. The label and the advertising can be written in a way that the consumer can interpret that 80 percent of the product to be "organic," when in truth only 16 percent (80 percent of the 20 percent) of the total formulation is.

Regretfully, given present regulatory practices, consumers have no easy way of distinguishing which organic cosmetics are most "truthfully" organic.

pH—refers to the level of acidity or alkalinity of a given chemical
   ingredient or product. As the hydrogen in a substance deter-
   mines the ingredient or product's level of acidity or alkalinity, the symbol *pH* stands for the power (p) of the hydrogen
   molecule (H). The pH of acids ranges between 0 and 6.9 and
   of alkalis between 7.1 and 14. A pH of 7 is considered neutral. The importance of a product's pH is based on its correlation to the skin's pH. Human skin has a pH in the acidic
   range, varying from 4.4 to 5.6 depending on the individual
   and the area of skin tested. The value of the surface pH
   is due to acids present in the stratum corneum. External
   factors, such as perspiration, tend to make the skin more
   acidic. The higher the skin's pH number the less acidic it is,
   and the greater its sensitivity reaction to very acidic compounds, often sensed as burning or redness. The lower the
   skin's numeric pH the more acidic it is, and thus it will be
   less sensitive to acid compounds such as peelings and other
   exfoliants. As a practical example, skin with a pH of 5 will
   be more sensitive to an AHA product with a pH of 3.8 than
   will skin with a pH of 4.4.

parabens—a family of synthetic preservatives widely used in
   cosmetics around the world since the 1920s because of
   their efficacy, low risk of irritation, and stability. This family includes butylparaben, ethylparaben, methylparaben,
   and propylparaben, with the last two being the most commonly used. All of these parabens are effective against a
   broad spectrum of microorganisms, including most fungi
   and most bacteria. They prevent the growth of other possible contaminants such as yeast and mold. They are used in
   quantities of 0.1 to 0.5 percent of total formulation, and it
   is estimated that 30 percent or less of the total amount of
   paraben used (0.03 percent to 0.15 percent) may penetrate
   the skin.

   In 2004, the safety of parabens as preservatives became an
   issue. This was the result of a UK study that focused on the
   use of paraben-containing deodorants. It evaluated if long-
   term use of parabens was biocumulative and thus somehow
   related to breast cancer. Since then, cosmetic chemists who
   are familiar with the skin-penetration activity of parabens
   maintain that an accumulation of parabens from topical application is not possible because once parabens enter the
   skin, they form metabolites that are incapable of mimicking
   estrogen. Other studies indicate that after entering the skin,

parabens are metabolized to para-hydroxybenzoic acid with only a small percentage remaining as the original paraben.

The most recently conducted studies seem to invalidate the claim of potential breast cancer risk when using cosmetics with parabens. Studies have shown that parabens are 1,000 to 1,000,000 times less estrogenic than estradiol, the major estrogenic compound in the body. Methylparaben has the weakest estogenic effect, approximately 2.5 million times less potent than 17-B estradiol, followed by ethylparaben. Phytoestrogens, substances from plants that have estrogen-like qualities including soybeans, clover, strawberries, sage, dong quai, red clover, pumpkin, and rosehips (among others), are considered to have natural estrogenic effects 1,000 to 1,000,000 times stronger than parabens.

The U.S. Food and Drug Administration (FDA) has stated: "FDA is aware that estrogenic activity in the body is associated with certain forms of breast cancer. Although parabens can act similarly to estrogen, they have been shown to have much less estrogenic activity than the body's naturally occurring estrogen." Despite this statement, the use of parabens in cosmetics remains controversial. More comprehensive studies are needed to conclusively determine the true scope of the potential harm caused by prolonged exposure to parabens resulting from daily use of cosmetics.

While the parabens used in cosmetics and toiletries are synthetically manufactured, parabens are naturally formed from an acid (p-hydroxy-benzoic acid) reportedly found in raspberries and blackberries.

peptides—short polymers formed by linking alpha amino acids. When such an amino acid chain is small, the molecule is called a peptide. When it is larger, it is called a polypeptide. Proteins are polypeptide molecules. While proteins cannot penetrate the skin, smaller peptides can be absorbed.

The ability to link different numbers of amino acids, thereby forming different peptides and polypeptides, gives these ingredients a variety of beneficial properties when incorporated into cosmetic products. These benefits include increased skin elasticity and smoothness to improvements in the appearance of wrinkles, a reduction of inflammation, and tissue repair. There are also claims that peptides can activate regenerative skin functions, increase collagen, and synthesize other epidermal components.

For cosmetic application, natural peptides are derived from cotton, rice, wheat, casein, and whey. They have various applications in hair and skin care formulations based on their molecular weight distributions, amino acid content, solubility, and odor profiles. Peptides can be natural or synthetic.

phytotherapy—refers to the use of plants or plant extracts for their therapeutic value in the cosmetic product. It includes the use of plant extracts, distilled waters, and essential oils.

phytoestrogen—a plant constitutent that has estrogenic efficacy. Estrogen stimulates the fibroblast to produce collagen and hyaluronic acid and thus, phytoestrogen-containing plants are claimed to improve collagen formation and hyaluronic acid. Blackberry, lily extract, spinach, red clover, and soy isoflavones have estrogenic efficacy.

polymers—large molecules constructed of smaller molecules of the same substance. In cosmetics, polymers are part of the encapsulation concept used for a sustained and controlled release effect of active ingredients. Polymers improve the delivery of lubricants and skin protectants and the duration of skin moisturization. They also act as emulsifiers. *See also* controlled release.

polyphenols—a family of very powerful botanical antioxidants. Polyphenols also reinforce collagen and elastin while preventing the degradation of fundamental tissue elements required for healthy skin. The polyphenols present in green tea include but are not limited to catechins, such as epigallocatechin gallate (EGCG), epigallocatechin (EGC), epicatechin 3-gallate (ECG), and epicatechin (EC). There are antioxidants in nature that also act as anti-inflammatory and anticarcinogenic agents. The stabilized grapeseed polyphenol works with essential fatty acids to protect cells against free-radicals. Polyphenols are claimed to treat and/or prevent skin conditions, including fine lines and wrinkles, acne rosacea, surface irregularities of the skin, and hyperpigmentation.

precipitate—small particles (above 1 micron) that have settled out of a suspension due to gravity or as a result of electrical discharge.

precursors—intermediate compounds of high biological potential that, when activated, are converted to another specific substance. This is the case, for example, of ergosterol (provitamin D_2), which is changed by ultraviolet radiation to vitamin D. Carotene (provitamin A) is a precursor that can be transformed into vitamin A.

Biological precursors are also defined as small molecules capable of penetrating the skin and, once in the skin—through a chemical reaction with skin's own chemicals and/or enzymes—convert into another, related compound that could have not penetrated in its original state because of molecular size or affinity problems. One example is retinyl palmitate. When applied to the skin, a percentage of it converts, through an enzymatic process, to retinol. Some substances labeled as biological precursors are said to stimulate the synthesis of collagen, elastin, proteoglycans, and structural glycoproteins.

preservative—ingredient added to a formulation, to ensure microbiological safety and stability. Preservatives guard products during consumer use from undesirable microorganisms (usually seen as mold growth) that can be introduced into an open container and become a possible health hazard. This is especially true for products that contain plant extracts. Without preservatives, these everyday items would become overloaded with bacteria, mold, and fungus.

An ideal preservative should include a broad antibacterial/antifungal spectrum; be nontoxic, nonirritating, and free of other sensitizing effects; be compatible with other products in the formulation; and be compatible with the product's packaging. While only some preservatives may cause irritation and sensitization, people tend to believe this is the case with most or all preservatives. This has led to "preservative-free" cosmetics. In reality, "preservative-free" products do not lack a preservative system. They are considered "self-preserving" based on a low pH value, the surfactants and antioxidants incorporated, aroma chemicals, alcohols, and some essential oils and other ingredients used to make the growth and survival of microorganisms difficult. The idea that preservative-free cosmetics are safer than those with preservatives is not necessarily true. The use of preservatives in cosmetics is a regulatory requirement.

protein—chain of amino acids join by peptide bonds. Incorporating proteins into skin care preparations can provide such benefits as film-forming and moisturizing, regenerating, stimulating cell proliferation, and reducing the irritation potential of certain surfactants. Originally, most of the proteins used were animal derived. These are now generally replaced with those of vegetable origin. Common and suitable sources for vegetable proteins include almond, oat, rice, soybean, and wheat.

reactive oxygen species—*see* free radicals.

retinoids—refer to ingredients derived from vitamin A, and include retinol, retinyl esters, and retinyl palmitate. Retinoids play an important role in repairing damaged and photodamaged skin. Retinoid treatment can result in the regeneration of the dermal collagen tissue by inhibiting excessive formation of collagenase enzyme responsible for the breakdown of dermal collagen and by also promoting collagen synthesis. The ability of retinoids to increase collagen types I and II makes them helpful in the prevention of bruising, tearing, and ulceration in mature skin. Retinol has become the preferred retinoid for cosmetic use.

sensitizer—refers to an ingredient(s) that can provoke a sensitivity reaction such as skin redness, swelling, itching, or any other adverse reaction.

skin conditioner—a general term referring to an ingredient's ability to help keep the skin in an optimal state. A skin conditioner might help improve skin tone, texture, softness, smoothness, and overall appearance.

solubilizer—helps dissolve normally insoluble materials such as fragrances and oils.

sun protection factor (SPF)—a measurement of the time that it takes the skin to turn red when exposed to ultraviolet energy. It refers *only* to UVB protection. It does not apply to UVA protection. A sunscreen's SPF number identifies the exposure time required to produce a minimal redness or minimal erythema dose (MED) on unprotected skin. Therefore, an SPF of 15, for example, means that the sunscreen offers 15 times greater protection against redness from exposure to UVB rays than if no sunscreen were applied. Because MED response varies by individual, the SPF value time varies accordingly.

In November 2007, the FDA proposed a new rule for sunscreen products. This rule expanded the established product performance categories from SPF 30 to SPF 50+. It established that any product with an SPF of at least 2 and no more than 12 is considered to offer *minimal sunburn protection*. Products with an SPF between 12 and 30 is considered to offer *moderate sunburn protection*. Products with an SPF between 30 and now 50+ are considered to offer *high sunburn protection*. This change was based on the argument that SPF 50 offers more UVB protection than the lower SPF values.

In addition, the 2007 proposed rule created a UVA rating system. This system would be based on a scale of one to four stars, with one star representing low UVA protection, two stars representing medium protection, three stars representing high protection, and four stars representing the highest UVA protection available for an over-the-counter (OTC) sunscreen product. If a sunscreen product does not provide at least a low-level (one star) protection, the FDA proposes to require a "no UVA protection" label on the front of the product, near the SPF values. This new rule may come into effect during 2009.

sunblock—a term not incorporated into the FDA's May 1999 final monograph, rendering it "non-monograph." This means that the term sunblock cannot appear anywhere on product labeling or promotional materials. *See* sunscreen.

sunscreen—as a technical term, refers to specific chemicals or compounds designed to protect the skin from harmful ultraviolet (UV) rays. Sunscreens can absorb, reflect, and/or scatter UV radiation, shielding skin from the sun's damaging effects. More loosely, however, the term is used to name a special class of personal-care products containing sunscreen ingredients. Unlike regular skin care or other cosmetics, in the United States, these products are classified as drugs and are therefore regulated by the Food and Drug Administration (FDA).

Sunscreens should absorb and/or reflect both UVB *and* UVA rays. This is very important because while UV light is responsible for tanning and UVB causes sunburn, both UVA and UVB damage the skin and increase the risk of skin cancer. The formulation of an effective UVA/UVB sunscreen requires the use of several sunscreen chemicals since those that are most effective against UVB rays are not necessarily effective against UVA. Daily protection against UVA is very important, as UVA radiation is a constant, year-round phenomenon.

The last final monograph for sunscreens released by the FDA was in May 1999. It established the conditions under which OTC sunscreen products are generally recognized as safe and effective, and not misbranded. Category I ingredients are those which the FDA classifies as Generally

Recognized as Safe and Effective. In the case of sunscreen chemicals, the following Category I table was approved by the FDA and implemented in 2001. Since then, only minor changes have taken place in the United States, while the list of approved sunscreen chemicals has been expanded significantly in the European Union.

Category I Active Sunscreen Ingredients and Maximum Concentrations Allowed in Finished Formulations

21 CFR 352.10	INCI Name	Maximum Concentration	Alternate or Drug Name
(a)	PABA	up to 15%	aminobenzoic
(b)	avobenzone	up to 3%	butyl methoxy-dibenzolmethane
(c)	cinoxate	up to 3%	cinoxate
(d)	(reserved)		
(e)	benzophenone-8	up to 3%	dioxybenzone
(f)	homosalate	up to 15%	homosalate
(g)	(reserved)		
(h)	methyl anthranilate	up to 5%	meradimate
(i)	octocrylene	up to 10%	octocrylene
(j)	ethylhexyl methoxy-cinnamate[1]	up to 7.5%	octinoxate
(k)	ethylhexyl salicylate[2]	up to 5%	octisalate
(l)	benzophenone-3	up to 6%	oxybenzone
(m)	ethylhexyl dimethyl PABA[3]	up to 8%	padimate O
(n)	phenylbenzi midazole sulfonic acid	up to 4%	ensilizole
(o)	benzophenone-4	up to 10%	sulisobenzone
(p)	titanium dioxide	up to 25%	titanium dioxide
(q)	TEA-salicylate	up to 12%	trolamine salicylate
(r)	zinc oxide	up to 25%	zinc oxide

[1] the new (INCI) name for octyl methoxycinnamate
[2] the new (INCI) name for octyl salicylate
[3] the new (INCI) name for octyl dimethyl PABA
From *Cosmetics & Toiletries,* 113(3), March 2000, p. 69.

Achieving a higher sun protection factor (SPF) product is not necessarily a question of dropping in more sunscreen chemicals, as this may increase the cost and irritation potential of the finished product. Alternatives are necessary.

Several of the chemicals listed above are generally used together in a sunscreen formulation in order to provide wide spectrum protection. FDA approval is required for sunscreen ingredient combinations. In the proposed 2007 rule, two new sunscreen chemical combinations have been approved: avobenzone with phenybenzimidazole sulfonic acid (ensilizole), and avobenzone with zinc oxide.

There is also the need for consumer education. Sunscreen efficacy is not only dependent on the ingredients used. It also depends on the adequacy of sunscreen application by the user. Sunscreen products must be applied evenly and in sufficient amounts to achieve adequate protection. A sunscreen's stated SPF is based on regulated laboratory testing of the product when it is applied at an even thickness of 2 mg/cm^2. Compare this to 0.5 mg/cm^2, the average thickness of sunscreen applied by the average person. Note that in the case of typical use, the average thickness of sunscreen application on individual sites can vary—ranging from 0 to 1.2 mg/cm^2! Also, sunscreens are a category of product that must remain on the surface of the skin for optimal protection. Thus, it is not correct to massage the sunscreen during application to ensure "penetration." Sunscreen application should be evenly spread on the skin's surface with gentle tapping motions. *See also* UV absorbers.

surfactant (surface active agent)—ingredient that lowers the surface tension of cosmetics and aids in the spreadability of products when applied on the skin. Surfactants are often found in cleansing agents, emulsifiers, foaming agents, solubilizers, and wetting agents. There are almost 2,000 different surfactants available to the cosmetic formulator. The present work in the cosmetic field is to develop low irritation surfactants that achieve a maximum emulsifying, solubilizing, and dispersing effect while causing minimal reaction with epidermal cells. The damaging effects of surfactants on the skin manifest themselves as dryness, roughness, scaling, and redness.

Irritation by surfactants accounts for a large number of adverse skin reactions. The level of irritation depends on the type of surfactant used, its concentration, and duration of the contact with the skin. Exaggerated use of surfactants coupled with preexisting sensitivity, extremes of temperature or pH, low humidity, or the combined use of other potential irritants such as abrasives, bleaches, or lipid solvents can bring about reactions such as skin irritation, inflammation, chapping, and roughness.

thickening/gelling agent—provides "body" to cosmetics, increases their stability, improves suspending action, and contributes to product feel and ease of application. Some thickening/gelling agents have film-forming characteristics, impart skin affinity, and can act as carriers/releasers for active ingredients. Most thickeners are synthetic, with only approximately 10 percent being of natural origin.

ultraviolet radiation—a form of energy from the sun traveling through space in the form of visible light. Sunlight is composed of many wavelengths spread across the electromagnetic spectrum. As these solar rays pass through the Earth's atmosphere, some of the wavelengths are filtered out. The remaining wavelengths reach Earth as UV and infrared light, and are grouped into three categories: UVA, UVB, and UVC. The atmosphere filters almost all light in the UVC range, but not in the UVA or UVB ranges. UVA penetrates deeply into the skin and can cause a phototoxic effect at the dermal level. UVB, with a shorter wavelength, is primarily responsible for causing skin redness, as its penetration and concentration is almost exclusively in the epidermis. Overall, UV light can cause a wide range of reactions including mild skin burn, edema and hyperpigmentation, premature aging, DNA damage, and skin cancer. In addition, UV light can trigger the production in the skin of secondary chemicals (e.g., collagenase enzyme) with capabilities to accelerate aging and damage normal skin function. *See also* UVA; UVB; UVC.

UVA—light composed of wavelengths ranging between 400–340 nm. UVA has the lowest energy potential but penetrates deeply into the skin, interacting with more skin structures and damaging collagen and elastin through the production of secondary chemicals that digest the elastin and collagen, leading to wrinkles. UVA may also damage cellular structure, cause DNA mutations or deletions, and inactivate some DNA repair mechanisms. UVA is a particularly potent carcinogenesis promoter, and it also promotes immunosuppression. UVA damage is cumulative, and is evidenced in wrinkles, sagging skin, and other visible signs of aging. UVA light accounts for about 95 percent of all UV radiation that penetrates the skin. UVA rays also come from sun lamps and sunbeds and thus is *just as damaging* as those rays which come directly from the sun.

UVB—light composed of wavelengths ranging between 340–280nm. This is called the burning or erythemal region because it can penetrate through the stratum corneum and epidermis, causing skin redness and sunburn. Directly absorbed by DNA molecules, UVB is a complete carcinogen in the skin and, in conjunction with certain chemical agents, can act as both a tumor initiator and tumor promoter.

UVC—light composed of wavelengths ranging between 280–200nm. UVC has the lowest wavelength and the highest energy since wavelength and energy are inversely related. Almost all of the light in this range is filtered out by Earth's atmosphere.

UV absorbers (UV filters)—another term for chemical compounds able to absorb UV light, remitting or reabsorbing it in a harmless form, and thus defusing its damaging energy. When UV light strikes a molecule of a UV absorber, the molecule is stimulated to a higher energy level. When it returns to its original energy state, the excess energy that was absorbed is emitted as light with a different energy state. Each sunscreen molecule can repeat this absorption–emission cycle multiple times before it decays. Common UV absorbers include organic compounds. Inorganic sunscreens are insoluble particles that lie on the skin surface and are not absorbed by the skin layers. Common UV absorbers include the following families of chemicals:

- *benzophenones*—these absorb UV light that goes beyond the 320nm range. Unfortunately, as materials, they are solids, which make them difficult to handle and hard to incorporate into cosmetic products.

- *cinnamates*—early sunscreen compounds, particularly benzyl cinnamate. They have good UV absorption in the 305 nm range. Currently, ethylhexyl methoxycinnamate (formerly octyl methoxycinnamate) is preferred because it is insoluble in water, making it ideal for waterproof products.

- *physical blockers*—compounds able to reflect UV light, thereby preventing it from reaching the skin. Titanium dioxide and zinc oxide are the two most common and popular physical blockers. Innovations in the manufacturing technology of zinc oxide and titanium dioxide have created micronized versions where UV light is not reflected but rather scattered, and which do not leave a noticeable film on the skin.

- *salicylates*—the first sunscreen chemicals to be widely used in commercial preparations. Benzyl salicylate, ethylhexyl salicylate (formerly octyl salicylate), and homomethyl salicylate are among the most popular. Salicylates are ideal for use in UVB sunscreens because they absorb UV rays falling between the 310–300 nm range. They also have an excellent safety profile. *See also* sunscreen.

UV filters—*see* UV absorbers.

vehicle (carrier)—cosmetic compound used to dilute an active ingredient, regulate its penetration into the skin, and/or help its surface application. It has been observed that the degree of ingredient effectiveness varies according to the vehicle used. This is called the "vehicle effect." In sunscreens, for example, the same amount of an active material in an oil or alcohol vehicle is less effective than the same material in a lotion vehicle, and this in turn is less effective than using a cream vehicle. The term vehicle also refers to components used in a cosmetic that provide the formulation with stability or consistency. A formulation can have one or more vehicles. Many times, a vehicle may also be an active principle (for example, alcohol).

vitamins—a group of substances essential for normal cell function, growth and development. Vitamins are grouped into two categories: fat-soluble, which are stored in the body's fatty tissues; and water-soluble, which are used by the body right away. Chemical and cosmetic research into the impact of vitamins in skin care has resulted in validating and increasing the role that certain vitamins play in cosmetic products. Vitamin A and its derivatives are key among the antiaging ingredients; vitamins E and C are superb antioxidants with synergistic effects; and other vitamins such as B, F, H, and P have been used as cosmetic ingredients at different times. Presently, vitamins A, C, and E are scientifically established as having greatest cosmetic value.

Though most consumers consider vitamins to be natural materials, in cosmetics they can be either naturally derived or synthetically produced. Most of the vitamin ingredients currently used in cosmetic formulations are synthetic versions of vitamins, vitamin derivatives, or some specific - vitamin element.

PART II

Product Ingredients

Introduction

This dictionary represents an analysis of cosmetic ingredients presently found on labels of skin care products. To compile this information, the authors requested ingredient labels from U.S. manufacturers and importers of skin care products. These ingredients, plus others noted for use in skin care product formulation, were then alphabetically listed. Ingredient functions were analyzed based on published data (print and electronic media), information provided by manufacturers, and interviews with cosmetic chemists from ingredient manufacturing companies. No data on product performance was directly obtained from cosmetic companies. This was done specifically to avoid the risk of describing product performance based on marketing claims.

To maintain uniformity, botanicals have been listed and described by their frequently used common or English name whenever possible, with most other names listed immediately after. Acacia, for example, can be found listed under A, as acacia (acacia gum; black catechu; gum acacia; gum arabic. . . .). To assist the reader with a botanical's Latin name, an alphabetical cross-reference has been compiled in the appendix at the end of this dictionary. For example, listed under A is *Acacia senegal*—acacia. Another example is horse chestnut with its Latin name *Aesculus hippocastanum*. It is listed and described in the main body of the dictionary under H for horse chestnut but found in the appendix under A for *Aesculus hippocastanum*.

The cosmetic industry is rapidly standardizing how ingredients are listed in order to facilitate ingredient-name recognition by the consumer. Manufacturers from the U.S., the European Union, Japan, and other countries are using a compound or chemical's

International Nomenclature of Cosmetic Ingredients (INCI) names when listing cosmetic ingredients on their product labels. Exceptions to the use of INCI names include some botanicals, coloring agents, and those INCI names that would not be accepted by consumers or the government of a specific market.

INCI names have helped reduce inconsistencies found in the past. These inconsistencies included the word order; the use of a full name by one manufacturer and an abbreviation or partial abbreviation by another; the use of the Latin name for botanicals by some and the common names by others, etc. INCI names are considered universal and therefore are often not translated into local languages, though individual governments can require translation.

Regardless of INCI standardization, occasionally ingredients will be listed by some form of abbreviation or an abbreviation and a chemical name: EDTA and DMDM hydantoin are examples. Often, such abbreviations are INCI standard. This dictionary has cross-referenced as many instances of this as feasible. Also, some cosmetics list a trade name designated by the manufacturer to protect the proprietary nature of the ingredient and/or formulation. Trade names are not found in INCI listings. Chemicals can also be listed by a marketing name that prevents the identification of its chemical composition.

An effort has been made in this edition to use INCI names whenever possible. When there has been a significant name change, both names—the original name and INCI name—are listed in their appropriate alphabetical order. The ingredient function, however, is discussed under the INCI name or its current most common form of reference. Other names for the same chemical are listed with a note to refer to the chemical's listed INCI name for description. For example, butylated hydroxyanisole is commonly known and referred to as BHA. This ingredient is listed under both forms of reference but described only under BHA since this is the most common. Another example is benzophenone-3, also known as oxybenzone. It is listed and described under benzophenone-3 but can also be found under oxybenzone with a reference to the first ingredient for description.

Ingredients listed under a company trade name are referenced both ways and described under their chemical name whenever the chemical component was disclosed or could be determined. An example is Ajidew. This is a trade name for sodium PCA (the INCI name). In this case, Ajidew is listed under A with a reference to sodium PCA for the description of ingredient properties.

In some instances, certain ingredients perform very similar functions. Their inclusion in a formulation is determined by their reaction with other ingredients present, formulator's preference, and/or cost. In such cases, a description is presented under one ingredient and all others are referenced to it. This is the case with certain PEGs and laureths. For example, PEG-10 sorbitan laurate is a cleansing and solubilizing solution agent. PEG-40 sorbitan laurate, PEG-44 sorbitan laurate, PEG-75 sorbitan laurate, and PEG-80 sorbitan laurate are all referred to as PEG-10 sorbitan laurate since they have a similar function.

Some ingredients are listed for marketing effect. Take, for example, fango mud. *Fango* is the term for mud in Italian; its description is found under mud. Other listings leave room for broad interpretation without real identification of the ingredient(s). Vague and marketing-oriented terms, whenever obvious, are noted in the dictionary. An example is active botanical fractions listed under A. This is a description involving two or more unidentified plant extracts, which precludes determining the ingredient's performance.

For some ingredients, minute quantities and low concentrations are an absolute requirement for appropriate skin response. For others, low concentrations render them ineffective. In addition, other ingredients present in a formulation may impact the performance and bioavailability of certain active components. When it comes to the value of effectiveness as stated on labels or promotional material, in some cases, the only way to be sure is based on the reputation and reliability of the cosmetic's manufacturer. Neither this book's authors nor an ingredient label reader is in a position to determine ingredient or product effectiveness based on the sequence of ingredients listed.

COSMETIC INGREDIENT LABELING REGULATIONS

Cosmetic ingredient labeling regulations were established by the FDA in 1977. They require ingredients to be listed in descending order of predominance by the nomenclature established in reference sources of ingredient names. Today, the dominant reference source is the *International Cosmetic Ingredient Dictionary and Handbook*, in which INCI names are listed. Flavor and fragrance ingredients need to be identified by the terms *flavor* and/or *fragrance*, as appropriate. Exempt from label disclosure under these regulations are the names of trade secret ingredients. A mechanism has been provided for the review of petitions for trade secret exemption. These regulations apply only to products for retail sale.

Cosmetics used at professional establishments such as salons or skin care clinics, or samples distributed free of charge, cannot fall under the requirement of ingredient declaration. Ingredient listings are printed on or affixed to product packaging. If a product is packaged in two containers, commonly bottle, tube, or jar housed in a box, it is required that the ingredients be printed on the package label of the outside container. Consider a cleanser sold in a box: the ingredient listing needs to appear on the box. Any listing on the bottle is optional. However, if an outer container is not used, then the listing needs to appear on the main container, in this case, on the cleanser bottle. Such listings may appear on any information panel of a package displayed under customer conditions of purchase or on a tag, tape, or card firmly attached to the external packaging. The regulation specifies that the information must be prominent, conspicuous, and clear.

Ingredients listed must be identified by the name established by the commissioner of the FDA for the purpose of ingredient labeling. If a name has not been established by the commissioner, it must be identified by the name adopted for the ingredient in the editions and supplements of the following sources (listed in descending order of priority utilization):

- *International Cosmetic Ingredient Dictionary & Handbook**
- *United States Pharmacopoeia*
- *National Formulary*
- *Food Chemical Codex*
- *USAN and the USP Dictionary of Drug Names*

Theoretically, if an ingredient name is not listed in any of these sources, the name generally recognized by consumers, or a chemical or technical name or description must be used. European regulations, however, require ingredients to be listed by their common name and that common name, with few exceptions, is the INCI name.

The original confusion surrounding herbal compounds is decreasing with INCI standardization. In the past, there were many cases where botanicals were listed by their botanical (Latin) name by some, and by their common name by others. For the most part, INCI names are Latin and often unrecognizable to the consumer. To manage this, manufacturers are opting to list the botanical

---

*The *CTFA Cosmetic Ingredient Dictionary* formerly served the same function and has been replaced by this new publication as most INCI terminology is based on the original CTFA listings.

name followed by the common name in parenthesis. Therefore, grapefruit extract could be found listed as *Citrus paradisi* (grapefruit) *extract.* The issue can be further complicated by the way cosmetic manufacturing companies choose to spell the ingredients used; again, this is becoming increasingly standardized, however.

To comply with the Fair Packaging and Labeling (FP&L) Act, ingredients in a formulation must be listed in descending order of predominance. One exception is that if a cosmetic is also a drug, the active drug ingredient(s) must be listed before the cosmetic ones. Each drug ingredient must be declared as an "active ingredient" and identified by its established drug name. The second exception to the order of the predominance rule is that if an ingredient is accorded confidentiality as a trade secret by the FDA, a listing of "other ingredients" instead of the ingredient's actual name(s) may be used at the end of the declaration. Rather than list "other ingredients," some companies list an ingredient or group of ingredients that are considered proprietary under an assumed company name which does not allow its identification through any of the listed sources. Companies must submit an application to the FDA for their ingredient(s) to have trade secret status. The Freedom of Information Act states, "A trade secret may consist of any formula, pattern, device or compilation of information which is used in one's business and which gives him an opportunity to obtain an advantage over competitors who do not know or use it." In other words, a trade secret is information of value not known to others and that cannot be readily ascertained.

The labeling regulation permits ingredients present at 1 percent concentrations or lower to be listed in any order, as long as they appear after the ingredients present at higher concentrations in their order of predominance. Color additives present at any concentration may be listed in any order after the listing of ingredients that are not color additives.

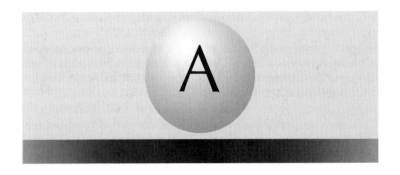

A

acacia (Acacia senegal) (acacia gum; black catechu; gum acacia; gum Arabic)—commonly used in traditional remedies as a soothing and anti-inflammatory agent. It is also used as a vegetable gum for product thickening. In extract form, acacia is recommended for dry, sensitive, or delicate skin. Acacia is the dried gummy sap from the stems and branches of various species of the African acacia tree. It may cause skin rashes in cases of allergy.

acacia gum—*see* acacia.

açaí (Euterpe oleracea) pulp oil—appears to have powerful antioxidant properties and an ability to help regulate skin lipids, thereby promoting skin repair activities. Derived from the berries of the Açai tree (part of the palm family); its constituents include essential fatty acids (omega-6 and omega-9), vitamin C, polyphenols, and phytosterols. It is recommended for use in moisturizers, after-sun products, and cosmetic preparations destined to improve skin softness.

acerola extract—credited with antioxidant and free-radical scavenging properties due to its high ascorbic acid content. It is also hydrating and said to enhance capillary strength. Acerola is derived from the ripe fruit of the West Indies or Barbados cherry variety.

acetamide MEA (ethanol acetamide)—a humectant recommended for use in emulsions. According to manufacturers, it has counterirritant properties.

acetate—a salt of acetic acid. Although listed on labels as acetate, to determine its appropriate action, it needs to be followed or preceded by another name (for example, tocopherol acetate), as this other name will indicate the compound's function.

acetone—a solvent considered to be a noncomedogenic ingredient, occasionally used in skin toners. It could be drying and very irritating to the skin depending on the concentration and frequency of use.

acetyl hexapeptide-1—a melanin-regulating peptide that appears to stimulate the skin's production of melanin. It is said to mimic the skin's own natural defense mechanism against UVB. Found in sun-protection products and those products that treat age or sun spots.

acetyl hexapeptide-3—a peptide claimed to intercept and stop the transmission of the chemical signal responsible for the muscle contractions that can lead to fine line and wrinkle formation, while also helping reduce the appearance of existing wrinkles. Found primarily in antiaging and antiwrinkle creams, as well as in eye creams.

acetyl hexapeptide-8—an antiwrinkle peptide. Synthetically produced and considered to be highly effective, clinical studies indicate it can reduce the depth of existing wrinkles. May be incorporated into products marketed as having a topical-BOTOX® or "wrinkle erasing" effect.

n-acetyl-l-cysteine—a skin conditioner. It may also have an antiaging application due to a demonstrated ability to regulate skin atrophy and reduce the appearance of fine lines and wrinkles. *See also* cysteine.

acetylated lanolin—an emollient that helps form water-repellent films on the skin.

acetylated lanolin alcohol—exhibits skin-softening and anti-allergenic properties. This is an ester that resembles steroids generally found on the skin. Considered highly comedogenic by some sources, with only a mild irritancy potential.

achillea extract—see yarrow extract.

acrylamide copolymer—has a film-forming capability and is similar to acrylates copolymer.

acrylamide/sodium acryloyldimethyl taurate copolymer—used as a thickener and/or stabilizer. Considered non-irritating. *See also* polymer.

acrylates—see acrylates copolymer.

acrylates copolymer—able to absorb skin secretions, thereby reducing skin shine and providing an improved skin surface for makeup application. Acrylates copolymer also imparts a pleasant feel to the cosmetic preparation and helps reduce any feeling of oiliness the product may have. Its various applications include incorporation into skin cleansers, oil control treatments, makeup, and loose and compressed powders. Used with a variety of other ingredients, including glycerine, cyclomethicone, retinyl palmitate, and vegetable oils, acrylates copolymer prolongs the availability of these other ingredients to the skin through a time-release type of activity. It also helps counteract some negative properties when applied to the skin, or further enhance positive ones. For example, acrylates copolymer reduces the tackiness and greasiness of glycerine while prolonging its availability in the interstitial network of the skin. When present with retinyl palmitate, acrylates copolymer improves the stability of the formulation and increases its skin contact time.

acrylates/C$_{10-30}$ alkyl acrylate crosspolymer—an emulsifier for oil-in-water emulsions with thickening and formula-stabilizing properties similar to a carbomer. Considered a second generation to carbomers, it has better waterproofing capabilities. It allows for the release of the formulation's oil phase component immediately on rubbing the product into the skin. Used in moisturizer emulsions and creams, waterproof sunscreens, and fragrance emulsions. *See also* carbomer.

acrylates/dimethicone methacrylate copolymer—an emollient with film-forming capacities. It also prevents caking in cosmetic preparations.

acrylates/t-octylpropenaide copolymer—provides a barrier to moisture loss as well as waterproofing/water-repelling properties. It is commonly found in skin care products requiring a film-forming component, including waterproof sunscreens, smudge-proof eye products, and hand and body moisturizers. Studies indicate that it allows for the gradual release of active principles over a period of time. Other properties include rub-off resistance and fragrance retention.

acrylic acid/acrylonitrogens copolymer—used as a primary emulsifier given binding and viscosity controlling capacities. It can also contribute to a product's moisturizing properties by acting as a film former on the surface of the skin. It is often found in preparations requiring waterproofing properties.

acrylic acid polymers—can be employed as thickeners, dispersion stabilizers, and viscosity modifiers for cosmetics. Clinical studies indicate no dermal reactions or irritations.

A

active botanical fractions—this is a vague listing involving two or more unidentified botanical extracts, which precludes determining the ingredient's appropriate or actual value. However, this listing is accompanied by a claim that the mixture combines antielastase of active plant fractions and, therefore, can be used for preserving elastin.

Adansonia digitata—*see* baoab.

adenosine—studies indicate antiwrinkle and skin-smoothing capacities.

adenosine phosphate—a nucleotide (building blocks of nucleic acid) added to skin care products to bind water and moisture.

agrimony extract (Agrimonia eupatoria)—astringent. Considered a beneficial botanical ingredient for use in toners.

AHA—*see* alpha hydroxyacid.

Ajidew—*see* sodium PCA.

Ajidew A-100—*see* PCA.

Ajidew N-50—*see* sodium PCA.

alanine—an amino acid that can act as a skin-conditioning agent. Usually used in combination with other amino acids.

albumen—*see* egg protein.

albumen extract—*see* egg extract.

alchemilla extract (Alchemilla vulgaris) (lady's mantle)—according to contemporary phytotherapy, alchemilla is astringent and beneficial for wound healing and to stop bleeding. It is anti-inflammatory and soothing. In addition, it is credited with anti–free radical and UV-filtering properties. Its constituents include tannins, saponins, salicylic acid, fatty acids, sterols, and amino acids. The root, flowering stems, and leaves are the parts used. *See also* lady's mantle extract.

alcohol (alcohol SD-40; alcohol SDA-40; ethanol; ethyl alcohol)—widely used in the cosmetic industry as an antiseptic as well as a solvent given its strong grease-dissolving abilities. Often used in a variety of concentrations in skin toners for acne skin, aftershave lotions, perfumes, suntan lotions, and toilet waters. Alcohol is drying to the skin when used in high concentrations. It is manufactured by means of the fermentation of starch, sugar, and other carbohydrates.

alcohol, C_{12-16}—a mixture of fatty alcohols with an attached carbon series (12 to 16 carbons in length). This type of modification is sometimes used by cosmetic formulators to either facilitate the penetration of another ingredient into the skin or to simply create a larger molecule when required for formulatory purposes. *See also* alkyl benzoate, C_{12-13}.

alcohol, C_{14-22}/C_{12-20} alkylglucoside—an emulsifier suitable for spray-on preparations.

A

alcohol benzoate/C_{12-15}—*see* alkyl benzoate, C_{12-15}.

alcohol SD-40 (alcohol 40)—a high-grade version of ethyl alcohol designed especially for cosmetic use. It evaporates almost immediately, leaving the active ingredients on the surface of the skin. Antibacterial properties are ascribed to it. "SD" is the acronym for "specially denatured" and the number 40 does not relate to the percentage of alcohol in the formulation but rather to the alcohol's grade. *See also* alcohol.

alcohol SDA-40—another way of describing alcohol SD-40. This could be read as "alcohol, special denatured alcohol." *See also* alcohol SD-40.

aleppo gall (oak bud extract)—an active botanical substance used in sun products due to its anti–free radical, UV filter, and skin repair activities in cases of UV ray damage. Aleppo gall helps combat the harmful effects of UVA rays and protects the skin, thanks to its UVB-filtering abilities. It also has astringent and antiseptic properties, making it useful for treating burns and healing wounds. Traditionally, aleppo gall was also used in the treatment of eczema.

alfalfa extract (Medicago sativa)—a botanical considered to have tonic and decongestant properties. Alfalfa is a widely cultivated perennial plant that can also be found growing wild on the borders of fields and in low valleys. The extract is obtained from the leaves.

algae extract (seaweed extract)—an active substance used to normalize the skin's moisture content and provide suppleness and firmness to the epidermis. There are many types of algae and they exhibit different properties. Depending on the variety used, benefits to the skin can include immunological, anti-free radical activity, an improved dermal condition, restructuring, wrinkle reduction, and tissue renewal. Algae can also act as a film former, moisturizer, hydrator, and emollient. Cosmetic manufacturers rarely disclose the specific strain of algae employed. This often remains as a part of the formulation's "secret."

algae extract and pullulan—used as a skin tightener. Manufacturers claim an immediate and long-term skin tightening effect thanks to an ability to stimulate and strengthen the

A

skin's collagen fibers. This algae-based polysaccharide (pullulan is a natural sugar with film-forming and moisture retention capacities) can also have some antioxidant activity. Manufacturers indicate it as beneficial for antiaging and antiwrinkle formulations and cosmetics wishing to claim a "lifting" effect. Constituents include vitamins B12 and C.

algae oil—*see* algae extract; seaweed extract.

algae protein—studies note that some specific varieties are good substitutes for animal-derived collagen. They are also finding that algae protein has potentially better moisturizing benefits at lower levels of use, and a reduced feeling of tackiness often associated with the higher-use levels of animal-derived collagen. *See also* algae extract; seaweed extract.

algin (alginic acid; potassium alginate; sodium alginate)—used in cosmetic formulations as a thickener, stabilizer, and gelling agent. Obtained from different varieties of brown seaweed.

alginate—used as a thickening agent in cosmetic preparations. Alginate may be used as microcapsules and is obtained from marine extracts.

alginic acid—*see* algin.

alkyl benzoate, C_{12-15} (C_{12-15} alcohol benzoate)—an emulsifier used in sunscreens, it also acts as a solubilizer for oxybenzone, and provides a good skin feel. This is a mixture of synthetic alcohols.

allantoin—a botanical extract said to be healing, calming, and soothing, it can also help protect the skin from harmful external factors (e.g., wind burn). It is considered an excellent temporary anti-irritant and is believed to aid in the healing of damaged skin by stimulating new tissue growth. Allantoin is appropriate for sensitive, irritated, and acne skins. Derived from the comfrey root, it is considered nonallergenic.

allyl methacrylates crosspolymer—a polymer delivery system. According to the manufacturer, it is sufficiently versatile to deliver a wide range of reactive ingredients, such as retinol. It can also successfully deliver volatile ingredients, such as fragrances, and easily soluble ones, such as the sunscreen chemical avobenzone.

almond flour—used primarily in soaps for a thicker consistency and a scrubbing action.

almond meal—used in cosmetic scrubs to achieve exfoliation. It does not have any other direct effect on the skin. It comes

in different sieve sizes: #1, very fine, through #10, very
large. Almond meal is made from the almond shell.

almond oil, bitter *(Prunus amygdalus amara)*—serves as an emollient and a carrier, providing an elegant skin feel and promoting spreadability in creams, lotions, and bath oils. Obtained
from the bitter almond, it supposedly stays fresh longer than
oil obtained from sweet almonds. It is the volatile essential
oil distilled from almonds, and is also used in fragrance and
flavors. When used in high concentrations, it is known to
cause strong allergic reactions, including headaches.

almond oil, sweet *(Prunus amygdalus dulcis)*—serves as an emollient and a carrier, providing an elegant skin feel and promoting spreadability in creams, lotions, and bath oils. Sweet
almond oil's main constituent is olein with a small proportion of linoleic acid glyceride. Very similar in composition to
olive oil, it is obtained from sweet almonds that have under-
gone a cleaning and crushing process, leaving them in powder
form. The powder is then cold-pressed and left to "rest" for
one to two weeks. After the resting period, the almond oil is
filtered and often bleached. Sweet almond oil is the triglyceride oil (vegetable oil) derived from almonds.

almond powder—*see* almond flour.

almond protein—has moisture-binding properties. Derived from
almond meal.

almondermin—leaves skin with a velvety feel. It has moisturizing,
smoothing, and soothing properties. Almondermin is a botanical extract mixture of sweet almonds and marshmallow.

aloe extract—a popular botanical recognized for centuries as
having beneficial medicinal properties including antibiotic,
anti-inflammatory, and wound healing. These benefits have
been found to apply to skin care as well. Aloe vera is frequently used in cosmetic preparations due to its apparent
moisturizing, soothing, and calming properties. It is excellent for dry and sensitive skin, as well as for the treatment
of sunburns and other minor burns, insect bites, and skin
irritations. Aloe extract is obtained from aloe vera leaves and
is also referred to as aloe vera gel. *See also* aloe vera.

aloe juice—also referred to as aloe vera gel. Technically, the
term *aloe juice* applies to a diluted version of aloe vera gel.
See also aloe vera.

aloe vera *(Aloe vera)*—an emollient and film-forming gum resin
with hydrating, softening, healing, antimicrobial, and anti-
inflammatory properties. Its moisturizing ability is its most

A

A

widely recognized characteristic. Aloe vera supplies moisture directly to the skin tissue. Other properties include moisture regulation and an apparent ability to absorb UV light. It has a slightly relaxing effect on the skin, making it beneficial for sensitive, sunburned, and sun-exposed skins. Aloe vera was popular in folklore medicine as a remedy for burns. It is frequently used in gels as an effective refresher and relaxant for irritated skin, hence its popularity in sun preparations for cooling and soothing. In addition, it is found to be an effective component in emulsions formulated for regulating dry skin. Apparently, aloe vera also has a synergistic effect when used in conjunction with other anti-inflammatory substances. Concentrations over 50 percent have been shown to increase the blood supply to the area of application. Although aloe vera's important constituents are minerals, polysaccharides, amino acids, and carbohydrates, it is constituted of about 99.5 percent water. Its benefit in a skin care product depends on the appropriate concentration, as different concentrations result in different benefits and end products. An almost odorless and nearly colorless extract, it is derived from the sap of the aloe leaf. It is used in cosmetics in a gel form (also referred to as an extract) or in a diluted version referred to as aloe vera juice.

aloe vera gel—the mucilage obtained from aloe vera leaves. *See also* aloe vera.

alpha bisabolol—*see* bisabolol.

alpha hydroxyacid (AHA)—the family name for a group of naturally occurring acids often referred to as "fruit acids." AHAs are used in cosmetic products as moisturizers, emollients, and exfoliants. They are also employed to treat such conditions as photodamage and hyperpigmentation, and, at the medical level, eczema, and ichthyosis. Their activity and associated benefits are dependent on the type of AHA used, the concentration employed, and the pH of the formula. The benefits attributed to these active substances include a reduction of fine lines and superficial wrinkles, a lightening of surface pigmentation, and softer, suppler skin with improved hydration. These noted benefits are a result of AHA activity to normalize the stratum corneum by reducing its thickness through exfoliation, and the creation of a more compact structure; increased skin hydration due to the natural moisturizing properties; an ability to activate hyaluronic acid which, in turn, will retain a greater amount of moisture in the skin; and an increase in dermal thickness due to increased hydration and a normalization of skin functions. There are six key AHAs found in various plants and fruits: glycolic acid found in sugar cane juice; lactic acid from sour milk and tomato juice; malic acid found in apples; tartaric acid from grapes and wine; and citric acid found in lemons, pineapples, oranges, and other fruits. Pyruvic acid is also an AHA. AHAs used in cosmetic preparations are synthetically derived. The exfoliating and hyperkeratinization-reducing properties of some AHAs make them prime ingredients for acne-oriented products, for reducing actinic keratosis, and for improving the appearance of aging skin. Also, their emollient and hydration properties help dry and aged skin. Of all the AHAs, glycolic and lactic acid, and their salts, are the most popular for use in skin care. They are considered the most effective, with this efficacy validated through a large number of scientific studies. Between the two, glycolic acid is regarded as somewhat more effective for the normalization of skin functions. Controversy has surrounded the long-term use and effect of AHAs, primarily glycolic and lactic acids. This resulted in a 1998 statement issued by two leading cosmetic industry organizations and governing bodies, the Cosmetic Ingredient Review (CIR) and Cosmetic Toiletries and Fragrance Association (CTFA). They assert that glycolic and lactic acids, as well as their respective glycolate and lactate derivatives, can be safely incorporated into retail cosmetic products at concentrations less than or equal to 10 percent with the product's final pH not to be below 3.5. They also note that in their directions for use, manufacturers should include a statement about the daily use of sun protection.

Some Examples of AHAs

Glycolic Acid	Lactic Acid	Malic Acid	Tartaric Acid	Citric Acid
CH_2OH	CH_3	$COOH$	$COOH$	$COOH$
CH_2OH	$CHOH$	CH_2	$CHOH$	CH_2
	$COOH$	$CHOH$	$CHOH$	$HOC-COOH$
		$COOH$	$COOH$	CH_2
				$COOH$

Comparison of relative molecular size of key AHAs.

A

alpha hydroxyacetic acid—*see* glycolic acid.

alpha hydroxycaproic acid—when added to sunscreen preparations, it can prevent the skin peeling that results from excessive sun exposure.

alpha hydroxyethanoic acid—*see* glycolic acid.

alpha-isomethyl ionone—used to mask odor in a formulation.

alpha linolenic acid—also known as omega-3. *See* linolenic acid.

alpha lipoic acid (ALA)—also known as thioctic acid. A powerful and versatile antioxidant that acts by neutralizing free radicals. It also appears to demonstrate an antioxidant activity similar to that of vitamin C: it has the capacity to help revitalize other antioxidants (including vitamins C and E) as well as coenzyme Q10, thereby prolonging their activity. Some evidence exists that it may be able to activate cell signaling. While used medically in the management of diabetes, in skin care it is found in antioxidant and antiaging cosmetics.

alpha tocopherol—the most commonly employed form of vitamin E. *See* vitamin E.

alpha tocopheryl ferrulate—a depigmenting agent that may be particularly effective in lightening hyperpigmentation resulting from UV exposure. It is said to inhibit melanin formation by suppressing tyrosinase activity. Alpha tocopheryl ferrulate is obtained by reacting an alpha tocopherol ester with ferulic acid. Ferulic acid, like alpha tocopherol, is an antioxidant. It is also a UV absorber. *See also* tocopherol.

althea extract (Althaea officinalis) (marshmallow extract; marshmallow root extract)—a botanical that is said to have emollient, soothing, and healing capabilities when incorporated into skin care formulations. It is considered particularly beneficial in aftershave preparations and in products that treat sunburns and dry skin. This is a natural hydroglycolic plant extract from the althea root.

alum—*see* potassium alum.

aluminum PCA—has astringent and antiseptic properties.

aluminum acetate solution (Burow's solution)—has astringent and antiseptic properties, and is used in astringent lotions and protective creams. This is a mixture of alkali metal acetate, acetic acid, and dibasic aluminum acetate with boric acid as a formulation stabilizer. Some cosmetic companies try to avoid using this ingredient because of its metal content since the benefits of metal-based products on the skin are questioned by some manufacturers. Prolonged and continuous use can produce a skin rash and severe sloughing of the skin.

aluminum hydroxide—an inorganic compound used to make a product less transparent. It is also used by formulators as a humectant, and to soften, smooth, and protect the skin. In addition it helps control product viscosity. Often found in facial masks and make-up preparations.

aluminum magnesium hydroxystearate—an additive and formulation stabilizer generally used in water-in-oil emulsions. It helps improve the suspension of insoluble particles or pigments in formulations, and is particularly useful when manufacturers desire a colorless gel.

aluminum starch octenyl succinate—an SPF enhancer, particularly when used in combination with titanium dioxide. It is hydrophobic (lacking affinity for water) and can be used to reduce the feeling of greasiness in a product.

aluminum stearate—a saline form of stearic acid used as a thickener and emulsifier, and to regulate the stability and suspension of a cosmetic formulation.

aluminum sulfate—a common aluminum salt used in astringents. It is very similar to aluminum.

amino acid—used in cosmetic formulations to enhance water retention and skin moisturization. Because of their reduced size, amino acids can penetrate deeper into the stratum corneum's cell layers than proteins, such as collagen, with a higher molecular weight. The ingredient's "feel" on the skin will depend on the amino acid composition of the protein used. In the past, the most commonly used amino acids were derived from animal collagen. Today, due to consumer demand, new vegetable substitutes are being introduced, and ongoing investigations are seeking alternative sources. Although amino acids are fundamental skin components, the skin does not utilize topically applied amino acids to produce new skin as the role of amino acids in skin formation is an extremely complex process.

γ-amino-β-hydroxybutric acid (gamma amino beta hydroxybutric acid)—studies indicate that when used in conjunction with vitamin E, it has an antiaging effect. It appears to impact microcirculation which, in turn, accelerates the skin metabolism and generally improves skin condition.

p-aminobenzoic acid (PABA)—a sunscreen chemical. *See* PABA.

A

aminobutyric acid—an amino acid with water-binding properties and possible anti-inflammatory capacities.

aminoethyl propanol—an alcohol with antibacterial and topical antiseptic properties generally used as a pH adjuster in cosmetic formulations.

aminomethyl propanol—an alcohol used as a pH adjuster in cosmetic formulations, it also acts as an emulsifier and may be used as a gelling agent. Its primary application is in hair preparations.

aminoserine—*see* serine.

ammonium acryloyldimethyltaurate/VP copolymer—a thickener.

ammonium alpha hydroxyethanoate—*see* ammonium glycolate.

ammonium bituminosulfonate—also known as ichthyol; ichthammol; sodium shale oil sulfonate. *See* sodium shale oil sulfonate.

ammonium caseinate—a binder and emulsifier incorporated into cosmetics as a polymer. It is a water-soluble protein powder, derived from milk. *See also* polymer.

ammonium chloride—used as a thickener and as an additive in nonalcoholic toners. According to cosmetic formulators, the ammonium component provides the tingling or stinging sensation that some people associate with toners or aftershaves, and which, in regular toners, is usually provided by the alcohol content. Ammonium chloride's use is the result of preference in formulation feel.

ammonium cocoyl isethionate—a surfactant. Its mildness and high-foaming property give a formulation a lubricating lather and impart a soft skin feel. It is derived from natural coconut oil.

ammonium glycolate—a cleanser used in shampoos and liquid soaps. Ammonium glycolate is also a neutralized version of glycolic acid commonly incorporated in glycolic acid-based cosmetics to reduce the irritation typically associated with the use of free glycolic acid. Ammonium glycolate has moisturizing properties as well. *See also* glycolic acid.

ammonium glycyrrhizinate—a conditioner, it is also used as a flavoring agent, particularly for lipsticks.

ammonium hydroxide—used in cosmetic preparations as an alkali to neutralize excessive acidity in a formulation.

ammonium lactate—when topically applied, it is found to thicken the viable epidermis while reducing the thickness of the corneum layer. It is a neutralized version of lactic acid. *See also* lactic acid.

ammonium laureth sulfate—a surfactant with foaming capabilities. It can also be employed as an emulsifying agent and is frequently found in skin cleansers. As a member of the ether sulfate group, it is considered less irritating than its lauryl counterpart, ammonium lauryl sulfate.

ammonium lauryl sulfate—a surfactant with emulsifying capabilities. Given its detergent properties, it can be used, at mild acidic pH levels, as an anionic surfactant cleanser. It is considered one of the most irritating surfactants, causing dryness and skin redness. Today, it is either combined with anti-irritant ingredients to reduce sensitivity, or replaced with less irritating but similar surfactants, such as ammonium laureth sulfate.

ammonium polyacryldimethyltauramide—a thickener and stabilizer. It is particularly effective at the high pH required by water-soluble sunscreen formulations.

ammonium polyacryloyldimethyl taurate—a polymer used to stabilize emulsions and control formulation viscosity.

amniotic fluid—some consider this simply an animal protein serving as a surface film-forming agent with moisturizing properties. Others claim it is nourishing, has antitoxic properties, acts as an epithelial stimulant, and can diffuse through the skin. Research indicates that amniotic fluid seems to have a positive effect on wound healing and cellular regeneration. Advocates of its use point out that animal sacrifice is not required to obtain the substance since the amniotic fluid (the fluid surrounding the cow embryo in utero) can be extracted from live animals in their third to sixth month of gestation, supposedly without harm to the animal or fetus.

amodimethicone copolyol—a silicone product with skin-softening and conditioning properties.

amphoteric 2—an extremely mild surfactant commonly used in baby shampoos. It can also serve as an excellent emulsifier.

amydimethyl PABA—*see* pentyl dimethyl PABA.

amyl cinnamal—used as a fragrance. While naturally occurring in some plants, it is most often synthetically derive when used in cosmetic products.

anemone extract (*Anemone sp.*)—a botanical ingredient with soothing and anti-inflammatory properties, as well as an

A

ability to heal superficial wounds. These attributes would make it appropriate for sensitive, delicate, and acne skin. There are about 70 species of anemones. Most frequently used are wood anemone (*Anemone nemorosa*) and the pasque flower (*Anemone pulstilla*). Some varieties of anemone are known to cause swelling and blistering. The extract is obtained from the whole herb.

angelica (*Angelica sp.*)—in both extract and essential oil form, this botanical is described as tonic, detoxifying, and purifying for the blood and lymph systems. It is also considered soothing. Angelica's principal constituents are volatile oil (about 1 percent), valeric acid, angelic acid, sugar, a bitter principle, and a peculiar resin called angelicin that is stimulating to the skin. The essential oil of the root contains terebangelene and other terpenes. The oils of the seeds contain methyl-ethylacetic acid and hydroxymyristic acid. Angelica extracts are made from the seeds, and more often, the roots.

anhydrous lanolin—an emollient and emulsifying agent. Its level of comedogenicity depends on how it has been processed for cosmetic use. *See also* lanolin.

anise extract (*Pimpinella anisum*)—used as a fragrance. No therapeutic value has been ascribed to the external application of this botanical. Anise's composition is 80 to 90 percent anethole and methyl claricol. The extract is obtained by steam distillation of the anise seeds. The extract may cause allergic reactions and produce hives, scaling, and blisters when applied directly to the skin.

p-anisic acid—also known as 4-methoxybenzoic acid. Generally used as a fragrance, it also has preservative (antimicrobial) capacities. New clinical studies indicate it may also have some ability to inhibit tyrosinase. Naturally occurring in anise seed.

annatto extract (*Bixa orellana*)—used in creams and sun products as a colorant and a highlighter. The orange color it provides is obtained from the plant's dried fruit, specifically the pulp.

apple extract (*Pyrus malus*)—claimed to have soothing and anti-inflammatory properties and to be beneficial for dry skin. In addition to the enzyme aneylase, fresh apples and apple juice contain malic acid (up to 90–95 percent of the fruit's total acid content) and tartaric acid, both of which can provide a degree of natural exfoliating activity. As vitamin and enzymatic actions are easily destroyed, the value of the enzymatic action and vitamin content of the fruit in cosmetic preparations is totally dependent on the product's formulation.

apricot oil—*see* apricot kernel oil.

apricot kernel oil—an emollient with a nongreasy feel. It provides good slip and lubricity to a product. Primarily used as a carrier, apricot kernel oil is rapidly absorbed by the skin, and once absorbed, acts as a good occlusive and moisturizing agent. It is popular for use in cosmetics given its skin-softening action. This oil has a high vitamin E content (*see* vitamin E) that some claim can aid the skin in retaining elasticity, clarity, and suppleness. Apricot kernel oil is a triglyceride in the same category as avocado oil, olive oil, and sesame oil, and consists of approximately 75 percent oleic acid, 20 percent linoleic acid, and unsaturated fatty acids esterfied with glycerin. Apricot kernel oil is considered by some chemists to be a natural replacement for mineral oil. It is extracted from the apricot kernel by expression and is far less expensive than almond oil, which it very closely resembles and can, therefore, substitute.

apricot powder—a natural peeling material incorporated into soaps and scrubs.

apricot seeds—the seeds are ground and then incorporated into soaps and scrubs as a natural peeling material.

apricot stone (ground)—*see* apricot powder.

arachidonic acid—an ingredient with skin-smoothing, emollient, and healing properties. Arachidonic acid is an essential fatty acid present in the skin and considered critical for appropriate skin metabolism. A constituent of vitamin F.

arachidyl alcohol—an emollient and a thickener. Often incorporated into cosmetics to prevent moisture loss and improve skin smoothness.

arachidyl glucoside—an emulsifier that may also be used to enhance the quality of a cosmetic cream or lotion in terms of its smoothness, creaminess, and thickness.

arachidyl propionate—aids in the rapid spreadability of a cosmetic preparation. It has a nonoily feel and a high sheen. A noncomedogenic, semisolid ester that liquifies at body temperature. Some consider it a possible replacement for lanolin.

arachis oil (peanut oil)—a carrier oil used in cosmetic products designed for sensitive and delicate skin. *See also* peanut oil.

areca nut extract (Areca catechu) (betel nut)—described as astringent, antibacterial, and aromatic. It may also have

A

potential tissue regeneration capabilities. Key constituents include tannin, gallic acid, and a number of alkaloids. In skin care, it is said to tighten pores, help control oiliness, and increase capillary strength. It is claimed to be 25 percent more astringent than witch hazel. Areca nut extract is more often employed in oily skin products and skin toners.

argan oil—emollient and skin conditioning, it also protects and moisturizes the skin. Its constituents include tocopherol, phenolic acid, carotenes, and essential fatty acids. It is obtained from the nut of the argan tree.

l-arginine—an amino acid used as a skin conditioning agent. *See also* amino acid.

arginine PCA—in a cosmetic preparation, it appears to have the ability to increase the skin's oxygen consumption and to improve moisturization.

Arlacel (165)—very good, acid-stable emulsifier. It keeps the oil and water molecules together to maintain a product's integrity and has no effect on the skin. Arlacel is a trade name for a glyceryl stearate and PEG 100 stearate mixture, sometimes also listed as a combination of glyceryl monostearate and POE stearate.

armoise oil—a mixture of natural essential oils said to have antimicrobial properties and the ability to act as a cosmetic preservative. For this mixture to be effective in a cosmetic preparation, a 2 percent concentration is required. Mixtures such as this in leave-on products may cause skin sensitivity if not carefully formulated.

arnica extract (Arnica montana)—a botanical credited with a wide variety of properties, including antiseptic, astringent, antimicrobial, anti-inflammatory, anticoagulant, circulation-stimulating, healing, and stimulating. Some claim it promotes the removal of wastes from the skin, aids in the promotion of new tissue growth, and is antiallergic. Traditionally used at the appearance of couperose condition, arnica extract is also considered excellent for an acne condition. It is effective in gels and creams designed to treat damaged, reddened, or tired skin. Important constituents include arnicin, a volatile oil, tannin, phulin, sesquiterpenes, flavonoids, and coumarins. The flowers of this perennial herb are said to contain more arnicin than the rhizome and are the preferred segment of the plant used. Repeated applications may produce severe inflammation and great care must be exercised in its use as some people are particularly sensitive to the plant.

arnica oil—credited with healing properties. *See also* arnica extract.

artichoke extract (Cynara scolymus)—sources claim that artichoke extract helps heal skin irritations and is anti-inflammatory and beautifying. Studies also indicate that artichoke extract leaves dry skin more vital, smoother, and firmer with an improvement at the dermal level. In cases of oily skin, it seems to help regulate oiliness, clear the skin, and make pores appear smaller. It is also believed to help even out skin tone and improve blemished complexions. Important constituents include tannin, pectin, and glucoside compounds.

A

ascophyllum algae—a type of algae. *See* algae extract.

ascorbic acid (vitamin C)—ascorbic acid and its derivatives, such as ascorbyl linoleate, are said to have skin-lightening and antioxidant properties. Its stability is a main concern among formulators when incorporating it into cosmetic formulations. *See also* vitamin C.

l-ascorbic acid ethylene oxide—a compound with skin-lightening properties. Tests indicate that it inhibits melanin formation.

ascorbic acid phosphate magnesium salt—see magnesium ascorbyl phosphate.

ascorbyl glucoside—according to the manufacturer, it functions as a time-release version of vitamin C (ascorbic acid), and therefore is more stable than traditional ascorbic acid. It is considered to have skin-lightening and antihyperpigmentation properties, thanks to an ability to suppress melanin production. Its skin-brightening capacities are attributed to an apparent ability to reduce pre-existing melanin levels (as in the case of freckles or age spots). Ascorbyl glucoside could also help promote collagen synthesis and help reduce skin inflammation. It is found in antiaging, antiwrinkle, and sun care products. *See* also vitamin C.

ascorbyl linoleate—an ascorbic acid derivative. It serves as a skin-lightening agent or inhibits skin darkening by preventing melanin formation.

ascorbyl palmitate—used as a preservative and an antioxidant in cosmetic creams and lotions to prevent rancidity. Ascorbyl palmitate facilitates the incorporation of ingredients such as vitamins A, D, and C into cosmetic formulations. It has no known toxicity.

ascorbyl polypeptide—an ingredient that allows for better incorporation of vitamin C into cosmetic preparations.

A

ascorbyl tetraisopalmitate—an emollient, it is derived from
l-ascorbic acid (vitamin C), and also has antioxidant and
skin-conditioning properties.

asebiol—said to regulate excessive oil gland activity, aid in emulsifying excess sebum, possess skin-softening properties,
and promote surface skin peeling. This is a mixture based
on hydrolized yeast extract containing lipopeptides and
phospholipids to which sulfuric amino acids, water-soluble
vitamin B, urea, methionin, and cysterin have been added.

l-aspartic acid—an amino acid used as a skin-conditioning
agent. *See also* aspartic acid.

aspartic acid—an amino acid used to enhance skin smoothness. It is usually present in products for dry skin. Aspartic acid is a nonessential amino acid naturally occurring
in animals, plants, sugar cane, sugar beets, and molasses.
A synthetic version is more commonly used for commercial
applications.

astaxanthin—an antioxidant. Molecularly, astaxanthin is similar
to beta-carotene, but in clinical studies it appears to demonstrate stronger antioxidant properties, including an ability to
inhibit lipid peroxidation and an anti-inflammatory capacity. It is used in cosmetics for its antioxidant properties, and
for possible UV protection abilities. Astaxanthin is a naturally occurring pigment, part of the carotenoid group, and
found in many foods. It is what provides salmon and certain
crustaceans (e.g. shrimp, crab, lobster) with their reddish
tint. Astaxanthin can also be synthetically produced.

Astrocaryum sp. butter—emollient and skin conditioning, it has
film-forming capacities to help the skin retain moisture.

atelocollagen—a skin conditioner and moisturizing emollient,
it is a protein obtained when telopeptides are enzymatically removed from collagen. Its physical properties are almost identical to those of natural, unsolubilized collagen.

Australian tea tree oil *(Melaleuca alternifolia)*—*see* tea tree oil.

avens extract *(Geum urganum)*—a botanical credited with antiseptic and skin-clearing properties. For therapeutic properties, the extract is obtained from the roots of the herb.

avobenzone (BMDM, *butyl methoxydibenzoylmethane)*—a sunscreen chemical that offers broad-range protection against
UVA rays. It is associated with some photoinstability, which
can be overcome in the overall sunscreen formulation. It is
approved for use up to 3 percent in the United States and

5 percent in the European Union. Avobenzone is noted to rarely be photosensitizing. *See also* butyl methoxydibenzoylmethane.

avocado oil—can function as an emollient and as a carrier oil in a cosmetic preparation, helping transport active substances into the skin. It is bactericidal and soothing, particularly to sensitive skin. Current speculation among researchers is that avocado oil may mobilize and increase the collagen of connective tissue. This would keep the skin moist and smooth, in addition to having a favorable influence in the treatment for minor skin conditions. Avocado oil has also demonstrated sunscreening characteristics and has been given the highest ranking by the *Encyclopedia of Chemical Technology* for sunscreen effectiveness when compared to other naturally derived oils such as peanut, olive, and coconut. In cosmetic formulations, it is also employed to help stabilize oil-in-water emulsions and can be effectively used in cleansing creams, moisturizers, lipsticks, makeup bases, bath oils, sunscreen, and suntan preparations. Avocado oil enjoys the highest penetration rate among similar oils (corn, soybean, olive, and almond). It consists mostly of oleic, linoleic, and linolenic acids. Other constituents include palmitic and palmitoleic acids, lecithin, phytosterol, carotinoids, and a high concentration of vitamins A, D, and E. This oil is obtained from the ripe avocado fruit and is generally expressed from the seed.

avocado oil (*unsaponifiable****)***—has excellent penetration and sunscreening properties. *See also* avocado oil.

azulene—renowned as an anti-inflammatory, calming, and soothing agent. Excellent for sensitive skin, azulene is a German chamomile derivative with a characteristic deep blue color. Careful, it stains! *See also* chamomile.

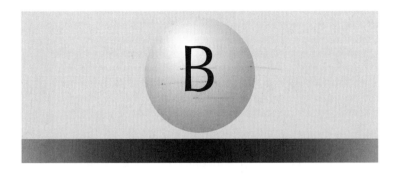

babassu oil—also known as babaçu oil. A superior emollient, babassu oil is recommended for use in sunscreen products. It can also benefit combination skin as it is appropriate for dry skin areas and does not exacerbate the oiliness of an already oily T-zone.

bacaba pulp oil—emollient and moisturizing, this botanical has a high oleic acid content, as well as omega-6 (linoleic acid).

baking soda—*see* sodium bicarbonate.

balm—*see* balm mint extract.

balm of Gilead (*Commiphora meccanensis, Commiphora opobalsamum****)***—helps in treatment of eczema and dry skin.

balm mint extract (*Melissa officinalis****) (balm; melissa)***—folklore ascribes the following properties to balm: "revivifying a man completely, effective for treating nervous disorders, strengthen the brain, relieves languishing nature."[1] Modern research, on the other hand, is a bit more specific, attributing calming, soothing, healing, antispasmodic, tightening, antibactericidal, and circulation stimulating properties to balm mint. It can be beneficially incorporated into acne treatment formulations and post-sun preparations, with positive action in products for blemished or sensitive skins as well. Balm mint's effectiveness is due to its constituents, which include citral, citronella, linalol, geraliol, and aldehydes. Its strong aroma makes it a popular fragrance component. Derived from the plant's leaves or leaf juice.

---

[1] Mrs. M. Grieve, *A Modern Herbal* (New York: Dover Publications, Inc., 1971).

B

balm mint oil (lemon balm; melissa oil)—the general effects attributed to this oil include sedative, antispasmodic, and antiseptic. Its use is indicated for acne skin and for individuals with dermatitis and eczema. Constituents include caffeic acid, rosemary acid, salicylic acid, luteoin, apigenin, glucose, maltose, and amino acids such as proline, asparogine, glutonine acid, valien, serine, alanine, and methionine. The recommended use level for this oil is 1 to 10 percent of a formulation's total composition. Balm mint oil has a very low yield and thus is very expensive. Because of this, it is widely adulterated, usually with citronella and lemongrass. The oil is obtained from the leaves and tops of *Melissa officinalis*. There are some indications that balm mint oil may cause skin irritation.

balsam Peru (Myroxylon pereirae)—a botanical to which strong medicinal actions are attributed. It is considered antibacterial, antifungal, and antiparasitic, and is preferred by some to sulfur ointments. It is recommended for cases of scabies and skin problems such as acne and eczema. Balsam Peru can also be employed in a cosmetic to mask odor, lending vanilla and cinnamon-like scent to a preparation. Its main constituents are a colorless, aromatic, oily liquid called cinnamein; a dark resin known as peruviol; a small quantity of vanillin; and cinnamic acid. It is extracted from the trunk of a large and beautiful tree, akin to mahogany. Every part of the tree, including the leaves, abounds in a resinous juice. It may cause skin irritation.

balsam tolu oil (Myrospermum toluiferum)—valuable to perfumers as a fixative. Its botanical actions are mostly indicated for internal use and its value in external applications is not clear. It is described as a stimulant. This oil is constituted of about 80 percent amorphous resin, with cinnamic acid and a little vanillin, benzyl benzoate, and benzyl cinnamate. It is sometimes used instead of balsam Peru. It is obtained by making V-shaped cuts in the tree.

bamboo extract—used in cosmetics for its moisture-binding properties.

banana oil (plantain fruit)—a carrier oil. The banana family is of more interest for its nutritional value rather than for its botanical properties. The use of plantain juice as an antidote for snake bites has been reported in parts of Southeast Asia since 1916.

baoab (Adansonia digitata)—highly emollient and soothing, it is said to enhance skin elasticity and have an immediate skin firming effect. The seed oil or an extract obtained from the pulp, seed, or plant leaf are often used in cosmetic formulations.

barberry extract *(Berberis vulgaris)*—its herbal properties have been reported as anti-inflammatory, antiseptic, and beneficial for application to cutaneous eruptions. The common barberry is a bushy shrub cultivated for its fruit, but the stembark and rootbark are used for cosmetic applications. Barberry bark's main constituent is berberine, a bitter alkaloid. Other constituents include oxyacanthine, bergamine, other alkaloidal matter, a little tannin, wax, resin, fat, albumin, gum, and starch.

bardane extract *(burdock)*—*see* burdock root extract.

barium sulfate—an emulsion stabilizer for sunscreen formulations. Outside of sunscreen preparations, this inorganic salt is most commonly used in noncosmetic soaps.

barley oil *(Hordeum vulgare)*—a carrier oil with soothing properties.

basil oil *(Ocimum basilicum)*—its properties are noted to include stimulating, tonic, purifying, and antimicrobial. Basil oil's constituents include methyl chavicol, eucalyptol, linalool, and estragol. It is often used as a carrier oil and for fragrance, and may have some application in acne preparations.

bayberry *(Myrica cerifera)*—its properties are described as astringent, antibacterial, and stimulant. Bayberry's application is primarily for acne and damaged skin. The parts of the plant used are the dried bark of the root and the wax. Volatile oil, starch, lignin, gum, albumen, extractive, tannic and gallic acids, acrid and astringent resins, a red coloring substance, and an acid resembling saponin are all constituents that have been found in the stembark and the root. The wax consists of the glycerides of stearic, palmitic, and myristic acids, and a small quantity of oleaic acid. Bayberry is another name for the wild cinnamon found in the West Indies and South America that yields oil of bayberry.

bean oil *(Phaseolus vulgaris)*—a carrier. Found to be soothing and relieve itching. Bean oil is said to be good for skin with an acne condition.

bearberry extract *(Arctostaphylos uva-urusi)*—the leaves have a powerful astringency and probably also an antiseptic and anti-inflammatory effect. Some sources cite skin-lightening properties as well. The main constituent of bearberry leaves is a crystallizable glucoside called arbutin. Other constituents

B

include methyl-arbutin, ericolin, ursone, gallic acid, ellagic acid, and probably also myriceting. The bearberry plant is a small shrub, and the dried leaves are the only part of the plant used in cosmetics.

beech tree extract *(Fagus sylvatica)*—it is claimed by herbologists that, when used in proper form, beech tree extract increases protein synthesis and enzymatic activity of keratinocytes. Other properties, such as stimulation and antiseptic, are also attributed to the beech tar, making it of value for application in various skin diseases. The oil is used in the same fashion as other fixed oils and is considered a carrier. Well-ripened beech nuts, called "mast," yield 17 to 20 percent of a non-drying oil similar to hazel and cottonseed oils.

beer yeast (natural)—*see* yeast.

bee pollen wax—*see* beeswax.

beeswax—one of the oldest raw ingredients used in cosmetic preparations. It is traditionally used as an emulsifier for water-in-oil emulsions and is now also used to regulate a formulation's consistency. Beeswax is used as part of the wax composition of solid and paste products such as creams, lipsticks, and pomades. When on the skin's surface, it can form a network rather than a film, as is the case with petroleum. Though there is no scientific proof for it, beeswax is credited with anti-inflammatory, antiallergic, antioxidant, antibactericidal, germicidal, skin-softening, and elasticity-enhancing properties. As an antioxidant, beeswax has some free-radical scavenging ability. Depending on its source, beeswax can be considered a noncomedogenic ingredient. It rarely causes sensitivity, and allergic reactions to beeswax are low.

beeswax (white)—regular beeswax that has been bleached. Unbleached beeswax is yellow. *See also* beeswax.

beeswax (liquid paraffin)—*see* beeswax.

beet powder *(Beta vulgaris)*—used mostly for color.

behenic acid—a long-chain fatty acid used in product formulations to form a viscous emulsion. Considered a noncomedogenic raw material.

behenoxy dimethicone—an emollient, pigment dispersant, lubricant, and moisture barrier silicone. It is used in small quantities to give smooth slip on the skin.

behenyl alcohol—a binder and an emulsion stabilizer. Used also to increase a formulation's viscosity. This is a mixture of fatty alcohols.

behenyl erucate—an occlusive skin-conditioning agent. Considered noncomedogenic.

behenoyl stearic acid—an emulsifier.

behenyl triglyceride—a skin-conditioning agent. Considered a noncomedogenic raw material.

bentonite (bentonite clay)—used to regulate the viscosity and suspension properties of a cosmetic formulation. It also acts as an overall formula stabilizer. Bentonite's water-absorption capabilities allow it to form a gelatinous mass. It is used in face masks because of its properties as a suspending agent. Considered a noncomedogenic raw material, bentonite is a colloidal aluminum silicate clay.

bentonite clay—see bentonite.

benzalkonium chloride—a preservative with antimicrobial and deodorant properties. It can also be used as a surfactant. With continuous use, it may cause occasional allergic reactions.

benzethonium chloride—a preservative that works against algae, bacteria, and fungi. In skin care preparations, it is safe for use at concentrations of 0.5 percent.

benzoic acid—a preservative primarily for use against molds and yeasts. Its performance is classified only as fair against bacteria. Benzoic acid is used in concentrations of 0.05 to 0.1 percent. Although it has a low sensitizing rate, it may cause an allergic reaction in persons sensitive to similar chemicals.

benzoin—a fragrant essential oil with bactericidal, anti-irritation, and anti-itching properties. It is considered a good ingredient for reducing skin redness and is a preservative of fats. While its primary constituent is benzoic acid, it also contains canillin and an oily aromatic liquid. This balsamic resin is extracted by cutting deeply into the trunks of trees that grow primarily in Indonesia and Thailand.

benzophenone-2—a sunscreen chemical with UV-absorbing properties.

benzophenone-3 (oxybenzone)—an oil-soluble UV absorber with absorption rates within the UVA and UVB peak ranges, it has an approved usage level of up to 6 percent in the United States and 10 percent in the European Union. Its popularity in sunscreen formulations is increasing as manufacturers become more concerned with potential safety problems associated with more traditional sunscreen chemicals. Benzophenone-3 enhances SPF and is popular among sunscreen formulators. However, some reports associate it with causing photocontact allergy. Considered a noncomedogenic raw material.

benzophenone-4 (sulisobenzone)—a commonly used, FDA-approved sunscreen chemical with UVA-absorbing properties and an approved usage level of 5 to 10 percent. Also considered an antiphoto-oxidant.

benzophenone-8 (dioxybenzone)—an FDA-approved sunscreen chemical with UVA-absorption capabilities. It has an approved usage level of 3 percent in the United States.

benzoyl peroxide—an antibacterial ingredient commonly used in acne treatments. It functions by forcing an oxidant (peroxide in this case) into the philosebaceous orifice where it releases oxygen, thereby diminishing the *P. acnes* population. This reduces the level of free fatty acids and the level of skin infection. Benzoyl peroxide may cause skin irritation in people with sensitive skin.

benzyl alcohol—a preservative against bacteria, used in concentrations of 1.0 to 3.0 percent. It can cause skin irritation.

benzyl laurate—an emollient ester that is easily emulsified and leaves the skin feeling silky. It is nontoxic, nonirritating, nonviscous, and nonoily. It also reduces the oiliness of mineral oil and solubilizes sunscreen actives.

benzyl nicotinate—can increase skin oxygenation—thanks to vasodilatation properties—and help stimulate the healing process of wounded skin. It is an ester form of niacin (vitamin B) of benzyl alcohol and nicotinic acid.

benzyl salicylate—a fragrance found naturally occurring in carnations and in certain members of the primrose family. While it can be derived for cosmetic use from natural essential oils, such as jasmine oil, neroli, and ylang-ylang, it can also be synthetically manufactured.

3-benzylidene camphor—a sunscreen chemical with UVB-filtering and absorption capacities with an approved usage level of up to 2 percent (in the European Union).

benzylidene camphor sulfonic acid—a UV filter and UV absorber with approval for use in the European Union with an approved usage level of up to 6 percent (in the European Union).

bergamot oil (Citrus bergamia, Monarda didyma)—considered an antiseptic and bacterial growth inhibitor. It is also considered good for oily and acne skin, and for seborrheic conditions. Sun exposure after applying pure bergamot oil, or a compound with a high bergamot oil concentration to the skin, may cause hyperpigmentation and a skin rash. When used in perfumes, the photosensitizing properties of bergamot are responsible for the hyperpigmentation seen behind the ear and on the neck area near the ear. The oil extracted from the rind of citrus fruits is referred to as bergamot orange. Regular bergamot is from the monarda plant, of which there are several varieties.

beta-carotene—a known antioxidant, it has demonstrated photoprotection properties particularly when taken internally. It is also used as a yellow-orange color additive. Beta-carotene is a caratinoid and a precursor to vitamin A. It is beneficial for dry and flaking skin. It is naturally occurring in fruits and vegetables that contain orange-yellow pigment, such as apricots, carrots, mangos, and oranges, but can also be synthetically manufactured.

B

beta-glucan—said to stimulate the formation of collagen. Incorporated into antiaging cosmetics in order to reduce the appearance of fine lines and wrinkles. *See also* glucans; polyglucan.

18 beta-glycerrhentinic acid (glycyrrhetic acid)—a triterpenic acid credited with anti-inflammatory, decongestant, and redness-reducing properties. It can also act as an epithelial regenerator. Used effectively in milks, creams, and gels for the treatment of sensitive skins. Obtained from the hydrolysis of glycyrrhizic acid. *See also* glycyrrhizic acid.

beta hydroxyacid (BHA)—refines skin texture by reducing stratum corneum thickness through surface exfoliation. BHAs are excellent for use in acne products due to their ability to exfoliate excessive dead cell accumulation around the orifice of the sebaceous follicle. Salicylic acid is the most commonly used example of a beta hydroxyacid. *See also* salicylic acid.

betaine—a surfactant and an excellent conditioner, viscosity builder, and foam booster. It is found mostly in skin cleansers, shampoos, and bath products.

beta-lipohydroxy acid—also known as LHA. A salicylic acid derivative that can help acne skin, particularly to prevent relapses when acne has been successfully treated. It is a keratolytic that helps prevent the formation of microcomedones. Beta-lipohydroxy acid also appears to improve the skin's tolerance to tretinoin when used in conjunction with the retinoid.

betony extract *(Stachys officialis)*—traditionally used in dermatological disorders as a soothing and anti-itching treatment. It is recommended for problem prone skin.

BHA *(butylated hydroxyanisole)*—a preservative with antioxident capabilities, not to be confused with beta hydroxyacids (BHAs).

BHA—*see* beta hydroxyacid.

BHT—also known as butylated hydroxytoluene. An antioxidant that also has preservative and masking capabilities.

bilberry fruit extract *(Vaccinium myrtillus)*—also known as European blueberry; huckleberry. It is astringent, anti-inflammatory, antioxidant, has a slight muscle-relaxing capacity, and in clinical studies it has shown an ability to protect collagen against degradation. Much of this action is attributed to its anthocyanin content. Anthocyanin (also known as an anthocyanoside) is a blue, red, or violet flavonoid (also found in currants, grapes, beets, and eggplant). Anthocyanin-containing plant extracts demonstrate powerful antioxidant activity, an ability to promote collagen biosynthesis and prevent collagen degradation. They also appear to reinforce capillaries, reducing their permeability and fragility. The anti-inflammatory properties come from an apparent ability to prevent the production of inflammatory chemicals such as histamines. In addition to anthocyanins, the plant's constituents include sugars, a variety of vitamins, tannins, pectins, quercetin, catechins, and acids. One formulatory challenge is the fact that as the fruit ripens, the anthocyanin seems to increase while the activity of the leaf constituents seems to fall.

bioflavonoid—a category of plant constituent with therapeutic attributes. Bioflavonoids have antioxidant properties, allowing them to absorb oxygen radicals that may cause skin oxidation. They are also antimicrobial, which may aid in anti-inflammatory activity against microbially caused skin irritations. A generic ingredient listing of this sort fails to identify the specific botanical(s) involved and may then refer to a group of compounds.

Biophytex—a manufacturer's name for a combination of plant extracts, including butchers broom, horse chestnut, and Indian water nave. Reported to have calming, desensitizing, and minor healing properties.

biosaccharide gum-1—skin conditioning and humectant. This is a derivative of sorbitol. *See also* sorbitol.

B

biotin (biotine; vitamin B₇/vitamin H)—antiseborrhoeic, some cosmetic manufacturers claim biotin has healing properties and as such, is a good ingredient for acne skin. Biotin is also part of the B complex group of vitamins (specifically vitamin B_7). A deficiency of this vitamin has been associated with greasy scalp and baldness. Its deficiency in humans is considered extremely rare, and the value of external applications through the use of cosmetic products is questionable.

biotine—*see* biotin.

birch (Betula sp.)—birch and birch derivatives have been described as astringent, antiseptic, cleansing, softening, and circulation stimulating, and they are believed to have curative properties in cases of skin diseases. In folklore, birch has been used for its healing effects on rashes and in cases of hair loss. Birch's important constituents include glanonoids, hyperoside, tannin, saponins, and quercetin. Even though some manufacturers list this ingredient as simply "birch," a proper description should be more specific, such as birch bark extract, birch leaf extract, or birch sap. Actual clinical data is scant in substantiating its therapeutic effects, as well as those of its derivatives. *See also* birch bark extract.

birch bark extract—described as having anti-irritant and antiseptic properties, and effective in acne treatment and sunburn products, soothing lotions, and aftershaves. The oil is astringent and is mainly used for its curative effects, especially in cases of acne and eczema. In folkloric medicine, birch bark extract was considered good for bathing skin eruptions. Destructive distillation of the bark's white epidermis yields an empyreumatic oil known as oil of birch tar, *Oleum rusci*, or dagget. This is a thick, bituminous, brownish-black liquid with a pungent, balsamic odor. It contains a high percentage of methylsalicilate, creosol, and guaiacol. It is almost identical to wintergreen oil.

birch leaf extract—believed to have antiseptic and astringent properties and to help heal skin irritations. It is used in traditional medicine for skin rashes. The leaves, which have a peculiar, aromatic, yet agreeable odor and a bitter taste, secrete a resinous substance with acid properties. They contain flavonoids, tannins, and essential oils.

birch sap—claimed to help retain moisture in the skin.

bisabolol—a botanical used for its anti-inflammatory and soothing properties. It is derived from chamomile and/or yarrow.

B

bis-digylceryl polyacryladipate-2—a synthetic substitute for lanolin, it is a skin softener.

bishydroxyethyl bicetyl malonamide—a skin conditioner.

bismuth oxychloride—an inorganic color additive. It is used mostly in makeup manufacturing and rarely in skin care formulations. It may also be used for pearlization in cosmetics.

bismuth oxychloride and mica and silica—a combination of minerals that diffuse and scatter light. May be used in makeup and cosmetic preparations, such as eye creams, to provide a "blurring" effect, thereby reducing the visibility of wrinkles, skin imperfections, and dark circles around the eyes, for example.

bitter almond extract—an emollient and a carrier, it may cause irritation and negative skin reactions. *See also* almond oil, bitter.

bitter orange extract (Citrus aurantium)—a botanical credited with soothing properties. It is obtained from the peel of bitter oranges, and it has a more delicate fragrance than sweet orange. *See also* orange extract.

black catechu—*see* acacia.

black cohosh extract (Cimicifuga racemosa) (black snakeroot, rattleroot, squaw root, bugbane)—said to have astringent, calming, skin protecting, antimicrobial, humectant, emollient, anti-inflammatory and antispasmodic properties. Cosmetic ingredient suppliers indicate it for use in anti-aging preparations. Black cohosh's primary constituent is a resin known as cimicifugin or macrotin; it also contains recemostin. Therapeutic properties come from the use of its root, and this is the plant component most often used.

black currant extract (Ribes nigrum)—its can be used in cosmetic products for astringent and skin-smoothing activities, as well as for its perfuming and emollient properties. Some report it to be anti-inflammatory. While the whole plant may be used, including the fruit, leaves, bark, and roots, the properties of the exact can depend on the part of the plant from which the extract is derived.

black currant seed oil—may be an effective ingredient for enhancing the skin's ability to develop normal barrier functions and the protective effect of the corneum layer. Black currant seed oil contains fatty, linoleic, and linolenic acids. When applied to dry skin, it may increase the skin's own content of these previously lacking components.

black pepper oil—its cosmetic application is unclear, though it may be used on skin inflammations and superficial wounds. This oil is obtained from a small-grain black pepper shrub found primarily in the hilly parts of Jamaica.

black tang—*see* seaweed extract.

black tea extract—*see* tea extract.

black walnut extract—an antiseptic, noncomedogenic raw material. *See also* walnut.

black willow bark extract (Salix nigra)—used as an exfoliating ingredient, given its salicylic acid content. *See also* willow extract.

blackberry extract (Rubus villosus)—regarded as excellent for its astringent and tonic properties due to the high tannin content of the root bark and the leaves. The leaf extract can be beneficially used for acne conditions.

blackthorn (Prunus spinosa)—the ability to identify its activity in a cosmetic formation depends on the part of the plant and form used. For example, the flower extract has emollient, moisturizing, and general skin-conditioning properties. The flower water is considered tonic. If the fruit's juice is used, the activity can be tonic, as well as astringent and skin conditioning. Finally, the wood bark extract is where blackthorn's antioxidant (free-radical scavenging) properties lie, and is astringent, like other parts of the plant. Blackthorn is also considered to be healing and soothing for the skin. Its constituents include flavonoids, sugar, tannin, organic acids, vitamin C, pectin, and trace elements.

bladderwrack—*see* seaweed extract.

blessed thistle extract (holy thistle)—tonic and stimulating properties have been attributed to this herb. It is an effective extract for problem-prone skin, such as skin with papules and pustules. In antiquity, this plant was believed to aid in the healing of skin sores and to reduce itching. Blessed thistle contains a volatile oil and a bitter, crystalline neutral body called cnicin, said to be analogous to salicin in its properties. One of many varieties of thistle.

bloodroot—*see* tetterwort extract.

blue centaury extract—*see* cornflower extract.

BMDM—*see* avobenzone; butyl methoxydibenzoylmethane.

bois de rose oil—a fragrance with a light camphor scent. This essential oil is obtained by means of steam distillation of

B

the chipped wood from the tropical rosewood tree. *Bois de rose* oil has no known toxicity.

boldine—attributed with strong antioxidant properties. It has also demonstrated an ability to protect against UVB rays. Boldine is a constituent of the boldo plant (*Peumus boldus* Mol.) native to Chile, and is found in the plant's leaves and bark.

borage extract (Borago officinalis) (borago)—its topical application is described as anti-inflammatory. It is beneficial for sensitive skin and allergic reactions. Borage contains potassium and calcium, combined with mineral acids. This is a hardy annual plant of which the leaves—and to a lesser degree, the flowers—are used.

borage seed oil (borage oil)—an effective anti-irritant, it has demonstrated hydrating properties and an ability to improve cases of pruritis and xerosis. It is a rich source of gamma-linolenic acid. *See also* borage extract.

boric acid—an effective preservative against yeast. It is used in concentrations of 0.01 to 1.0 percent and has fair to good antiseptic properties. It may also be used as a buffer and denaturant. Boric acid is prepared from sulfuric acid and natural borax. It can cause skin rashes and irritation if used in high concentrations. The use of boric acid in cosmetic preparations is no longer very popular.

borneol—utilized in perfumery for its peppery odor. Borneol is a naturally occurring substance found in coriander, ginger oil, oil of lime, rosemary, strawberries, thyme, citronella, and nutmeg. Its toxicity is similar to that of camphor. *See also* camphor.

boron nitride—a synthetically manufactured white, talc-like powder that can reflect light, giving a product a sparkle effect. It is primarily used in color cosmetics to provide subtle shimmer; however, it can also be found in skin care formulations for enhancing product smoothness and slip.

boxwood (Buxus sempervirens)—skin conditioning, it also has absorbent properties. Boxwood's constituents include saponins, chlorophyll, tannin, and wax. The sap can cause itching or irritation.

bran extract—used in peels and scrubs for its mild abrasive qualities.

Brazilian babassu nut oil—*see* babassu oil.

brewer's yeast—*see* yeast.

brewing grain extracts—said to be anti-inflammatory with some anti-irritant properties. Brewing grain extracts are reported to inhibit certain types of erythema, relieve skin itching, and provide an antimycotic effect. The grains include barley and wheat.

British gum—see dextrin.

2-bromo-2 nitro-1,3 propane diol—also known as bronopol. This preservative is effective against a broad range of microorganisms but performs best against fungi and yeast. Used in concentrations of 0.01 to 0.1 percent, it is nontoxic, nonirritating, and nonsensitizing to humans. Safe as a cosmetic ingredient up to and including 0.1 percent concentrations, except under circumstances where its reaction with amines and amides can result in the formation of nitrosamines or nitrosamides. It has a slightly higher-than-moderate sensitizing potential in leave-on cosmetic preparations. Unstable at high temperatures and inactive in sulfur-containing formulations.

bronopol—see 2-bromo-2 nitro-1,3 propane diol.

brown seaweed—see seaweed.

buckthorn—see cascara sagrada extract.

burdock—see burdock root extract.

burdock root extract (Arctium lappa)—credited with antibacterial and antifungal properties and an apparent ability to help regulate/normalize oil production. Traditionally used in the treatment of mild acne conditions. When applied externally as a compress, burdock leaves are considered highly effective for relieving bruises and inflammation. Burdock's constituents include inulin, mucilage, sugar, a crystalline glucoside called lappin, fixed and volatile oils, and some tannic acid. Extracts from the fruit (commonly though mistakenly referred to as the seeds) are also considered beneficial for chronic skin diseases. The dried root and root extract are the official therapeutic segments of burdock.

buriti pulp oil—also known as *Mauritia flexuosa.* Emollient, antioxidant and free-radical scavenging. Rich in carotenoids (including beta-carotene) and essential fatty acids (particularly oleic and palmitic acids), it is often used to help regenerate the skin's hydrolipid barrier. Beneficial for use on burned or sunburned skin, it is also said to be nourishing, moisturizing, and able to improve skin elasticity. Incorporated into products for aging, dry and very dry skin, eczema, sun care preparations, and lip and hair care products.

Burow's solution—see aluminum acetate solution.

butchers broom extract *(Ruscus aculeatus)*—no clear benefit for skin care application has been attributed to this botanical. Some sources cite it as having slimming and anticellulite effects, as well as diuretic and anti-itching properties. Butchers broom is a low, shrubby evergreen plant of which the herb and the root are used.

butyl alcohol—an emulsion stabilizer and occlusive skin-conditioning agent. The mono-octadecyl ether of glycerin.

butyl methoxydibenzoylmethane (BMDM, avobenzone)—when incorporated as an active ingredient, butyl methoxydibenzoylmethane is listed as avobenzone, a sunscreening agent with broad-range UVA protection. However, when listed among other ingredients, either with the full nomenclature or the abbreviation BMDM, it is most likely being used as a UV absorber, helping maintain a product's stability in face of UV exposure. For example, when placed in clear glass or plastic containers, the color of some emulsions will fade due to UV penetration through the container's clear material. By adding BMDM, a formulator can help reduce or eliminate the possibility of a product's fading or succumbing to other associated UV instability. *See also* avobenzone.

butyl oleate—an ester of butyl alcohol and oleic acid with lubricant, moisturizer, and emollient properties.

butyl paraben—a preservative against fungi and yeast, with little sensitizing effect. It is generally used in combination with other preservatives to increase the preservative activity spectrum. Butyl paraben is only effective in the acid pH range. *See also* parabens.

butyl phenyl methylpropional—a fragrance.

butyl stearate—a stearic acid used in very small quantities in cosmetic preparations as an emulsifier for creams and lotions. It has been shown to cause allergic reactions.

butylated hydroxyanisole—*see* BHA.

butylated hydroxytoluene—*see* BHT.

butyldiadipate—an emollient and pH-adjusting agent with good penetrating properties.

butylene glycol—a solvent with good antimicrobial action. It enhances the preservative activity of parabens. Butylene glycol also serves as a humectant and viscosity controller, and to mask odor.

1,3 butylene glycol—a solvent and viscosity-decreasing agent commonly used in cosmetic and toiletry preparations.

B

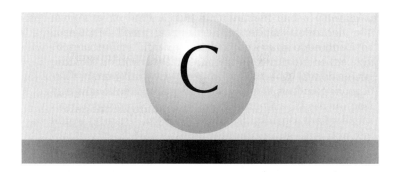

cactus extract—an emulsifier for creams and lotions that, as an active substance, is described as good for sunburns and other minor burns, insect bites, skin irritations, swelling, and inflammation. It has been used in folklore medicine for edema. Its sticky, gelatinous quality makes it valuable for face masks, particularly the clear, peel-off types. The main constituents of cactus include cactin, flavonoids, amino acids, and polysaccharides.

caffeine—able to break down lipids, it has a lipolytic effect on fatty cells. Given this ability and its draining properties, caffeine is used for skin firming and tightening. Among its constituents are tannin and the alkaloid methylxanthine. This bitter-tasting, odorless white powder occurs naturally in coffee, cola, guana paste, kola nuts, and tea. Caffeine is obtained as a by-product of decaffeinated coffee. It is often incorporated into body product formulations targeting cellulite and slimming, as well as in eye creams that claim to reduce puffiness.

cajeput oil (*Melaleuca leucadendron*)—healing, antiseptic, stimulating, and mildly counterirritant properties. It is used externally for acne and other skin problems, such as psoriasis and eczema. The principal constituent of this oil is cineol, at an average level of 45 to 55 percent. Also present is solid terpineol as well as several aldehydes, such as valeric, butyric, and benzoic. It is similar in odor to camphor and eucalyptus. Cajeput oil is extracted from the leaves and twigs of the cajeput tree.

calamine—has mildly astringent and cooling qualities, and is particularly useful for sunburned or irritated skin. Calamine is a mineral solution consisting primarily of zinc oxide with the addition of approximately 0.5 percent ferric oxide.

calamint (Calamintha officinalis) (calamintha)—considered to reduce bruising. Calamint contains a camphoraceous, volatile, stimulating oil in common with the other mints. Obtained from a bushy plant closely related to the thyme family and ground ivy.

calamintha—*see* calamint.

calcium alginate—used as a visual accent in cosmetics. This is an alginate gel impregnated with an oily core material that can be pigmented or neutral in color.

calcium chloride—a compound that helps improve the reaction among certain ingredients used in cosmetic formulations. This inorganic salt is now rarely used in skin care products and is being replaced with potassium chloride.

calcium hydroxide—an inorganic base employed as a topical astringent and alkali in solutions or lotions. It can burn the skin and eyes.

calcium pantetheine sulfonate—a versatile ingredient that can be used to boost UV protection in a sunscreen. It also has anti-inflammatory properties, and serves as a skin whitener or lightener. Clinical studies indicate an ability to inhibit tyrosinase activity and melanin synthesis. It is most commonly used in moisturizers and antiaging and SPF products.

calcium pantothenate—used as an emollient and to enrich creams and lotions in hair care preparations. This is the calcium salt of pantothenic acid found in liver, rice, bran, and molasses. It is also found in large amounts in royal jelly.

calcium thioglycolate—used almost exclusively in depilatory creams and hair products, this is a calcium salt of thioglycolic acid. It may cause skin irritation.

calendula extract (Calendula officinalis) (marigold)—an emollient said to have healing, wound-healing, soothing, antiseptic, anti-itching, and anti-inflammatory properties. It can be effectively used in cases of oily and/or delicate skin as well as for acne. The extract is obtained from the calendula blossom. *See also* marigold extract.

calendula hydrolysates—a calendula derivative. *See* calendula extract.

calophyllum inophyllum seed oil—an antioxidant with UV-absorption capacities. It can also be used as an antimicrobial

C

and a skin conditioner. Its properties are said to include the improvement of cell regeneration. Often incorporated into antiaging and regenerating creams, sun and post-sun creams. In the same family as *Calophyllum tacamahaca. See also* tamanu oil.

calophyllum tacamahaca seed oil—*see* tamanu oil.

camelina sativa seed oil—emollient and skin conditioning, it is used in antiaging cosmetic products for its reported ability to improve skin elasticity and suppleness. Among its constituents are alpha-linolenic acid, linoleic acid, and tocopherol.

camellia oil—used as a nongreasy emollient for skin care products. Camellia oil plays an important role in antioxidation as a result of its high content of oleic acid. Derived from the seeds of *Thea sasanqua nois.*

camellia seed powder—an ingredient from Asia used for its abrasive action.

camellia sinensis leaf extract—*see* green tea extract.

camphor (Cinnamomum camphora)—credited with anesthetic, anti-inflammatory, antiseptic, astringent, cooling, and refreshing properties, and thought to be slightly stimulating to blood circulation and function. Once absorbed by the subcutaneous tissue, it combines in the body with glucoronic acid and is released through the urine in this condition. Camphor is effective for oily and acne skin treatment, and has a scent similar to eucalyptus. In high concentrations, it can be an irritant and numb the peripheral sensory nerves. Natural camphor is derived from an evergreen tree indigenous to Asia, although now its synthetic substitute is often used.

camphor benzalkonium methosulfate—a UV filter and UV absorber. It also has antimicrobial properties.

camphor oil—*see* camphor.

candelilla wax (Euphorbia cerifera)—binds oils and waxes, and gives body to a formulation. It is also used as a film former. Obtained from candelilla plants, it is similar to carnauba wax.

candlenut—*see* kukui nut oil.

canola oil—has good emolliency and lubricity. Canola oil is a rapeseed oil extract considered to be a natural replacement for mineral oil.

capryl isostearate—an emollient.

caprylic/capric triglyceride (Tricaprylin)—an emollient with good spreading properties. It promotes penetration and does not leave visible traces of oiliness on the skin. It is effectively used in creams, lotions, and oil formulations.

caprylol collagen amino acids—a liquid with an antiacne effect. *See also* amino acid; collagen.

capryloyl collagenic acid—this lipoamino acid is found to have similar antibacterial properties as benzoyl peroxide when tested against *S. aureus*, *S. epidermidis*, and *P. acnes* bacteria. Test results show it to be most effective and helpful in treating mild cases of acne vulgaris, though it demonstrates some positive results against moderate and severe acne cases as well. While it reduces inflammatory lesions, it does not affect comedones and cysts. When treatment is suspended, there is a mild relapse of the acne lesions.

capryloyl salicylic acid—a skin conditioner. This is an ester of salicylic and caprylic acids.

caprylyl/capryl glucoside—a surfactant used in cleansing preparations, primarily shampoos.

caprylyl glycol—an emollient with moisturizing properties that may also be used as a cosmetic stabilizer. When found in combination with phenoxyethanol these two ingredients work together as an antimicrobial.

caramel—used as a coloring agent. It provides products with a slight touch of brown. Some sources also state that it acts as a soothing agent in some skin care preparations. Caramel is a concentrated solution obtained from heating sugar or glucose solutions.

caraway oil (Carum carvi)—a carrier oil credited with the ability to alleviate bruises, and believed to have tissue-regenerating properties. It is said to be beneficial for acne and oily skin. Caraway is a member of the group of aromatic, umbelliferous plants, such as anise, cumin, dill, and fennel, characterized by carminative properties. Carvene (also found in dill and cumin oils), an oxygenated oil, and carvol are the principal constituents of caraway oil. Caraway oil is obtained from the distillation of the seeds, and may cause allergic reactions and skin irritation.

carbocysteine—an amino acid used in cosmetic formulations. *See also* amino acid.

carbomer 934, 940, 941, 980, 981—these high molecular-weight, cross-linked polymers are used as thickening and suspending agents, and as emulsion stabilizers in cosmetic formulations. They are often used with triethanolamine, sodium hydroxide, or other alkaline compounds to crosslink the polymer. White, slightly acidic powders, carbomers react with fat particles to form thick, stable emulsions of oils in water.

Carbopol—a trade name for carbomer. *See also* carbomer.

carboxyethy-y-aminobutyric acid—described as an ingredient promoting cellular growth. May be used in antiaging preparations.

carboxymethyl cellulose (cellulose gum)—a thickener. Used in cosmetic formulations when a reactant is not required or desired. Often used in bath preparations, beauty masks, hand creams, and shampoos. It is considered a noncomedogenic raw material.

carboxymethyl chitin—moisturizing. Derived from the exoskeleton of shrimp and crab. *See* chitin.

carboxypolymethylene—*see* carbomer.

carboxyvinyl polymer—provides viscosity, and is suitable for both thickening and stabilizing emulsions or dispersions in cosmetics. Its incorporation into cosmetic formulations results in very clear gel preparations. A synthetic resin.

C

cardamom oil (Elettaria cardamomum)—credited with antiseptic, stimulating, and deodorant properties. This is a large perennial herb that yields cardamom seeds containing volatile oil, fixed oil, salt of potassium, a coloring principle, starch, nitrogenous mucilage, ligneous fiber, an acrid resin, and ash. The volatile oil contains terpenes, terpineol, and cineol.

carmine—a crimson pigment. This is the aluminum lake of the coloring agent cochineal, a natural pigment derived from the dried female insect *Coccus cacti*. Carmine may cause allergic reactions.

carnauba wax—used to firm and texturize cosmetic preparations, and give them a less fluid consistency. Carnauba wax also forms a protective layer on the skin's surface. It has the highest melting point among natural plant waxes and does not usually cause allergic reactions. This wax is obtained from leaves and leaf buds of the Brazilian wax palm.

carnitine—a skin-conditioning agent, surfactant, and formulation viscosity-increasing substance. Carnitine is used primarily in hand and body preparations.

carnitine hydroxycitrate—said to help break down fat stored in the cells more effectively than caffeine, making it beneficial for use in slimming and body contouring products.

carnosine—an antioxidant that works to prevent cellular damage due to free radical activity. Studies indicate an ability to boost the immunological functions. Carnosine is a naturally occurring amino acid. In cosmetics, it has antiaging and skin-conditioning applications.

carob extract *(Jacaranda procera, Caroba balsam)*—its botanical property is reported as anti-infectious. In the small leaves—carob extract's source—caroborelinic acid, carobic acid, steocarobic acid, carobon, and carobin have been found.

carotene—used to provide a red-orange color in cosmetic formulations. It is the primary yellow coloring component of butter, carrots, and egg yolk. Carotene is found in plants as well as in many animal tissues. *See also* beta-carotene.

carotene oil—a red-orange colored oil containing carotene, used for coloring. A carrot extract.

carrageenan—*see* carrageen extract.

carrageen extract *(Chondrus crispus)* **(Irish moss)**—a very common thickener that, in its sodium salt form, has jellifying properties. It can help maintain the skin feeling soft and in good condition. Carrageen is a polysaccharide of red algae origin with a seaweed-like odor and is considered nontoxic. *See also* seaweed extract.

carreghane extract (red algae)—*see* seaweed extract.

carrot extract *(Daucus carota)*—there are some indications that, when obtained from carrot leaves, the extract may have cleansing and healing properties due to its strong antiseptic qualities. The root contains no less than 89 percent water. The juice also contains sugar, a little starch, extractine gluen, albumen, volatile oil, vegetable jelly or pectin, saline matter, malic acid, and carotin. Carrot's botanical properties depend on its volatile oil.

carrot oil—used since the 16th century for skin diseases due to its believed cleansing, purifying, and draining properties. This carotene-rich emollient has been indicated for acne skin conditions, dermatitis, skin irritation, skin rashes, and wrinkles. Derived from the carrot root.

carrot oleoresin—has good conditioning properties. This ingredient is found more often in hair care products.

cascara sagrada extract *(Rhamnus purshiana)* **(buckthorn; sacred bark)**—used to add a skin-soothing factor in lotions and creams. The assertion has been made that the bark contains flucosides. The extract is prepared from this shrub's bark.

casein amino acids—hydrolyzed milk protein. Used as an emulsifier in many cosmetics. It also binds water for moisturization. *See also* amino acids; milk protein.

castor isostearate succinate—used by cosmetic formulators as a replacement for lanolin. Classified as a natural ingredient.

castor oil—a highly emollient carrier oil that penetrates the skin easily, leaving it soft and supple. It also serves to bind the different ingredients of a cosmetic formulation together. Castor oil is high in glycerin esters of ricinoleic acid. It is rarely, if ever, associated with irritation of the skin or allergic reactions. Obtained through cold-pressing from seeds or beans of the *Ricinus communis* (castor oil) plant. Impure castor oil may cause irritation, as the seeds contain a toxic substance that is eliminated during processing. Its unpleasant odor makes it difficult to use in cosmetics.

caviar—*see* roe extract.

cedar—*see* cedarwood oil.

cedarwood oil (Thuja occidentalis) (cedar; thuja)—credited with antiseptic, sedative, and astringent properties. It is used as a fixative in fragrances because it blends well with other oils. This clear oil is also valuable for use on skin eruptions and to relieve itching. It is good for acne and oily skin, and could be helpful in cases of dermatitis, eczema, and psoriasis. Two types of cedarwood oil exist: Atlas cedarwood oil from Morocco (*Cedrus atlantica*) and one derived from the *Juniperus virginiana* (or red cedar) that is actually a juniper of the United States (its oil, however, is very similar to true cedarwood). The oil may cause skin irritation when used in high concentrations. Cedarwood oil is obtained from recently dried, leafy, young twigs.

celandine (Chelidonium majus)—also known as tetterwort. Attributed with antispasmodic properties, and can help reduce inflammation. It can, however, also cause irritation. Celandine contains numerous alkaloids, including chelidonine, sanguinarin, alpha- and beta-homo chelidonine, berberine, and cheleryhrine, some of which may help improve blood flow. Among its other constituents are resin and protease enzymes. It has also been used for dying purposes, and hence may also serve as a "natural" colorant. It is a member of the poppy family. It may be incorporated into eye care products to improve the appearance of tired eyes.

cellular protein—*see* protein.

C

cellulose—a thickener and an emulsifier. Obtained from plants.

cellulose (microcrystalline)—used as an emulsifier in cosmetic creams. It is the chief constituent of plant fiber.

cellulose fiber—used as a thickener, suspending agent, and binder.

cellulose gum—a thickener and an emulsifier equivalent to cellulose fiber. It is resistant to bacterial decomposition and provides a product with uniform viscosity. Constituents are any of several fibrous substances consisting of the chief part of a plant's cell walls. *See also* carboxymethyl cellulose.

cera alba—*see* beeswax (white); beeswax.

ceramides—the name for a family of naturally occurring lipids that act primarily in the skin's uppermost layer, forming a protective barrier and reducing natural transepidermal water loss. Ceramides repair the stratum corneum layer in cases of dry skin, improve skin hydration, and increase the feeling of softness. They are beneficial for stressed, sensitive, scaly, rough, dry, aged, and sun-damaged skin. Ceramides play an essential role in the structure of superficial epidermal layers and form an integral part of the intercellular membrane network. They help generate and sustain the skin's barrier function. This is extremely important: if the stratum corneum's hydration is maintained, then it functions more normally in terms of flexibility and desquamation, its integrity is upheld, and the skin is less susceptible to irritation. Ceramide production decreases with age, accentuating any tendency to dry skin. When incorporated into a skin care preparation, the topical application of ceramides could benefit the stratum corneum if the ceramides manage to fill the intercellular spaces and if they are hydrolyzed by the correct extracellular enzymes on the skin. Such application also can stimulate ceramide production in the skin, thereby increasing the skin's natural lipid content and reinforcing the skin's protective barrier, measured through transepidermal water loss. Topically applied ceramides have been shown to capture and bind the water, necessary for the skin to remain supple, smooth, and hydrated. Natural ceramides are obtained from animals and plants. Ceramides can also be synthetically manufactured, however, it is hard to synthesize ceramides identical to those found in nature, making them expensive raw materials.

C

cereal lipoplastidins—coconut oil that has been mixed with a number of cereal grain extracts such as rice, bran, and/ or oat.

cereal germ oil—a carrier.

cereal seed oil—a carrier.

ceresin—incorporated into skin care formulations in order to regulate the viscosity, suspension properties, and overall stability of a preparation. Used in protective creams as a beeswax and paraffin substitute. This white to yellow waxy mixture of hydrocarbons is obtained by the purification of ozokerite. Ceresin is a waxy material that may cause allergic reactions.

ceresin wax (ceresin)—a thickener and a binder with noncomedogenic properties. *See also* ceresin.

ceteareth, ceteareth 4, 12, 19, 20, 30—all are used for their emollient, emulsifying, antifoaming, and/or lubricant properties in cosmetic formulations. Ceteareth is obtained from a combination of cetyl alcohol and stearyl alcohol. Ceteareth-4 is the polyethylene glycol ether of cetearyl alcohol, and ceteareths-20 and -30 are also good solubilizing agents.

cetearyl alcohol (cetostearyl alcohol)—an emulsifying and stabilizing wax produced from the reduction of plant oils and natural waxes. Also used as an emollient and to give high viscosity to a finished product. Cetearyl alcohol is a mixture of fatty alcohols consisting primarily of cetyl and stearyl alcohols.

cetearyl glucoside—an emulsifier and surfactant.

cetearyl isononandate—an emollient with a high hydrophobic effect.

cetearyl octanoate—an emollient. This ingredient can be either a palm kernel or coconut derivative, and has a high degree of water repellency. It is used in noncomedogenic moisturizers. In nature, it occurs on the feathers of water birds.

cetearyl olivate—an olive-oil derived emulsifier. Said to also reduce transepidermal water loss. Often used in conjunction with sorbitan olivate.

cetearyl palmitate—an emollient. When incorporated into a skin care product, it leaves the skin with a velvety feel. This ingredient has replaced spermaceti wax.

ceteth—used as a surface active agent in cosmetics. A ceteth is a compound of derivatives of cetyl, lauryl, stearyl, and oleyl alcohols mixed with ethylene oxide.

C

ceteth 20—an emulsifier for oil-in-water creams and lotions.

cetostearyl alcohol—*see* cetearyl alcohol.

cetrimonium bromide—*see* cetyl trimethylammonium bromide.

cetyl alcohol—a versatile ingredient that can serve as an emollient, emulsifier, thickener, binder, foam booster, or emulsion stabilizer, depending on the formulation and need. It is derived from coconut or palm oil as well as being synthetically manufactured. Considered by some sources to be a noncomedogenic material.

cetyl alcohol 40—a preservative and carrier similar to cetyl alcohol.

cetyl dimethicone—an emollient and occlusive skin-conditioning agent based on silicones.

cetyl dimethicone copolyol—an emulsifier and emollient used in cosmetic preparations to form water-in-oil emulsions that have viscosity but also rub out easily. These types of preparations are used in sunscreen formulations where good spreadability and waterproofing are valued characteristics. Used in moisturizers, these emulsions provide a good moisture barrier and reduce the speed of transepidermal water loss.

cetyl esters—used in formulations to give body to emulsions. They are also formulation stabilizers and thickeners. Cetyl esters are generally indistinguishable from natural spermaceti wax in terms of composition and properties. Cetyl esters are made from a combination of various fatty esters with cetyl palmitate.

cetyl hydroxyethyl cellulose—similar to hydroxyethyl cellulose, but might yield slightly different thickness and absorption properties within a formulation. *See also* hydroxyethyl cellulose.

cetyl palmitate (synthetic spermaceti)—its chemical structure is the same as whale spermaceti. It may be used to thicken, produce viscose emulsions, give stability, and add texture to emulsions. It is similar to cetearyl palmitate.

cetyl phosphate—a mild emulsifier with a low irritancy potential.

cetyl ricinoleate—an emollient and emulsion stabilizer considered to be a noncomedogenic ester.

cetyl trimethylammonium bromide (cetrimonium bromide)—a cosmetic biocide and an emulsifying agent. A quaternary ammonium salt.

chamomile extract (Anthemis nobilis; Matricaria chamomilla)—has clinically proven anti-inflammatory and repairer properties. It is also considered bactericidal, anti-itching, soothing, antiseptic, purifying, refreshing, and hypoallergenic with the ability to neutralize skin irritants. There are various forms of chamomile, including Roman chamomile (*Anthemis nobilis*) and German chamomile (*Matricaria chamomilla*). German chamomile tends to be more potent than Roman due to its higher azulene content. Active constituents include azulene, bisabolol, and phytosterol. The chamomile plant is aromatic, and its flower heads are used to obtain aqueous-alcoholic extracts and the blue chamomile oil. Chamomile is considered a noncomedogenic raw material and can be beneficially used in aftershaves and eye treatment preparations, as well as in products for dry skin.

chamomile oil—considered a capillary wall constrictor, antiallergenic agent, and antiseptic, cooling, analgesic, emollient, and healing. It has been found to be good for treating burns and skin inflammations as well as dermatitis. It is beneficial for use with acne, dry, or supersensitive skin. The active principles are a pale blue volatile oil (which can turn yellow with time), a little anthemic acid, tannic acid, and a glucoside. The volatile oil obtained through distillation is lost in the preparation of the extract. The whole plant is odoriferous and of value, but the flower heads are primarily credited with therapeutic benefits. Because the chief botanical virtue of the plant lies in the central disk of the yellow florets and in the cultivated double form of the white florets, the botanical properties of the single, wild chamomile are considered to be the most powerful.

chamomile flower oil—see chamomile oil.

chaparral extract (Larrea divaricata)—attributed with anti-inflammatory, antioxidant, and antimicrobial properties, it can also be used for fragrance. This desert shrub, native to the southwestern United States, produces a sticky resin on its stems and leaves that provide natural UV protection for the plant. It is uncertain whether this translates to a skin benefit. Some sources, however, cite UV-protection capacities. Used in products that treat acne, eczema, psoriasis and contact dermatitis. Chaparral's primary constituent is nordihydroguaiaretic acid (NDGA), an antioxidant.

chaulmoogra oil (Taraktogenos kurzii)—a soothing and anti-inflammatory oil. It is considered by some to be healing, with good application in acne cases. It contains chaulmoogric acid and palmitic acid. Its fatty oil constituent has

C

been found to yield glycerol, a very small quantity of phytosterol, and a mixture of fatty acids. Chaulmoogra oil can be irritating and have an unpleasant odor. It is obtained from the seeds of *Taraktogenos kurzii*.

chestnut extract *(Castanea sativa)*—due to its high tannin content, the extract from the bark is claimed to have an astringent effect when applied topically.

China clay—*see* kaolin.

Chinese angelica root—*see* angelica.

chitin (chitine)—a moisture retainer and film-forming agent. This is a polysaccharide that is naturally occurring in the shells of crustaceans, such as shrimp and crab, as well as in some fungi and algae. *See also* chitosan.

chitine—*see* chitin.

chitosan—a film-forming polysaccharide that can aid the skin's moisture-retention capacity. In addition, it appears to help bind other ingredients (for example, to increase liposome stability), thereby increasing the availability of active ingredients to the skin. Antibacterial properties are also associated with chitosan. Some studies show that it can help improve the water-resistance properties of sun protection creams and lotions, as well as the longevity of a fragrance's scent (the perfume adheres more strongly to the skin and evaporates more slowly, over a longer period). Chitosan also appears to improve the microbiological stability of a preparation. It functions similarly to hyaluronic acid and collagen in helping prevent transepidermal water loss, thus also helping increase the skin's moisture content. It acts as a skin conditioner, improving skin softness and suppleness. It may be found in moisturizers, sunscreens, and acne preparations, in addition to hair care products. It is the decarboxylated form of chiten and can hold water without creating a feeling of tackiness in a cosmetic preparation. According to some chitosan suppliers, the use of shrimp shells is one of the most important sources. They consist of 30–35 percent protein, 30–35 percent minerals, 15–20 percent chitin, with some traces of lipids, dyes, and soluble proteins. *See also* chitin.

chitosan ascorbate—a synthetically produced ingredient that combines the film-forming and binding properties of chitosan with the antioxidant properties of ascorbic acid. It is synthetically produced by combining chitosan with ascorbic acid and sodium. *See also* chitosan and ascorbic acid.

C

chlorhexidine—used as a topical antiseptic in liquid cosmetics. It is strongly alkaline and may cause irritation.

chlorhexidine digluconate—a preservative generally used in concentrations of 0.01 to 0.1 percent to protect against bacteria. It is unstable to high temperatures. Chlorhexidine digluconate is more widely used in Europe than in the United States. *See also* chlorhexidine.

5 chloro-2 methyl-4 isothiazolin 3 one and 2-methyl 4 5-hydroxy-2styryl-4-pyrones—a skin-lightening agent due to its ability to inhibit melanin formation. It is stable and nonirritating to the skin.

chlorophenesin—a preservative with fungistatic and bactericidal properties.

chlorophyll—used as a natural coloring agent. It is credited with skin-soothing and healing properties, thanks to its phytol content, and has a mild deodorizing effect. Chlorophyll is the green coloring matter found in all living plants and seen in plant leaves.

chlorophyllin copper complex—a color additive obtained from chlorophyll. *See also* chlorophyll.

chloroxyethanol—a preservative with low sensitizing potential.

chloresteric esters—a cholesterol derivative. *See also* cholesterol.

cholesterol—a moisturizer and emollient that acts as a powerful emulsifier in water-in-oil systems. Cholesterol is a fatlike substance found in plant and animal cells. It is also present in the secretion of the sebaceous glands and, therefore, is a component of the fat on the skin's surface. Considered a noncomedogenic raw material. It may sometimes be obtained from sheep's wool wax.

choleth 24—an emulsifying agent, considered a noncomedogenic raw material. It is often employed for its moisturizing action. A polyethylene glycol ether of cholesterol.

chondroitin sulfate—reported to increase water-binding properties when used with hydrolyzed protein and to enhance the moisturizing effects of creams and lotions. In the skin, chondroitin sulfate is a component of the natural glycosaminoglycans.

Chondrus crispus extract (brown seaweed)—*see* seaweed extract.

chromium compounds—these are oxides used primarily for green eye shadows and greenish mascaras. Chromium compounds may cause allergic reactions when applied to the skin.

C

chromium hydroxide green—a color additive used primarily in makeup preparations. *See also* chromium compounds.

chromium oxide green—a color additive used primarily in makeup preparations. *See also* chromium compounds.

cimicifuga racemosa root extract—*see* black cohosh extract.

cinchena—*see* cinchona extract.

cinchona extract (Cinchona ledgeriana) (cinchena; quinquina)—a major source of quinine. Cinchona extract has long been known for its tonic, antiseptic, and astringent properties. It also has been used commonly as a remedy for malaria and fever in tropical areas. It is obtained from the bark of various Latin American plant species belonging to the *Linnaean* genus. If used in large quantities, cinchona will cause headaches and nausea in those allergic to it.

cinnamic acid—has sunscreen capabilities. Some manufacturers use it to replace PABA due to its lower allergic and phototoxic reaction incidence. Cinnamic acid is found in cinnamon leaves and cocoa leaves, and is an essential oil of certain mushrooms. It may cause allergic skin rashes.

cinnamon oil (Cinnamomum zeylanicum)—said to have a stimulating effect on the skin. It can also be used for fragrance. Widely recognized for its tonic and antiseptic properties, cinnamon oil is very important in traditional pharmacopoeia. Cinnamon oil is used in a wide variety of skin care and make-up preparations. It is obtained from distillation of the plant's leaves. It can cause irritation if used in high doses.

cinnamon bark oil—has similar properties to those of cinnamon oil, but this distillation of the plant's bark is considered of much higher quality than extractions from leaves. Use in high doses or in high concentrations could produce skin irritations. *See also* cinnamon oil.

cinnamyl alcohol—naturally occurring in cinnamon bark. Can be used as a fragrance.

cinoxate (2-hydroxy-p-methoxycinnamate)—an FDA-approved sunscreen chemical with an approved usage level of 1 to 3 percent. Studies indicate it causes photosensitivity. *See also* cinnamic acid.

cinquefoil extract (Potentilla anserina) (five leaf grass; silverweed)—an astringent ingredient incorporated into formulations for its anti-inflammatory and healing properties. It can be of value for problem skin. Cinquefoil is a creeping

C

plant with large yellow flowers. The extract is obtained from the herb and root of the plant.

citral—a naturally occurring aroma compound used to provide a lemon-type fragrance. Citral is a constituent of lemon oil, lemongrass oil, lime oil, ginger oil, verbena oil, and other plant-derived essential oils.

citric acid—has astringent and antioxidant properties. It can also be used as a preservative with a low sensitizing potential. It is not usually irritating to normal skin, but it can cause burning and redness when applied to chapped, cracked, or otherwise inflamed skin. Derived from citrus fruits.

citric oils—refers to one or a combination of oils from citrus fruits such as orange oil, lemon oil, grapefruit oil, and the like.

citronella—used primarily as a fragrance (perfuming and masking), it also has tonic properties. It is derived from the essential oil of the *Cymbopogon nardus* plant, and its constituents include geraniol (approximately 60 percent), citronellal, camphene, limonene, linalool, and borneol.

citronella java oil—antiseptic and widely used in soaps and deodorizers. It may also have insect repellent properties. This herb distillation may cause a skin rash when used in cosmetics.

citronellol—a constituent of plant essential oils. Found abundantly in eucalyptus oil. It is used for masking odor or providing a fragrance component to a cosmetic product.

Citrus aurantium amara—also known as bitter orange. *See* bitter orange.

clary sage oil (Salvia sclarea) (sclary sage oil)—could be beneficial in products designed for use around the eyes due to its soothing and anti-inflammatory properties. Its fragrance may have aromatherapeutic value, such as promoting cell regeneration for normal, dry, and sensitive skin types.

clay—as a general ingredient category, it may include bentonite, beetum, and China clay. Most frequently used for its ability to absorb oil or water, it is also employed as a bulking, stabilizing, and viscosity-controlling agent. Clay can help clarify liquids, act as an emollient, and serve as a poultice. It is found as a color component in face powders, face masks, body powders, and makeup foundations. It does not cause skin allergies.

clay-earth—*see* clay.

clay sediments—*see* clay.

***cleavers extract** (Galium aparine)*—said to be useful in treating eczema. Cleavers extract is recommended for normal to dry skins.

clematis—the extract from the plant's roots and stems has anti-inflammatory action. However, the leaves and flowers, when crushed, irritate the eyes and produce inflammation when applied directly to the skin. Clematis is a perennial plant.

climbing ivy extract—*see* ivy.

***clove oil** (Eugenia caryophyllus, Caryophyllus aromaticus, Syzygium aromaticum)*—considered a powerful antiseptic and wound-healing agent with a strong germicidal effect. Clove oil is also indicated as a topical, local anesthetic. Depending on the part of the plant from which the oil is derived (buds, flowers, leaves, or stems) it may also be tonic, astringent, improve skin texture and feel, and help mask odor. Eugenol is a key constituent of clove oil and is associated with many of its therapeutic benefits. This oil is obtained from the buds, flowers, stems, and leaves of a small evergreen tree. It may cause strong skin irritation when used in high concentrations, although in diluted forms, it is generally harmless.

clove bud oil—has similar properties to clove oil, though it is most often used for its odor-masking properties. Distillates from dried buds are considered of higher quality than those obtained from the stems and leaves. Clove oil derived from the plant's leaves is sometimes used to adulterate the oil obtained from the bud.

***clover extract** (Trifolium sp.)*—the fluid extract is used as an antispasmodic. A short-lived perennial plant, clover produces abundant blossoms that are used in herbal oils and extracts. Extract obtained from clover leaf and clover root is considered antioxidant and able to improve the skin's general condition.

clover blossom extract—credited with astringent properties and an ability to mask odor. *See also* clover.

***club moss extract** (Lycopodium clavatum)*—the spores of club moss have traditionally been used as an external dusting powder for various skin diseases and wounded surfaces. The tops of the plants are cut as the spikes approach maturity, and the powder is shaken out and separated with a sieve.

C

cocamide DEA—a thickener and viscosity builder for cosmetic surfactant systems. It is added to liquid cleansers of the lauryl sulfate variety to help stabilize the lather and improve foam formation.

cocamidopropyl PG-dimonium chloride phosphate—an antimicrobial and antifungal that is very mild to the skin. *See also* coconut oil.

cocamidopropyl betaine—a surfactant derived from a coconut oil salt. It is particularly effective in shampoos, foam baths, shower foams, and other preparations where a high, creamy foam and good skin tolerance are desired. *See also* coconut oil.

cocoa butter—softens and lubricates the skin. This yellowish vegetable fat is solid at room temperature but liquifies at temperatures between 90°–100°F (32.2°–37.8°C). Thus, it is frequently used in lip balms and massage creams due to its favorable melting point (i.e., close to body temperature). Cocoa butter is considered comedogenic and may cause allergic reactions.

coco-caprylate/caprate—a light and cosmetically elegant emollient obtained from vegetable sources.

cocoamidopropylamine oxide—a conditioner, viscosity builder, and foam booster. Derived from coconut oil.

cocoampho carboxyglycinate—used as a skin softener and lubricant, and commonly incorporated into soaps and creams. It is a solid fat from cocoa plant seeds.

cocoglucoside—a very mild cleansing agent, naturally derived from coconut oil and fruit sugar.

cocoglyceride—used for its emollient, emulsifying, and skin-conditioning properties. *See also* hydrogenated cocoglyceride.

coconut alcohol—a multi-function ingredient that may be incorporated into a cosmetic as an emollient, emulsifier, stabilizer, or surfactant, or to help control a product's viscosity. Its actual function in a product will depend on the specific formulation.

coconut oil—used as a cream base. A raw material in soaps, ointments, massage creams, and in sunscreen formulations. Soft white or slightly yellow in color and semisolid in consistency, coconut oil is a grouping of primarily short-chain fatty acids bonded with glycerin and expressed from coconut kernels. It is stable when exposed to air. Coconut oil may be irritating to the skin and cause skin rashes. It is also considered comedogenic.

cocoyl sarcosine—its application in skin care products is not clear. It is formed from caffeine through decomposition with barium hydroxide.

coenzyme Q10—*see* ubiquinone.

Coffea arabica fruit extract—also known as CoffeeBerry® extract. A powerful, natural antioxidant with antiaging and skin-lightening properties. The extract is obtained from the whole fruit, rather than from the seed or bean, as in the case of coffee seed oil (*Coffea arabica* seed oil).

coffee seed oil (Coffea arabica)—extracted from green coffee beans, it is rich in essential fatty acids including linoleic acid. It can also be used as a masking agent for odor. Depending on how the ingredient is used, coffee seed oil may also be beneficial for draining and slimming. The oil is obtained from the seed/bean. *See also* caffeine.

Coleus barbatus extract (coleus)—a botanical that appears to have cleansing and soothing properties. It is a tropical plant, and in traditional medicine was used to relieve scorpion bites and centipede stings.

collagen—very popular in skin care formulations for its great hydration potential and its ability to bind and retain many times its weight in water. This water-binding and retention ability makes collagen effective for use in skin moisturizers as a skin-protecting agent. It will not leave a feeling of tackiness or dryness on the skin, especially when used in hydrolyzed or soluble forms. As a film former, collagen aids in reducing natural moisture loss, thereby helping hydrate the skin. In skin care preparations, it enhances the humectancy of a topical product, contributes sheen, builds viscosity, and leaves the skin smooth and soft. Collagen is not water soluble, and has been very popular in cosmetic formulations for more than 30 years. Collagen is considered a "commercially pure" protein found in animal connective tissue, and it is similar to the collagen produced by the body in the skin and bones. Also considered an anti-irritant, collagen does not cause allergic reactions when used on the skin. It is very stable, bland in odor, and light in color. This is one of the most effective and economical proteins available to cosmetic formulators.

collagen amino acids—has a higher moisture-binding capacity than collagen alone, thereby improving the moisturizing efficacy of skin creams and lotions. Collagen amino acid is a mixture of amino acids resulting from the complete hydrolysis of collagen. Its moisture-binding capacity is due to the very large number of hydrophilic groups per unit weight. *See also* collagen.

collagen amino-polysiloxane hydrolyzate—*see* collagen.

collagen fiber—anti-irritant and hydrating. When used in particular sponge versions, it can serve as a delivery system for active ingredients. Its lack of solubility in water and other commonly used cosmetic ingredients has restricted its range of application.

collagen hydrolysates (hydrolyzed animal protein; hydrolyzed collagen)—collagen processed to achieve a lower molecular weight than regular collagen, which facilitates its use in cosmetic formulations and improves the properties of regular collagen. This is one of the most common forms of collagen used in cosmetic formulations. *See also* collagen.

collagen (soluble)—demonstrates enhanced moisture uptake and, therefore, is more effective than collagen. This is a clear liquid form of collagen preferred for use in cosmetics because, when incorporated into a formulation, it will not separate as regular collagen would. When incorporated into detergents, soluble collagen significantly reduces the amount of amino acids extracted from the skin when washing with the detergents and water. Soluble collagen is perhaps the most widely used and recognized high molecular-weight protein in skin care formulations. *See also* collagen.

colloidal oatmeal—an anti-itching skin protectant with soothing properties. Its lipid content gives it enhanced lubricity and emolliency. Colloidal oatmeal has consistently been recommended for use on infants, adults, and the aged in bath, lotion, and poultice preparations designed for topical application on damaged skin. The addition of colloidal oatmeal into bath water diminishes inflammation and irritation that frequently occur in eczema cases when bathing with soap alone. It is used in cleansing creams, soaps, and bath products. *See also* oat.

colloidal sulfur—*see* sulfur.

colostrum—a naturally occurring substance, colostrum is a fluid secreted by the mammary glands just after giving birth. When combined with elastin, it leaves a colloidal film that mimics the natural elastin.

C

coltsfoot extract (Tussilago farfara)—has astringent, emollient, conditioning, and moisturizing properties. Studies indicate a possible skin-lightening effect. Coltsfoot extract contains a high concentration of mucilage, making it useful for soothing delicate and/or easily inflamed skin. The leaves are the primary plant part used, but the flower stems are also utilized. Cystine is among its noted constituents.

comfrey extract (Symphytum officinale)—contains allantoin and is credited with healing, astringent, and emollient properties. It is used in cases of swelling and bruising, cuts, papules, and pustules. Comfrey extract was traditionally used topically for soothing and anti-itching treatment, as well as for eczema and sunburns. The whole plant is considered excellent for soothing pain in any tender, inflamed, or suppurating part. Comfrey root's chief and most important constituent is mucilage. It also contains from 0.6 to 0.8 percent of allantoin and a bit of tannin. Some say that certain alkaloids found in comfrey are toxic. The roots and leaves are generally collected from wild plants.

C

coneflower extract (Echinacea angustifolia)—*see* echinacea.

copper—copper-based ingredients are often used as coloring agents in cosmetics. Copper itself is nontoxic, but soluble copper salts, notably copper sulfite, are skin irritants. In the body, copper combines with certain proteins to produce a variety of enzymes, which in turn serve as catalysts for different functions. For example, copper plays a role in the keratinization process. In normal skin, this catalytic action is completed in 8 to 12 hours, however more than three days may be required in cases of copper deficiency. Through such enzymatic activity, copper is involved in melanin production, as decreased pigmentation has been observed in cases of copper deficiency. Such enzyme-based action also links copper to maintaining and repairing the skin's connective tissues (collagen and elastin), as well as to wound healing.

copper aspartate—*see* copper.

copper gluconate—*see* copper.

copra oil—*see* coconut oil.

coriander oil (Coriandrum sativum)—used in the appropriate mixture and dosage, it can work with other natural oils and extracts as a preservative. It also serves as a deodorant. Coriander oil is produced from the distillation of the fruit (the so-called seeds), which contains about 1 percent of volatile oil, the active constituent. The fruit also contains malic acid. Coriander oil can cause allergic reactions.

corn cob meal—used in face and bath powders. Made from the ear of Indian corn.

corn germ oil—a skin softener derived from the germ of the seed of the corn plant.

corn meal—used as a thickening agent. It is a coarse corn flour prepared by milling the corn kernel. *See also* corn starch.

corn oil—used as a carrier. This vegetable oil has average emollient properties. Although not particularly prone to cause allergies, it is also not widely used in cosmetic formulations. It is considered somewhat comedogenic. Corn oil is obtained from the wet milling of corn.

corn seed extract—found in creams, lotions, and revitalizing ampules. *See also* corn seed fraction.

corn seed fraction—credited with increasing skin metabolism. It is rich in amino acids, sugar, vitamin B, and phytates. Can be used in creams, lotions, and post-sun preparations.

C

corn starch—used as a thickener in cosmetics and in face powders. Corn starch absorbs water and is soothing to the skin. It can cause allergic reactions such as inflamed eyes, stuffy nose, and perennial hay fever. A natural material obtained from corn kernels.

cornflower extract (Centaurea cyanus)—used in folklore as a tonic and stimulant with action similar to that of blessed thistle. A water distilled from cornflower petals was formerly thought of as a remedy for weak eyes. Cornflower extract has been used in Europe since ancient times to treat bites. Considered beneficial for normal skin and skin care products designed for use around the eyes. Healing properties, particularly in cases of bruises, are attributed to cornflower extract obtained from the plant leaves. Important constituents include gentiopicrin, erythrocentaurine, nicotinic acid compounds, essential oil, and oleanolic acid.

cornflower water—*see* cornflower extract.

cotton seed oil (hydrogenated)—a carrier. This oil is used in the manufacture of soaps, creams, and baby creams. Although it is known to cause allergies and be mildly irritating, it is widely used in cosmetics. Considered somewhat comedogenic. Expressed from various species of cotton.

coumarin—considered a blood thinner, it can also increase blood flow. Some sources cite antioxidant capacities, as well. It is a specific plant constituent and is what creates the fragrance of freshly mowed hay. Coumarin is found in such plants as cherries, lavender, licorice, and sweet clover.

crambe abyssinica seed oil—a nongreasy emollient, it improves skin feel and moisturization. A member of the mustard family.

cranberry seed oil (Vaccinium macrocarpon)—plays a role in skin moisturization by helping protect the skin's lipid barrier. It is also nourishing, and said to help promote the absorption of fatty acids by the skin. Its constituents include vitamins A and E, omegas-3, -6, and -9, and phospholipids and phytosterols. Its application includes use in cosmetic creams or lotions for dry, dehydrated, and aging skin.

crane's bill extract (Geranium maculatum)—credited with astringent and tonic properties. Constituents include gallic and tannic acids. The leaves and roots are the parts used.

cream—contains lecithin, sterols, and oils plus 18 to 40 percent butterfat. It is the yellowish part of cow's milk.

cresin—*see* ozokerite.

cryolidone—a PCA derivative. Cryolidone increases resistance to heat following UV radiation. As it provides a cooling effect on the skin, it is suggested as an ingredient for post-sun and aftershave products.

cucumber extract (Cucumis sativus)—credited with moisture-binding, moisture-regulating, soothing, tightening, anti-itching, refreshing, softening, healing, and anti-inflammatory properties. It contains amino acids and organic acids that are claimed to strengthen the skin's acid mantle. This extract can be used in aftershave preparations, eye treatment products, and treatments for oily skin. It is also effective in emulsions as a tightening agent for tired, stressed skin, and in sun preparations as a refresher. Important constituents include minerals, mucins, and amino acids. The fruit is the part used.

Cucumis melo—the Latin name for melon, including honeydew, cantaloupe, and sugar melon. Cantaloupe also has astringent properties. The fruit, root, or seed extracts—as well as the juice and water of melon—are all known to maintain the skin in good condition. Melon water is also humectant, while melon juice is considered to have soothing properties. Among the constituents of melon are vitamins A and C, pectin, flavonoids, volatile oils, and fructose (a sugar).

cupuassu butter—also known as cupuaçu butter; *Theobroma grandiflorum* seed butter. Emollient and moisturizing, it also improves skin softness. Cupuassu butter contains phytosterols, and appears able to regulate the balance and activity of stratum corneum lipids. It is also reported to have a high water-absorption capacity, making it particularly beneficial for dry skin. The butter is extracted from the seeds of the Cupuassu tree, native to Brazil.

curcumin—*see* turmeric.

cyclohexasiloxane—a silicone-based emollient.

cyclomethicone—provides a silky, smooth feel to skin care products, and is considered a noncomedogenic emollient. This is a form of silicone that can deliver active ingredients and also serve as a vehicle for delivering fragrance.

cyclopentasiloxane—incorporated into a formulation for its emollient and solvent activity.

cyclotetrasiloxane—a silicone-based emollient. *See also* cyclomethicone.

Cymbopogon nardus—*see* citronella.

O-cymen 5-OL—a bactericide used in hand and body preparations. A phenol derivative.

cypress extract (Cupressus sp.)—an extract derived from the leaves and twigs of the cypress tree. *See also* cypress oil.

cypress oil—said to have antiseptic, astringent, healing, soothing, and antispasmodic properties. Cypress oil is also claimed to be useful in treating acne and in inhibiting oil gland secretion. It can also be used as a fragrance. This oil, which can range from clear to yellow to brown, is generally obtained from a distillation of cypress cones.

cysteic acid—an amino acid that is used in skin care cosmetics as a skin conditioner.

cysteine—an essential amino acid obtained by fermentation. Cysteine is a component of the skin's natural moisturizing factor and can help normalize oil gland secretion due to its sulfur content. It is also said to promote wound healing. In addition, studies indicate that cysteine helps increase levels of glutathione (an antioxidant) in the body. It is considered beneficial in treating oily skin.

C

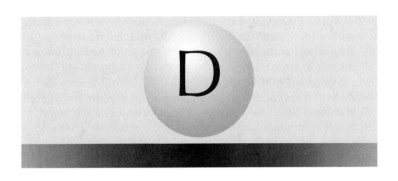

D

D&C colors—refer to color entry in Chapter 4.

D-alpha-tocopherol—*see* vitamin E.

daisy extract (Bellis perennis)—said to be tonic and skin conditioning. Daisy was a component in a popular 14th century wound ointment. This application continued through the centuries, using daisy alone or in combination with ox-eye daisy. The flowers and leaves are found to have a certain amount of oil and ammoniacal salts.

damiana leaves extract (Turnera aphrodisiaca)—the cosmetic properties of this spicy, aromatic extract are not clear, but they could be tonic, astringent, and potentially antispasmodic. The leaves, which are the part used, produce a greenish volatile oil that smells like chamomile and damianin, an amorphous bitter principle, resins, and tannin.

dandelion extract (Taraxacum officinale)—has tonic properties, refreshes the skin, and corrects pH balance. It apparently also aids in increasing the respiratory capacity of skin tissue. Dandelion extract is said to be beneficial for dry skin and can also be found in acne preparations. The plant root, rather than the flower, is used in cosmetic preparations as the juice of the root is the more powerful part of the plant. The main constituents of dandelion root are taraxacin, a crystalline, bitter substance; and taraxacerin, an acrid resin. Other constituents include inulin, gluten gum, potash, citric acid, sterols, and vitamins B and C. Dandelion is used in many patented medicines.

DEA (diethanolamine)—an organic alkali used in formulations to neutralize organic acids. Usually listed on ingredient labels preceding the compound that it is neutralizing. Oleth-3 phosphate, for example, is a powerful emulsifier, but it is very acidic when it is made, so manufacturers use DEA to neutralize it. The organic alkali improves the nature of a formulation.

DEA cetyl phosphate—an emulsifying agent that gives a rich, velvety feel to a product. It can be used as a primary or secondary emulsifier, depending on the concentration. This is the diethanolamine salt of cetyl phosphate.

DEA dihydroxypalmityl phosphate—an emulsifier.

DEA oleth-3 phosphate—an emulsifier. This is the diethanolamine salt of a complex mixture of phosophoric acid esters and oleth-3.

DEA oleth-10 phosphate—an emulsifying agent used primarily in moisturizing preparations. This is the diethunolamine salt of a complex mixture of phosphoric acid esters and oleth-10.

DEA p-methoxycinnamate (octocrylene)—a chemical UV absorber that exhibits excellent UV absorption and has an approved usage level of 8 to 10 percent. Because of its water solubility, it is not generally used in waterproof formulations.

decaglyceryl dipalmitate—*see* polyglyceryl-10 dipalmitate.

decene/butene copolymer—used to control product viscosity.

decyl alcohol—serves as an intermediate for surface-active agents. It is also an antifoam agent and a fixative in perfumes. Decyl alcohol occurs naturally in sweet orange and ambrette seed. It is also derived commercially from liquid paraffin.

decyl glucoside—a mild, foaming cleansing agent.

decyl oleate—an emollient with good penetrating properties that facilitates product spreadability and provides a formulation with good feel on the skin. A component of the sebum of human skin, it is also produced synthetically and from olive oil.

decyl polyglucose—a nonionic surfactant with good foaming properties. It is extremely mild to the eyes and skin. It can be obtained from naturally derived raw materials from renewable sources, though this depends on the supplier.

dehydroacetic acid—a preservative with low sensitizing potential. This is a weak acid used as a fungi- and bacteria-destroying agent in cosmetics. The presence of organic matter decreases its effectiveness. It is not irritating or allergy causing when applied on the skin.

D

deoxyribonucleic acid—see DNA.

dermasomes—liposomal preparations containing cosmetic ingredients (usually actives) entrapped within lipid spheres. Dermasomes provide increased penetration and absorption, improved product efficiency at lower usage levels, and targeted and time-released delivery.

devil's claw (Harpagophytum procumbens)—said to have anti-inflammatory and moisture-binding capabilities. The plant's root contains mucilage.

dextran—a polysaccharide with water binding properties, it is also used to control product viscosity. Some studies indicate a capacity to enhance the antiaging activity of formulations containing weak acids, as well as to reduce possible skin irritation arising from such acids.

dextran sulfate—clinical studies indicate a possible capacity to reduce oedema. It is cited as a binder and skin conditioner.

dextrin (British gum; starch gum)—absorbs moisture. This powder, produced from corn starch and modified by means of a bacterial process, may cause an allergic reaction. Used as a binder in cosmetic form.

dextrose—see glucose.

DHA—see dihydroxyacetone.

DHPH—see dipalmitoyl hydroxyproline.

diatomaceous earth—in purified form, it is used for powders and as an abrasive agent in peeling formulations. If improperly formulated, it may be too abrasive as a peeling agent. Diatomaceous earth is a fine-grain, almost white powder consisting mostly of amorphous silicic that is obtained by crushing the silicic acid structures of monocellular sea algae.

diazolidinyl urea—an antiseptic and deodorizer. It is also a broad-spectrum preservative against bacteria and fungi. Generally, it is used in concentrations of 0.03 to 0.3 percent. It has been found that diazolidinyl urea is a stronger sensitizer than imidazolidinyl urea for people sensitive or allergic to formaldehyde.

dibehenyl fumarate—a wax with thickening and film-forming properties that is used as a coemulsifier.

di-C_{12-15} alkyl fumarate—an emollient.

dicaprylyl ether—a skin conditioning agent.

dicaprylyl maleate—a derivative of malic acid, with emollient and skin-conditioning properties. It can also be used

D

as a solvent in cosmetic preparations. It is synthetically manufactured.

dicetyl dilinoleate—a nonirritating emollient that provides slip, emollience, and a smooth, satiny feel to a cosmetic preparation. It leaves the skin feeling soft, supple, and without greasiness. It is claimed that dicetyl dilinoleate helps normalize the epidermal lipid structure and promotes the formation of soft, flexible, and healthy looking skin. It may also act as a vehicle for the delivery of active topical substances. This ingredient can be effectively incorporated into creams, lotions, skin oils, and makeup bases that contain sunscreens. Dicetyl dilinoleate can be used as a replacement for partially hydrogenated animal and vegetable tallows, cocoa butter, and isopropyl lanolate. It is based on omega-6 linoleic acid, a naturally occurring vegetable derivative.

dicetyl phosphate—used in cosmetic preparations as an emulsifier and surfactant.

dichlorobenzyl alcohol—a preservative and antimicrobial, particularly effective in protecting against yeasts and molds.

diethanolamine—*see* DEA.

diethanolamine p-methoxycinnamate—*see* DEA p-methoxycinnamate.

diethylamino hydroxybenzoyl hexyl benzoate—a UV filter that helps protect against UVA and demonstrates good photostability.

diethyl lauramide—*see* lauramide DEA.

diethylene glycol monoethylene ether—*see* ethoxydiglycol.

diethylhexyl butamido triazone—a sunscreen chemical that acts as a UV filter and absorber.

digalloyl trioleate—an FDA-approved sunscreen chemical with an approved usage level of 2 to 5 percent. A chemical UVB absorber, digalloyl trioleate, is no longer available as it apparently exhibits a poor UV absorption profile.

dihydroxyacetone (DHA)—a self-tanning agent used in cosmetics designed to provide a tanned appearance without the need for sun exposure. It is also a UV protector and a color additive. As a self-tanning agent, it reacts with amino acids found on the skin's epidermal layer. Its effects last only a few days as the color it provides fades with the natural shedding of the stained cells. Reportedly, it works best on slightly acidic skin. DHA, when combined with lawsone, becomes an FDA Category I (approved) UV protectant. In 1973, the FDA declared that DHA is safe and suitable for use in cosmetics or drugs that are applied to color the skin, and has exempted it from color additive certification.

2-dihydroxyethyl-2-hydroxy-6, 10,14-trimethylpentadecane—facilities the penetration of vitamin E into the skin. It has also demonstrated free-radical scavenging abilities and can function as a blocker of UV rays.

diisoarachidyl dilinoleate—a liquid wax emollient that provides good product spreadability. It may replace mineral oil in skin care preparations.

diisoarachidyl dodecanedioate—an emollient. This liquid wax provides a feel similar to heavy mineral oil but without the greasiness and oiliness associated with it. It may, therefore, be used as a partial or total replacement for mineral oil in formulations where improved tactile properties are sought. Diisoarachidyl diodecanedioate leaves a protective, though not completely occlusive, film on the skin. Its qualities suggest use in special cleansing preparations; rich, soft creams; and sunscreens. Considered a potentially excellent vehicle for the delivery of active topical substances. It is nonirritating in skin and eye tests.

diisocetyl dodecanedioate—an emollient that enhances skin feel and texture. It also may be incorporated into a cosmetic preparation for emulsifying or surfactant activity.

diisopropyl adipate—a low-viscosity emollient. It increases a preparation's spreadability.

diisopropyl dimerate—a chemical modifier that lowers the irritation potential of ingredients incorporated into a formulation.

diisopropyl sebacate—can be used in cosmetic formulations for its emollient properties. It is also used as a solvent, particularly for fragrances.

diisostearyl dimer dilinoleate—an occlusive skin-conditioning agent primarily used in makeup and hand and body preparations.

diisostearyl malate—a film former and a secondary emollient used mostly in makeup or other formulations involving suspensions.

dimethicone—a form of silicone used to give products lubricity, slip, and good feel. It can also serve as a formulation defoamer and help reduce the feeling of greasiness that some creams leave on the skin immediately upon application. It is also reported to protect the skin against moisture loss

D

when used in larger quantities. It improves product flow and spreadability. In combination with other ingredients, dimethicone becomes a good waterproofing material for sunscreen emulsions, and helps reduce the greasiness often seen in high-SPF preparations.

dimethicone copolyol—provides soft feel and helps reduce irritation caused by soap. Used to improve the skin feel of some sunscreen preparations. A modified form of dimethicone. *See also* dimethicone.

dimethicone copolyol isostearate—acts as a skin softener and gives a formulation high lubricity. *See also* dimethicone.

dimethicone copolyol phosphate—an emulsifier.

dimethicone copolyol polyacrylate—a water-resistant emulsifier with film-forming properties.

dimethicone/vinyl dimethicone crosspolymer—a thickener that can absorb skin oils, leaving a dry, silky feel.

dimethiconol esters—fatty wax that liquifies when rubbed on the skin. *See also* dimethicone.

dimethiconol hydroxystearate—an oil-phase compound with nonocclusive hydrophobic film formation on skin. *See also* dimethicone.

dimethiconol stearate—a nonocclusive hydrophobic waterproofing base used in sunscreens and other skin care applications. *See also* dimethicone.

dimethyl aminoethanol—*see* dimethyl MEA.

dimethyl MEA (DMAE)—also known as dimethyl aminoethanol. Appears to have firming properties. Is considered antiaging, anti-inflammatory and antioxidant.

dimethyl isosorbide—a carrier. Its particular skin penetrating ability opens the possibility of enhancing active substance efficacy in optical products. Its physical characteristics and solubility properties are superior to those of propylene glycol, glycerin, or ethyl alcohol.

dimethyl oxazolidine—a compound that improves the activity of a preservative present in a cosmetic formulation. It is nontoxic at approved cosmetic-use levels.

dimethyl siloxane—*see* dimethicone.

dimethylisosorbide—*see* dimethyl isosorbide.

dimethylsilanol hyaluronate—has very strong skin hydrating activity. It appears to provide regenerating, restructuring, and repairing action for tissue supplement and, therefore,

D

is said to improve skin elasticity and firmness. Finds application in antiaging products and those for skin maintenance such as night, sun, and protective creams.

di-n-octyl carbonate—functions as a solvent and can be used to facilitate solubility and spreadability of such sunscreen components as benzophenone-3 and methylbenzylidene camphor. Also a dispersing agent.

dioctyl adipate—an emollient. It allows transepidermal respiration through occlusive-type films. Has a very low irritancy level.

dioctyl malate—a light film former and emollient used in skin care formulations.

dioctyl maleate—a film former and emollient derived from maleic acid.

dioctylcyclohexane—an emollient used as a squalene substitute.

dioctyl sodium sulfosuccinate—a mild surfactant used as a cleansing agent.

dioxybenzone—*see* benzophenone-8.

dipalmitoyl hydroxyproline (DPHP)—an antiaging ingredient with moisturizing properties, it is said to enhance skin firmness and protect elastin fibers. Another function is to act as a carrier of hydroxyproline through the skin. A vegetal derivative. *See also* hydroxyproline.

dipotassium phosphate—used as a buffering agent to control the degree of acidity in solutions.

di-PPG myristyl ether adipate—an emollient with multiple beneficial properties. It can provide better delivery of active ingredients to the skin, and, through its film-forming capabilities, enhance the skin's ability to retain active ingredients. In addition, it can disperse physical sunscreens such as titanium dioxide and zinc oxide. It also provides excellent skin-softening action.

dipeptide-2—could help improve lymphatic drainage. Used in eye creams to help reduce puffiness and the appearance of dark circles. It is also used as a skin conditioner.

dipotassium glycyrrhizinate—a liquorice derivative that helps reduce skin redness and inflammation, thanks to its anti-irritant, calming, and soothing properties. It can be incorporated successfully into sensitive skin products, while also appearing to help improve oily skin.

dipropylene glycol monomethyl ether—*see* PPG 2 methyl ether acetate.

D

disodium EDTA—a preservative used in concentrations of 0.1 to 0.5 percent.

disodium laureth sulfosuccinate—a very mild surfactant, appropriate for baby and child care products. It reduces the irritation properties of high-foaming surfactants when used in the same product formulation.

disodium lauriminodipropionate—a surfactant with cleansing and foaming properties.

disodium mono-oleamido MIPA sulfosuccinanate—*see* dioctyl sodium, sulfosuccinate.

disodium phosphate—considered a moisturizer. This inorganic salt absorbs moisture from the air that is then supposed to be released to the skin. In dry climatic conditions, however, it may draw moisture from the skin and release it to the air, aggravating dryness. Without water, disodium phosphate may cause slight irritation.

DL-alpha-tocopherol—*see* vitamin E.

DMDM hydantoin—a popular preservative with moderate sensitizing potential, it is used to control against mold, mildew, and bacterial spoilage. This preservative is similar to imidazolidinyl urea, as both act by releasing formaldehyde into the formulation. Cosmetic expert panels have determined that DMDM hydantoin is safe for use in cosmetic products, and it has an excellent safety record for use in both leave-on and wash-off preparations. Maximum-use concentrations are set at 0.2 percent in the U.S. and 0.6 percent in the European Union. DMDM stands for dimethylimidazolidine, though in a listing the acronym is rarely spelled out.

DNA (freeze-dried) (pure biological) (pure vegetal) (deoxyribonucleic acid)—a surface film-forming protein with moisturizing action. DNA's large macromolecules do not enable it to penetrate the skin. In addition, its affinity with the corneum layer keeps it anchored to the skin's surface, where it serves to protect and retain skin moisture. While the use of DNA was particularly popular in the 1980s, its incorporation into cosmetic products since then has practically disappeared. It is usually used in a potassium salt form obtained from fish sperm.

drometrizole trisiloxane—a UV absorber/UV filter, it provides UVB- and some UVA-spectrum protection. It is approved for use as a sunscreen chemical in the European Union but not in the U.S. (at the time of writing).

D

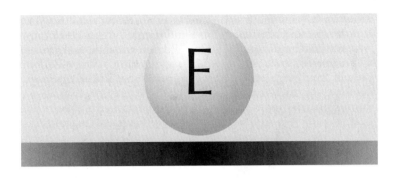

ECM—*see* extra cellular matrix.

EDTA—helps boost a formulation's preservative system and is also a chelating agent.

echinacea *(Echinacea angustifolia)*—also known as coneflower. Echinacea is well known for its ability to boost the body's immune system. It is described as having antiseptic and antibacterial properties rendering it helpful in treating skin lesions and in shortening skin healing time. It also has anti-itching, soothing, and moisturizing properties when used in skin care products. It is commonly used in acne preparations. The main constituents of both the oil and the resin, derived from the wood or bark of the plant, are inulin, inuloid, sucrose, sulose, betaine, phytosterols, and fatty acids such as oleic, cerotic, lizolic, and palmitic.

egg lecithin—emollient and particularly recommended for sensitive skin. *See also* egg protein; egg yolk extract.

egg oil—recommended for sensitive skins. It is extracted from the egg yolk using vegetable oil. *See also* egg protein; egg yolk extract.

egg protein—creates a film, thereby acting as a moisture-retention agent allowing the skin to build up a supply of water. This moisturization process tightens and softens the skin only temporarily as the skin cannot utilize the protein contained in an egg. Egg protein is primarily used in facial masks. It may cause skin rashes and other disorders in those with an allergy to eggs.

egg extract—a protein. Egg white provides emollient, humectant and skin-conditioning properties. Egg yolk has emulsifying

E

capabilities and may be used in products for sensitive skin. It contains lecithin sterols and vitamin A. Egg extract provides a temporary tightening effect on the skin. *See also* egg protein.

egg powder—used in many cosmetics, including face masks, creams, and bath preparations. It provides a temporary tightening effect on the skin. *See also* egg extract.

Egyptian rose extract—*see* rose extract.

eicosapentaenoic acid—also known as EPA. Emollient and skin conditioning, this omega-3 fatty acid helps repair and maintain the skin barrier functions. It is said to improve the structure and function of the skin cell membrane. In addition, it may also have anti-irritant and anti-inflammatory properties.

elastin—a surface protective agent used in cosmetics to alleviate the effects of dry skin, enhance skin flexibility, improve skin feel, increase and improve the tension of the skin, and influence the formation of tropocollagen fibers when used in combination with soluble collagen. Preparations containing elastin and peptides derived from it are reported to promote wound healing. Reportedly, in such systems, elastin can absorb lipids from the skin, and when applied to scars, increase the structural glycoproteins and elastin available in the scar tissue. Elastin is an elastic structural protein found in the dermis together with collagen, and is difficult to obtain in pure form. Collagen and elastin are similar, although elastin has a different amino acid composition and is found in lower concentrations. Its molecular size is also much smaller than collagen's, and as a result, there is a tendency to believe that it penetrates the surface epidermal layers, thereby improving overall skin appearance, softness, and suppleness. Often used in moisturizing products and those products for aging or mature skin.

E

elastin (hydrolyzed)—a modified form of elastin that, given its greater solubility, is more convenient for use in cosmetic formulations than regular elastin. *See also* elastin.

elastin hydrolysates—*see* elastin (hydrolyzed).

elastin polypeptides—an elastin derivative that can be used as an active ingredient carried by liposomes.

elder extract (*Sambucus sp.*)—an herb that is said to have astringent, antiseptic, and emollient properties. It is useful for problem or inflamed skin. Ointments made of elder leaves have been domestic remedies for bruises, swelling, and wounds. Elder leaves are also an ingredient in many cooling ointments. The bark, leaves, flowers, and berries have all been used botanically, though use of the bark is now considered obsolete. Manufacturers report that presently the flower is the preferred segment of the plant.

elder flower extract—mildly astringent and a gentle stimulant. It is principally used as a vehicle for eye and skin lotions. It is reported to be particularly beneficial in treatment of dry skin. In the 19th century, elder flower water was commonly used to clear the complexion of freckles and sunburn and to keep the skin in good condition. The most important constituent of elder flower is a trace of semisolid volatile oil, present in a very low percentage, which possesses the scent of the flower in a high degree. *See also* elder extract.

elecampane *(Inula helenium) (horseheal; scabwort)*—its herbal properties for topical use are described as astringent and antiseptic. In the past, it was used for treating skin problems in people and animals. Its common name, scabwort, comes from the belief that it cured sheep affected with the scab. It gets its other name, horseheal, from its reputed virtues in curing skin diseases suffered by horses. Elecampane's therapeutic value is attributed to its abundant content of inulin, a polysaccharide found in plants. It can also be used to mask odor. The extract used for therapeutic purposes is preferably obtained from the root of a two- to three-year-old plant. When the plant is older, the root becomes too woody for extraction.

elm bark *(Ulmus sp.)*—credited with astringent, healing, and soothing properties that could benefit surface skin problems.

elm extract—described as a problem skin extract due to its healing and reputed cicatrizant properties. Extracts from elm leaves have been recommended by herbologists to wash wounds, bruises, and sore eyes.

embryo extract (embryonic extract)—its use is based on the theory that its particular hormone content can rejuvenate the skin. This is a controversial concept, as some scientists deny its validity and professionals in esthetics claim otherwise. This notion becomes even more controversial when referring to retail cosmetics. It may cause an allergic reaction in people allergic to eggs. Embryo extract was used more frequently in the past. Given current cosmetic technology, it has been replaced with ingredients of nonanimal origin.

embryonic extract—*see* embryo extract.

emulsifying wax—an emulsifier and thickening agent used to give body to a formulation. Unlike some waxes (for example, beeswax), this is not a true wax. It is a chemical mixture of emulsifiers and fatty alcohols that permits the formulation of stable creams.

emulsifying wax NF—this is the same as emulsifying wax and is considered a noncomedogenic raw material. NF is the abbreviation for a reference called National Formulary. It denotes quality compliance with the pharmaceutical monogram.

English daisy extract—said to reduce swelling. *See also* daisy extract.

English oak extract—*see* oak bark extract.

enzymes—*see* enzyme entry in Chapter 4.

epidermal lipid extract—an example of a vague ingredient description found on some product labels. Literally, this would be an oil or fat extracted from the epidermis. It is not specific enough to allow one to determine if it refers to lipids that blend with those in the human skin or if lipids extracted from animal epidermis are being used.

ergocalciferol—*see* vitamin D.

erythrityl triethylhexanoate—can be incorporated into a skin care formula for a variety of purposes, including as an emollient and a solvent. It also can maintain the skin in good condition.

escin—a saponin occurring in the seed of the horse chestnut tree. *See also* horse chestnut extract.

esculin—used as a skin protectant in ointments and creams. This is a glucoside compound originally obtained from the leaves and bark of the horse chestnut tree. *See also* horse chestnut extract.

esculoside—utilized in formulations for the treatment of cellulite. Esculoside is apparently beneficial for impaired microcirculation.

ethanol—*see* ethyl alcohol.

ethanol acetamide—*see* acetamide MEA.

ethoxydiglycol—a solvent for essential oils, fragrance materials, and terpene oils. It is used often in nail enamels but can also be incorporated into skin care products as a humectant.

E

Ethoxydiglycol is nonirritating, nonpenetrating, and non-comedogenic when applied to the skin.

ethoxydiglycol behenate—used to enhance a product's final consistency and creaminess.

ethoxydiglycol oleate—an emollient.

ethoxyethanol—*see* ethylene glycol monomethyl ether.

ethoxylated plant sterols—*see* plant sterols.

ethyl alcohol—also known as ethanol. Commonly known as rubbing alcohol. Ethyl alcohol is ordinary alcohol and is used medicinally as a topical antiseptic, astringent, and antibacterial. At concentrations above 15 percent, it is also a broad-spectrum preservative against bacteria and fungi, and can boost the efficacy of other preservatives in a formulation. Cosmetic companies tend to use alcohol SD-40 in high-grade cosmetic manufacturing as they consider ethanol too strong and too drying for application on the skin. Obtained from grain distillation, it can also be synthetically manufactured. *See also* alcohol.

ethyl 4-(bis[hydroxypropyl]) aminobenzoate—an FDA-approved sunscreen chemical with an approved usage level of 1 to 5 percent.

ethyl arachidonate—an emollient with healing and smoothing properties. Reported for use in indoor tanning preparations. It is the ester of ethyl alcohol and arachidonic acid. A modified form of ethyl arachidonate can reduce the possibility of irritation that can result from using straight ethyl arachidonate.

ethyl cellulose—a binder, film former, and thickener. It is used in suntan gels, creams, and lotions. This is the ethyl ether of cellulose.

ethyl dihydroxypropyl PABA (ethyl dihydroxypropyl p-aminobenzoate)—an FDA-approved sunscreen chemical for UVB absorption. It exhibits the widest range of UV spectrum–absorption abilities among UVB absorbers. Its structure results in very limited solubility by commonly used cosmetic solvents, so it is not among the more frequently used chemicals in its class. Due to its limited popularity, it was withdrawn from the marketplace in the early 1990s and is no longer available.

ethyl dihydroxypropyl p-aminobenzoate—*see* ethyl dihydroxypropyl PABA.

E

ethyl ether—a solvent that may cause skin irritation. Although considered a noncomedogenic raw material, it is rarely used in cosmetics.

ethyl linoleate (vitamin F)—an emollient and an essential fatty acid. *See also* vitamin F.

ethyl linolenate—an emollient reportedly used in indoor tanning preparations. It is not very popular as it may pose rancidity problems.

ethyl paraben—a preservative with minimal sensitizing potential. *See also* parabens.

ethylene acrylate copolymer—a film former, binder, and viscosity-increasing agent. A synthetic polymer. *See also* acrylates.

ethylene glycol monomethyl ether (ethoxyethanol)—considered a noncomedogenic raw material. It is used as a solvent in nail products and as a stabilizer in cosmetic emulsions. It is able to penetrate the skin and may cause skin irritation.

ethylene glycol monostearate (glycol stearate)—a noncomedogenic raw material that provides a pearly look and consistency to clear preparations. *See also* glycol stearate.

ethylenediamine tetraacetic acid—*see* EDTA.

2-ethylhexyl 2-cyano-3, 3-diphenylacrylate—also known as octocrylene. A UV absorber. *See* octocrylene.

ethylhexyl dimethyl PABA—formerly referred to as octyl dimethyl PABA. Ethylhexyl dimethyl PABA is the International Nomenclature of Cosmetic Ingredients (INCI) listing. An FDA-approved sunscreen chemical with an approved usage level of 1.4 to 8 percent in both the U.S. and the European Union. In the 1970s, it was the most popular sunscreen chemical available as it is one of the best UVB absorbers. Its use, however, has been replaced by octyl-p-methoxycinnamate as a result of the PABA-free trend in sunscreen products. A PABA derivative, it can cause skin irritation and photocontact allergy.

ethylhexyl glycerin—a skin conditioner and preservative derived from glycerin.

2-ethylhexyl 2-hydroxybenzoate—*see* octyl salicylate.

2-ethylhexyl isostearate—a chemical reactant used in cosmetic formulations to reduce the amount of antioxidants needed for that particular formulation. Also an emollient for high-quality skin care preparations. This is an isosteric acid derivative.

E

2-ethylhexyl methoxycinnamate—*see* octyl methoxycinnamate.

ethylhexyl methoxycinnamate—also known as octinoxate and octyl methoxycinnamate. This is the INCI name for what has been listed in the past as octyl methoxycinnamate. Currently both nomenclatures are in use, though ethylhexyl methoxycinnamate will become the standard. *See* octyl methoxycinnamate.

ethylhexyl p-methoxycinnamate—provides excellent UVB protection with some limited UVA absorption, as well. *See also* octyl methoxycinnamate.

2-ethylhexyl p-methoxycinnamate—*see* octyl methoxycinnamate.

ethylhexyl-p—*see* octyl palmitate.

ethylhexyl palmitate—*see* octyl palmitate.

2-ethylhexyl salicylate—also known as ethylhexyl salicylate; octyl salicylate. A UVB absorber. *See* ethylhexyl salicylate.

ethylhexyl salicylate—the INCI name for octyl salicylate. An FDA-approved UVB sunscreen chemical, it absorbs within the entire UVB range. It has an approved usage level of 3 to 5 percent in both the U.S. and the European Union, and is a good solubilizer for benzophenone-3. In suntan lotions, it is used as a preservative and antimicrobial. This is a salt of salicylic acid occurring in wintergreen leaves and in other plants. It is also synthetically manufactured. Considered a noncomedogenic raw material.

ethylhexyl triazone—the INCI name for octyl triazone. A UV filter and absorber. Clinical studies show high photostability and very high UVB-absorption capacity, particularly when compared to other popular UV filters. Studies also indicate that even low concentrations of ethylhexyl triazone in a sun care preparation can contribute significantly to the final product's SPF. It appears to perform particularly well in synergy with zinc oxide.

eucalyptol—considered an antiseptic. This is a monoterpene compound that provides the fragrance associated with the essential oil of eucalyptus. Eucalyptol is also used to fragrance cosmetic preparations. *See also* cajeput oil; eucalyptus oil.

eucalyptus extract (Eucalyptus globulus)—possibly a mild astringent with antiseptic properties. It may also act as an insect repellent. *See also* eucalyptus oil.

eucalyptus oil—described as having antiseptic, disinfectant, antifungal, and blood-circulation activating properties. It is

E

also used as a fragrance. Native to Australia, it was regarded as a general cure-all by the Aborigines and later by the European settlers. It has a long tradition of use in medicine, and is considered one of the most powerful and versatile herbal remedies. It is said that eucalyptus oil's antiseptic properties and disinfectant action increase as the oil ages. The most important constituent of the oil is eucalyptol. The essential oil is obtained from eucalyptus leaves. Eucalyptus oil may cause allergic reactions.

eugenol—a botanical fraction. It is antibacterial, anti-inflammatory, and pain relieving. It can also be used as a local, topical anesthetic and antiseptic. In a cosmetic formulation, it can also be used to mask odor or provide fragrance. Eugenol is a yellow, oily liquid and is generally associated with clove oil. However, it is also found in nutmeg, cinnamon, and bay leaf.

Euterpe oleracea—*see* Açai pulp oil.

Euterpe oleracea pulp oil—*see* Açai pulp oil.

evening primrose oil (Oenothera biennis)—has therapeutic botanical properties described as astringent and helpful for skin irritations. Incorporated into certain preparations at a 10 percent concentration, it appears to improve cases of pruritis and xerosis. Evening primrose oil contains a high amount of gamma linoleic acid, which is one of the essential fatty acids vital for maintaining the normal functioning of the epithelial barrier membrane. Evening primrose oil improves the skin's hydration and its ability to develop normal barrier functions.

evergreen clematis (Clematis vitalba)—anti-inflammatory and astringent. Its constituents include mucilage, chlorophyll, and vitamins. Stems and leaves are the parts used.

everlasting oil (Gnaphalium polycephalum)—reported to decrease UVB-induced erythema on sunburned skin. If applied prior to sun exposure, it helps prevent the development of sunburn. The photoprotective activities of this oil are largely due to the action of its flavonoids content.

extra cellular matrix (ECM)—described as a mixture of bioactive substances including collagen, glycosaminoglycans, heparan sulfate, dermatan sulfate, chondroitin sulfate, and the glycoproteins laminin and fibronectin. It has the ability to stimulate the cells to actually help repair the skin. In general, it is believed to improve cellular function. Used primarily in products for wrinkled or mature skin.

E

eyebright extract (Euphrasia officinalis)—an herb credited with astringent, anti-inflammatory, and tonic properties. As indicated by its name, it has traditionally been used in eye care preparations to decrease and counteract eye area inflammation and potential irritations. Some manufacturers claim that when combined with horsetail and lady's mantle, it works to counter skin wrinkling around the eye area. Important constituents of eyebright extract include tannin, mineral salts, and iridic glycosides. The extract is prepared from the plant after it has been cut just above the root.

E

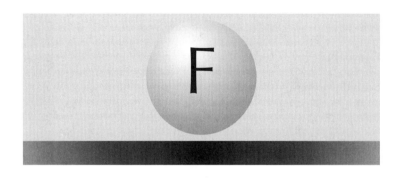

FD&C colors—refer to color entry in Chapter 4.

fango—*see* mud.

fango mud—a redundancy, as *fango* means mud in Italian.

farnesol—described as a substance of high biological potential, capable of acting in the skin as a true bioactivator. A biological precursor and fatty alcohol, farnesol is one component of vitamin K. Farnesol is said to help smooth wrinkles, normalize sebum secretion, and increase the skin's elasticity, tissue tension, and moisture-binding capability. It is able to penetrate the epidermis. In humans, it is found in the skin and is involved in sterol biosynthesis. It is also used for deodorant, odor masking, and skin-soothing properties. It is widely present in vegetables and found in many essential oils (for example, acacia, lilac, lily of the valley, rose, orange blossom, oak moss, and sandalwood).

farnesyl acetate—a tonic, it is also used for perfuming. A variety of beneficial effects on the skin's metabolic process have been noted with the use of compounds consisting of a mixture of farnesyl acetate, farnesol, and panthenyl triacetate.

fennel extract (Foeniculum vulgare)—described as a cleanser and detoxifier indicated for oily skin types. The principal constituents of fennel oil are anethol and fenchone, plus d-pinene, phellandrine, anisic acid, and anisic aldehyde. Anethol, also a main constituent of anise oil, may produce hives, scaling, and blisters when applied directly to the skin. The therapeutic properties of fennel oil are most probably due to fenchone, and so only the varieties of fennel that contain a good proportion of fenchone are suitable

F

for therapeutic use. Fennel oil is obtained from a distillation of the seeds.

fenugreek extract (Trigonella foenum-graecum)—considered an emollient, anti-inflammatory, and healing ingredient. It was traditionally used in treatments for irritated skin. The seeds of this annual herb have been used through the ages and were held in high regard among the Egyptians, Greeks, and Romans for medicinal and culinary purposes.

fern (Dryopteris sp.) (shield fern)—healing, cleansing, and skin conditioning. Its chief constituents include tannin, filicic acid, and filamaron. Fern oil and the powdery fern extract are obtained from the plant's rhizome.

ferric ferrocyanide—a blue color with no known toxicity. Used as a colorant.

ferulic acid—a plant-derived antioxidant and free-radical scavenger, it protects the skin against UVB-induced redness. When incorporated into formulas with ascorbic acid and tocopherol, ferulic acid can improve their stability and double the photoprotection capacities offered by the formulation. In clinical studies, ferulic acid exhibits good permeation capacities through the stratum corneum, which can be attributed to its lipophilic properties.

feverfew extract (Chrysanthemum parthenium)—used for its esters and borneol as a counterirritant. It is claimed to relieve the pain and swelling caused by insect bites. Feverfew is a perennial, herbaceous plant.

fibronectin—as a cosmetic ingredient, it is described as a surface protective agent with a moisturizing and protective effect. Fibronectin's function in the skin is to strengthen the attachments between collagen and elastin fibers, fibroblasts, and other cells in the dermis with connective tissues. Its presence may also be important to cell growth. Research suggests fibronectin plays a significant role in maintaining a healthy basal layer. There is also some evidence that fibronectin may act as a cell regenerator by reversing abnormal cell formation and growth. Fibronectin is a glycoprotein and an important component of the skin's basal layer. Produced by many types of cells, it is present in the skin primarily in the basal membranes. It constitutes 1 to 3 percent of the total cellular protein of fibroblasts.

F

fibronectin (hydrolyzed)—a humectant and moisturizing agent for skin creams and lotions. *See also* fibronectin.

field poppy extract—therapeutic properties are described as pain and spasm soothing.

figwort extract (Scrophularia nodosa)—traditionally used in cases of superficial burns, including sunburn, cutaneous eruptions, swelling, and inflammations. There are a number of varieties of figwort, including common, yellow, balm-leaved, water, and knotted, all appearing to have similar properties. The extract is obtained from the plant's leaves.

fir needle—*see* pine needle extract.

firmogen—provides an astringent, strengthening, and lightening effect. Its use in cosmetic formulations results in smoother skin feel. Firmogen is a biological substance, blending polysaccharides with hydrolyzed enzymatic proteins.

fish collagenic protein—a transparent, uncolored gel used in moisturizers.

fish glycerides—a fish oil used primarily in soaps.

five leaf grass—*see* cinquefoil extract.

flavonoids—a general category of plant derived antioxidants. *See also* bioflavonoids and full entry in Chapter 4.

flavonastaes—an enzyme. *See also* enzyme.

flowers extract—probably used as a fragrance. Such a listing is an all-encompassing statement that does not allow one to identify the type of flowers used and, therefore, prohibits one from determining any therapeutic value.

fluid oil—a play on words describing the physical state of the oil rather than the type of oil used. This does not allow one to identify the value or function of the oil in the cosmetic preparation.

folic acid—generally used as an emollient. In vitro and in vivo skin studies now indicate its capacity to aid in DNA synthesis and repair, promote cellular turnover, reduce wrinkles, and promote skin firmness. There is some indication that folic acid may also protect DNA from UV-induced damage. Folic acid is a member of the vitamin B complex and is naturally occurring in leafy greens.

fragrance—refer to fragrance entry in Chapter 4.

frankincense (Boswellia thurifera)—described as an anti-inflammatory agent and a mild antiseptic that brings relief to dry and sensitive skins and helps heal all types of wounds. Its astringent properties are said to help balance oily or overactive skin. This is one of the oldest essential oils in use, and dates back to ancient Egypt.

F

fructan—moisturizing and anti-inflammatory, it is also used to help improve skin barrier function. A fructose derivative. *See also* fructose.

fructose—a naturally occurring sugar in fruits and honey. It has moisture-binding and skin-softening properties.

fruit oil extract—a blend used in perfumery.

fucus—*see* seaweed extract.

fucus algae (Fucus vesiculosus) (fucus seaweed)—a succulent giant kelp with some preservative and fragrance value. Its essential oil exhibits antimicrobial activity, as it contains compounds similar to traditional preservatives.

fucus seaweed—*see* fucus algae.

fullerenes—also known as fullerines; buckyball. Fullerenes are soluble carbon molecules. They are the result of nanotechnology and its application in skin care. The most common form of fullerenes is C60; other forms include C70, C76, and C84. Generally incorporated into antiaging cosmetics, and studied for antioxidant and free-radical scavenging properties, fullerenes are most commonly used to minimize potential reactions through an interaction with the immune system.

fullerines—*see* fullerenes.

fumitory herb extract (Fumaria officinalis)—credited with curative properties due to its purifying powers. Historically, it was attributed with bleaching and skin-clearing properties as well. The leaves yield a juice credited with medicinal properties due to the presence of fumaric and malic acids. This is a small annual plant considered a common weed.

F

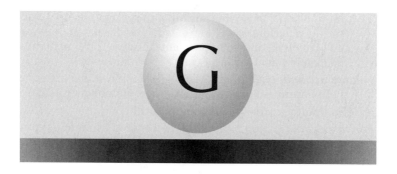

galactoarabinan (GA)—has humectant and exfoliating properties. It is also a film former, and as such can help reduce
transepidermal water loss. In aqueous solutions, GA can de-
posit a clear film, creating or helping to create an occlusive
environment which, in turn, can enhance the functionality
of a formulation's active ingredients. In humid conditions,
GA acts as a moisture binder, and in dry conditions, it is
able to retain moisture. Additionally, GA can improve the
uniformity of emulsion droplets resulting in a more stable
emulsion and potentially more efficacious formulation. In
vitro and in vivo studies indicate a possible beneficial impact to the immune system due to an ability to enhance
Langerhans cell proliferation and cytokine production. GA
has been shown to enhance AHA exfoliation activity without increasing skin irritation, and it also exhibits its own
exfoliant properties independent of AHA presence in a formulation. GA is a polysaccharide found in all plants and is
the dominant sugar of the western larch tree.

galactomannan—a polysaccharide. *See* senna.

galbanum (Ferula galbaniflua)—depending on the form used
(gum, gum extract, or resin oil), galbanum is perfuming
but can also exhibit antimicrobial and tonic properties.

gallic acid—a potential bleaching agent and antioxidant, it is also
astringent. Scientists are finding that gallic acid may serve as
a skin-lightening agent by inhibiting the action of the tyrosinase and peroxidase enzymes. Some studies indicate that it
is more effective than hydroquinone when combined with
the proper ingredients. It is also incorporated into antiaging

G

formulations, providing an ability to prevent mucopolysaccaride deterioration. It is a constituent of witch hazel and oak bark, among other plants; however, it is generally obtained from nutgalls for commercial purposes.

gamma aminobutyric acid (GABA)—an amino acid claimed to help improve skin elasticity. *See also* aminobutric acid.

gamma linoleic acid—*see* linoleic acid.

garlic extract *(Allium sativum)*—Recognized as an antiseptic and bactericide. It is sometimes externally applied in ointments and lotions to reduce hard swellings and to treat problem skin (for example, acne). The active properties of garlic depend on a pungent, volatile, essential oil that is obtained by distillation with water. This oil is a sulfide of the radical allyl present in the onion family, and it is rich in sulfur but contains no oxygen. The common garlic is included in the same group of plants as the onion.

garlic oil—considered a healing oil with bacteriostatic and bactericidal action. It is incorporated into skin care formulations for skin healing and to aid in clearing problems such as eczema and acne. *See also* garlic extract.

garlic sage—*see* germander extract.

gelatin—used as a natural sealant against moisture loss and as a formulation thickener. The films produced by gelatin are tacky when moist and hard, and brittle when dry. This is a product obtained by the partial hydrolysis of mature collagen derived from the skin, connective tissue, and bones of animals. It does not have the water-binding ability of soluble collagen.

gellan gum—used as a gelling agent, thickener, and stabilizer in cosmetic preparations.

genistein—an isoflavone commonly found in soy. It has demonstrated UV-protection properties through antioxidant activity. Studies indicate genistein can promote collagen synthesis, making it also applicable in antiaging cosmetics. *See also* isoflavones.

gentian extract *(Gentiana sp.)*—credited with cooling, antiseptic, and anti-inflammatory activity. Studies indicate that the gentian root also has skin-lightening capacities, thanks to an ability to inhibit melanocyte tyrosinase production. All known gentian species are remarkable for their intensely bitter properties but are considered valuable tonic medicines. The root is the principal part used for medicinal and cosmetic purposes. Dried gentian root contains gentian, gentiamarin, and bitter glucosides together with gentianic acid (gentisin) and gentiopicrin.

geraniol—perfuming and with tonic properties. It is a primary constituent in many essential oils, including citronella, lavender, lemongrass, orange flower, and ylang-ylang.

G

geranium oil *(Pelargonium sp.)*—its botanical properties are described as refreshing, anti-irritant, mildly tonic, and astringent. Although good for all skin types, it is of particular benefit to oily and acne skins, and to those with inflammatory tendencies. The cell-regenerating activities claimed for geranium would also make it useful for aged skin. Although there are many varieties of geranium, including wild geranium and English geranium, all belonging to the same botanical family, their uses may be somewhat different. Geranium oil is obtained by steam distillation from the entire plant, and is widely used in perfumery and cosmetics.

geranium burbon oil—*see* geranium oil.

Germall II—the trade name for imidazolidinyl urea, a preservative. *See also* imidazolidinyl urea.

germander extract *(Teucrium scorodonia) (garlic sage; wood sage)*—credited with astringent and tonic properties. Noted as useful for skin problems and wounds. The whole herb is used for manufacturing the extract.

GHPT—*see* guar hydroxypropyltrimonium chloride.

ginger root extract *(Zingiber officinale)*—healing, tonic, antiseptic and anti-inflammatory. It is also incorporated into cosmetic formulations for its odor masking properties.

ginkgo biloba extract (ginkgo extract)—credited with antioxidant properties, it also appears to aid fibroblast cells in the production of collagen and elastin. This ability is attributed to a number of flavonoid fractions, including quercetin, kaemphferol, and ginkgetin. Additionally, ginkgo is an anti-inflammatory and may help improve a couperose condition due to a protective effect on vascular walls. Ginkgo was used in folkloric medicine as a blood vessel dilator because of its ability to increase blood flow and stimulate tissue oxygen consumption. It is considered a beneficial antiaging ingredient. Ginkgo's key constituents include ginkgolide and bilobalide, catechin, tannin, quercetin, and luteolin.

ginkgo extract—*see* ginkgo biloba extract.

ginseng extract (Panax sp.)—considered tonic and to be nourishing due to its vitamin and hormone content. It seems to aid in diminishing wrinkles and helps dry skin. It is also said to aid in increasing skin elasticity, perhaps due to a stimulation of sterol and protein production. Other claims include skin rejuvenating, oxygenating, and stimulating. Folkloric remedies cite use for boils, bruises, sores, and swellings. This root's active components are called ginsenosides, and are said to be responsible for the revitalization and reactivation of epidermal cells. Important constituents include saponins, mucin, vitamin B, and ginsenoside. The extract comes from the root. Ginseng has been associated with many allergic skin reactions.

ginseng root extract—a redundancy, as the portion of the plant used therapeutically is the root. *See also* ginseng extract.

ginsenosides Rb₁—a manufacturer's composition said to provide elastin synthesis by dermal fibroblasts. The active components of this mixture are reported as gensenosides, basically ginseng varieties, including *Panax notoginseng* and *Panax quinquefolium*. This would most likely be used in antiaging and skin-toning products due to the apparent impact on skin elasticity. *See also* ginseng extract.

glucans—studies indicate an ability to stimulate immune system activity, thereby helping the body fight a variety of infectious diseases caused by bacterial, fungal, viral, and parasitic organisms. Glucans also seem to have antitumor activity. *See also* polyglucan.

glucoronic acid—a chelating agent, pH adjuster, and humectant that gives a smooth feel to the skin.

glucose—has moisture-binding properties and provides the skin with a soothing effect. It is a sugar that is generally obtained by the hydrolysis of starch.

glucose glutamate—a humectant for hand creams and lotions, and a skin conditioner and moisturizer that enhances lather in surfactant systems. Glucose glutamate is the ester of glucose and glutamic acid and is considered a noncomedogenic, nonirritating raw material.

Glucoviton—a trade name referring to a mixture of glucoronic acid and Hydroviton.

glutamic acid—a moisture binder and an antioxidant. Glutamic acid is an amino acid manufactured by means of fermentation, generally from a vegetable protein.

glutaral (glutardialdehyde)—a broad-spectrum preservative that can cause skin irritation. This is an amino acid occurring in green sugar beets.

glutardialdehyde—*see* glutaral.

G

glutathione—a peptide believed to enhance the skin's cellular metabolism and oxygen utilization. It has been found to protect the fibroblast against free-radical induced oxidation. Glutathione is naturally occurring in the body and is essential for the proper functioning of the immune system. A plant and animal tissue component.

glutathione monomethyl ester—an alkyl ester of glutathione. *See also* glutathione.

glutathione peroxidase—helps control inflammation. Its most frequent application is in shaving preparations. Glutatione peroxidase is an enzyme and a natural antioxidant.

glycereth-26—*see* glycerin

glyceridic oil (hydrogenated)—emollient and skin conditioning.

glycerin (glycerol; propanetriol)—a humectant used in moisturizers. It is water-binding and able to draw and absorb water from the air, thus helping the skin retain moisture. Glycerin has been studied extensively for its hydrating abilities. Some of its associated skin benefits are attributed to its ability to facilitate enzymatic reactions in the skin, promoting corneocyte desquamation. Based on the data available, glycerin has been established as a good skin-moisturizing agent. Glycerin also improves the spreading qualities of creams and lotions. It is a clear, syrupy liquid made by chemically combining water and fat that is usually derived from vegetable oil. While glycerin has not been shown to cause allergies, it may be comedogenic and irritating to the mucous membranes when used in concentrated solutions.

glycerin monostearate—*see* glyceryl monostearate.

glycerine—*see* glycerin.

glycerol—a glycerin alcohol. *See also* glycerin.

glycerol stearate lipophilic—*see* glycerin.

glyceryl—a glycerin ester. *See also* glycerin.

glyceryl aminobenzoate (glyceryl PABA, glyceryl p-aminobenzoate)—a sunscreen chemical for UVB absorption with an approved usage level of 2 to 3 percent. It is, however, too water soluble to be effectively used in waterproof formulations,

G

and its use raises safety concerns about the presence of benzocane.

glyceryl arachidonate—an emulsifier and emollient with moisturizing properties. It is reportedly used in suntan gels, creams, and lotions.

glyceryl behenate—derived from the glycerides of coconut fatty acids, it acts as an emollient, lubricant, and/or emulsifier in a cosmetic preparation.

glyceryl caprylate—a coemulsifier, solubilizer, and surfactant that promotes absorption and has bacteriostatic action in cosmetic formulations.

glyceryl dibehenate—an emollient and a lubricant, it is a glycerin derivative.

glyceryl isostearate—*see* glyceryl mono-isostearate.

glyceryl laurate—a coemulsifier for oil-in-water emulsions. It is also a superfattening agent that promotes absorption and has a bacteriostatic effect.

glyceryl linoleate—an emollient with moisturizing capabilities. It is synthetically produced from naturally derived ingredients.

glyceryl mono-isostearate (glyceryl isostearate)—an isostearic acid often incorporated into cosmetic formulations as an emollient.

glyceryl monostearate (glycerin monostearate; glyceryl stearate)—widely used in cosmetics. It functions as an emulsifying and solubilizing ingredient, dispersing agent, emollient, formula stabilizer, and surface-action agent for a wide variety of products. Employed in baby creams, face masks, foundation, and hand lotions. It is often derived from hydrogenated soybean oil. Glyceryl monostearate has little or no toxicity. *See also* glyceryl stearate.

glyceryl oleate—an emollient and stabilizer derived from olive oil. A water-in-oil emulsifier that allows for softer emulsions than glyceryl stearate.

glyceryl PABA—*see* glyceryl aminobenzoate.

glyceryl ricinoleate—an emollient and an emulsifier used in the preparation of creams and lotions.

glyceryl stearate—an emulsifier that assists in forming neutral, stable emulsions. It is also a solvent, humectant, and consistency regulator in water-in-oil and oil-in-water formulations. It may also be used as a skin lubricant and imparts a pleasant skin feel. Glyceryl stearate is a mixture of mono-, di-, and triglycerides of palmitic and stearic acids, and is made from glycerin and stearic fatty acids. Derived for cosmetic use from palm kernel or soy oil, it is also found in the human body. It is very mild with a low skin-irritation profile. A slight risk of irritation exists if products contain poor quality glyceryl stearate.

glyceryl stearate lipophilic—*see* glyceryl stearate.

glyceryl stearate SE—self-emulsifying glyceryl stearate. Provides a stable, uniform oil-in-water emulsion. *See also* glyceryl stearate.

glyceryl tribehenate—also known as tribehenin. *See* tribehenin.

glyceryl tri-isostearate (triisosteatin)—an emollient and emulsifier.

glyceryl trioctanoate—an emollient with skin-softening abilities.

glycine—an amino acid used as a texturizer in cosmetic formulations. It makes up approximately 30 percent of the collagen molecule.

glycoceramides—it is suggested that the topical application of glycoceramides helps replenish intercorneal lipids, and regulates the skin's ability to bind and retain moisture. In addition, it improves the ability of hydrophilic and hydrophobic materials to traverse the corneum layer (the movement of water into the skin and removal of by-products of cell metabolism from the skin). This ensures the intercellular regulatory balance and enhances and restores the barrier function. Glycoceramides can be incorporated into emulsions. *See also* ceramides.

glycocitrates—a combination of glycolic and citric acids used instead of AHAs in some preparations. This substitution is based on the premise that glycocitrates are milder than an AHA such as glycolic acid, and that they provide similar results. Their activity does not appear to be scientifically validated in a significant manner.

glycocoll—*see* glycine.

glycogen—a skin-conditioning agent. It is a high molecular-weight polymer distributed through the cell protoplasm.

glycol palmitate—an emulsion stabilizer, it can also make a product more opaque and act as a skin conditioner.

glycol propylene—*see* propylene glycol.

glycol stearate—can be utilized as a detergent, emulsifier, surfactant, thickener, stabilizer, and emollient in cosmetic formulations. It converts clear cleansers to ones that are pearly.

G

glycolic acid (hydroxyacetic acid)—reduces corenocyte cohesion and corneum layer thickening where excess dead skin cell buildup can be associated with many common skin problems, such as acne, dry and severely dry skin, and wrinkles. Glycolic acid acts by dissolving the internal cellular cement responsible for abnormal keratinization, facilitating the sloughing of dead skin cells. It also improves skin hydration by enhancing moisture uptake as well as increasing the skin's ability to bind water. This occurs in the cellular cement through an activation of glycolic acid and the skin's own hyaluronic acid content. Hyaluronic acid is known to retain an impressive amount of moisture and this capacity is enhanced by glycolic acid. As a result, the skin's own ability to raise its moisture content is increased. Glycolic acid is the simplest alpha hydroxyacid (AHA). It is also the AHA that scientists and formulators believe has greater penetration potential because of its smaller molecular weight. It is mildly irritating to the skin and mucous membranes if the formulation contains a high glycolic acid concentration and/or a low pH. Glycolic acid proves beneficial for acne-prone skin as it helps keep pores clear of excess keratinocytes. It is also used for diminishing the signs of age spots, as well as actinic keratosis. However, glycolic acid is most popularly employed in antiaging cosmetics due to its hydrating, moisturizing, and skin-normalizing abilities, leading to a reduction in the appearance of fine lines and wrinkles. Regardless of the skin type, glycolic acid use is associated with softer, smoother, healthier, and younger looking skin. Glycolic acid is naturally found in sugar cane. *See also* alpha hydroxyacid.

glycolipids—emulsifiers and moisturizers. *See also* glycoprotein (soluble).

glycoprotein—a skin-conditioning agent derived from carbohydrates and proteins. In the body, glycoproteins play a significant role in immune response. *See also* glycoprotein (soluble).

glycoproteins (soluble)—a group of proteins found in the intercellular layers, the best known of which is fibronectin. It is found in the cellular matrix of the dermis and plays a role in cell migration during wound healing. The mechanism by which it might provide cosmetic benefits has not yet been clearly established, although it could be related to the role of glycoproteins in immune response. *See also* fibronectin.

glycosaminoglycans—a group of chemically related polysaccharides that are major components of the extra cellular matrix (ECM) and of connective tissues. They are used in cosmetics for their ability to increase hydration and the elasticity and pliability of the skin. Glycosaminoglycans are credited with film-forming, moisturizing, and firming properties. They reportedly leave the skin smooth and with a pleasant, velvety softness and evenness, and minimize wrinkle appearance. They are easily accepted by the skin due to their high charge and affinity. This group of complex materials, formerly identified as mucopolysaccharides, includes such individual components as hyaluronic acid, chondroitin, chondroitin sulfate, chondroitin 6-sulfate, dermatan sulfate, heparin, and heparin sulfate. As proteoglycans, glycosaminoglycans are derived from cartilaginous fish. They can also be derived from various animal proteins as well as synthetically prepared. *See also* mucopolysaccharides.

glycoside/C-$_{12-16}$—a mixture of synthetic fatty alcohols with 12 to 16 carbons in the alkyl chain.

glycosphingolipids—said to replenish the lipids lost from the skin and renew the skin's barrier function and moisture-binding capacity. When incorporated into aftershave preparations, they also seem to help soothe nicks and cuts. Laboratory studies prove that glycosphingolipids can reduce transepidermal water loss when applied to the skin, even at 5 percent in a typical oil-in-water emulsion. Glycosphingolipids, a compound of lipids and sugars, are a class of molecules embedded in the membranes of cells throughout the body where they act to regulate the interaction of healthy cells with their environment.

glycyrrhetic acid—*see* 18 beta-glycerrhentinic acid.

glycyrrhetinic acid—anti-irritant, antiallergenic, anti-inflammatory, skin-lightening, and smoothing properties are attributed to this ingredient, which is also a carrier. It is the organic compound derived from glycyrrhizic acid or shredded licorice roots.

glycyrrhizic acid—a hydrolyzed glycyrrhizin. It is credited with anti-inflammatory and antiallergenic properties. Studies comparing glycyrrhizin with hydrocortisone found glycyrrhizin to be somewhat milder but longer lasting in effectiveness. Once the application of hydrocortisone is suspended, the symptoms return. This does not appear to be the case with glycyrrhizin. It does not have

G

side effects and is chemically stable so it can be safely used on a continuing basis. *See also* licorice extract.

goa powder *(Andira araroba)* **(araroba; bahia powder; brazil powder; goa)**—used in traditional medicine for treatment of skin diseases, including psoriasis and eczema. May have applications in cosmetics for dry skin. The powder's primary constituents include alkalis, benzene, chrysarobin (a reduced quinone), and resins. Its activity is attributed to a high chrysarobin content (approximately 80 percent). The *Andira araroba* tree is common to Bahia, Brazil.

goji berry *(Lycium barbarum)*—also known as matrimony vine. An antioxidant. *See* matrimony vine.

goldenrod extract *(Solidago sp.)*—considered to have antiseptic action and recommended for use in acne products to discourage the spread of infection through skin pustules. The extract is made from the leaves of various species of *Solidago*.

goldenseal extract *(Hydrastis canadensis)*—reported to be effective in the treatment of eczema, itching, and wounds. Native Americans valued the root for its general ulceration-healing properties. The extract is made from the plant's rhizomes. Goldenseal extract's main constituents are the alkaloids berberine, hydrastine, and canadine. The rhizome is said to be much more alkaloid-rich than the root.

gotu kola extract *(Centella asiatica)* **(hydrocotyl; Hydrocotyl asiatica; Indian pennywort)**—traditionally used for couperose condition. It was also used for soothing and anti-itching treatment in dermatological disorders. Gotu kola is a known inhibitor of keratinocyte proliferation, making it useful in the treatment of severely dry skin such as psoriasis. It may also promote circulation and serve as an anticellulite ingredient. In addition, gotu kola is considered healing. It is helpful against sunburns and other superficial, though not extensive, burns. Gotu kola's activity is due to such constituents as phytosterols, glycosides, tannins, and essential oils.

grape—used in extract form, it is described as tonic, with anti-inflammatory, redness-reducing, and decongestant properties. It is also an antioxidant. All of these traits make it particularly beneficial in antiaging, after-sun, and other sun care products. Grape's main constituent is a high proportion of berberin, with oxycanthin also present. Grapes contain vitamin C, chlorophyll, and enzymes. The value of these components to the skin is based on the method of extract processing and cosmetic manufacturing.

grapefruit extract (Citrus paradisi)—reported as having antiseptic properties. It is indicated as beneficial for oily skin. Fresh grapefruit juice contains vitamin C and is very acidic. As such, in high concentrations, it is too caustic to use on the skin and face. There should be no problem, however, at normal use levels. The extract obtained from the juice is preferred over that of the rind, as there is practically no vitamin C available in the rind. Furthermore, unless properly obtained and processed, fertilizers and insecticide residues on the rind may provoke blemishes and allergic reactions in sensitive people. As vitamin C is considered an unstable component, grapefruit extract's value in cosmetics depends on the method of extraction and the product's formulation.

G

grapefruit oil—used as a fragrance and also as an active component with anti-irritant properties. Grapefruit oil is indicated for work with the lymphatic system.

grapefruit seed extract—said to have antibacterial properties. This is the extract from the seeds of the grapefruit. *See also* grapefruit extract.

grapeseed extract—considered a counterirritant with soothing, antioxidant, and antibacterial properties. Grapeseed extract contains polyphenols and high levels of procyandins. *See also* grape.

grapeseed oil—has moisturizing and nourishing properties due to its high linoleic acid content. Grapeseed oil is the fixed oil obtained by pressing grapeseeds.

green apple extract—*see* apple extract.

green clay—*see* clay.

green tea extract (Camellia sinensis L.)—a powerful antioxidant due to its catechin content, it is also known to be an antibacterial, anti-inflammatory, and a stimulant. In clinical studies, green tea has demonstrated an ability to prevent or at least postpone the onset of such illnesses as cancer and heart disease. This is attributed to the catechin component's ability to penetrate into a cell, thereby protecting the cell from free radicals and associated damage. Because of its antioxidant properties, green tea is usually incorporated into antiaging formulations. When applied topically, it can also reduce skin swelling. In addition, it can be found in

G

sunscreens, given its ability to extend the product's SPF. The extract and its associated catechins can be obtained from both the plant and its dried leaves. Other constituents of green tea include caffeine and phenolic acids.

guaiac extract *(Guaiacum officinale)*—credited with antiseptic and stimulating properties. The resin, with therapeutic properties, is extracted from the hard wood of the guaiac tree.

guanine—color. It is mixed in water and used primarily in nail polish to achieve a pearlized effect. It has been greatly replaced by either synthetic pearl or aluminum and bronze particles. Guanine is obtained by scraping the scales of certain fish such as alewives and herring.

guar gum—has a coating action on the skin that allows for moisture retention. Often used as a thickener and emulsifier in cosmetic formulations, guar gum is a polysaccharide found in the seeds of a specific plant. It is the nutrient material required by the developing plant embryo during germination. When the endosperm, once separated from the hull and embryo, is ground to a powder form, it is marketed as guar gum.

guar hydroxypropyltrimonium chloride (GHPT)—an anti-irritant and anti-inflammatory that is also used as a thickening, conditioning, and antistatic agent. It helps maintain a product's smoothing action. Some manufacturers cite it as also having skin-softening capabilities. It imparts excellent skin conditioning in creams or lotions that otherwise may not be used on the face. It adds lubricity to a product when in contact with the skin. There is some evidence that it can enhance a formulation's viscosity and stability. A derivative of guar gum.

guarana seed extract *(Paullinia cupana)*—constituents include theophylline and caffeine, which makes it popular in anti-cellulite products for tonic and draining activity.

gum acacia—*see* acacia.

gum Arabic—*see* acacia.

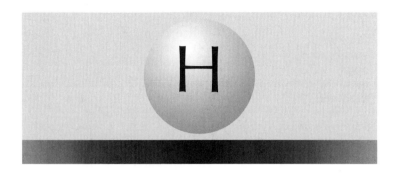

H

hamamelis (winterbloom; witch hazel)—*see* witch hazel.

hamamelis (dry) extract—claimed botanical properties include anti-free radical, UVB absorber, healing, soothing, and anti-itching activity. *See also* witch hazel.

hawthorn extract (*Crataegus oxyacantha*)—sources cite it as having active constituents with valuable therapeutic properties such as antispasmodic, vasodilator, and sedative. Obtained from the berries, flowers, and/or leaves of the hawthorn plant.

hayflower extract—reported to activate the circulatory system, have analgesic properties, and provide a tightening effect on the skin. Historically, hayflower extract was used in Europe to stimulate the circulation and for rheumatic complaints. Its many active constituents include essential oils, vitamin D, amino acids, carotinoids, caffeic acid, 4-methoxycinnnamic acid, and tannin. This extract has a faintly sweet fragrance. Hayflower is not a specific plant but rather a mixture that is formed by the leftover blossoms and leaves in a hay loft.

hazelnut extract—said to have astringent properties.

hazelnut oil—a carrier oil credited with nourishing properties. As a carrier, it imparts excellent lubricity, pale color, and low odor. This oil is used in products designed for dry skin. Obtained from the nuts of various species of the hazelnut tree.

hectorite—one of the principal constituents of bentonite clay. Used as a thickener and suspending agent in water-based systems in oil-in-water emulsions.

helichrysum oil—*see* everlasting oil.

henna extract *(Lawsonia insermis)*—primarily a colorant that provides a reddish-brown hue to products. It is also a conditioner. Henna's properties are described as antiseptic and astringent. Important constituents include mucins, phytosterols, and naptho-quinones. Generally, the extract is obtained from the leaves.

heptane—a solvent and viscosity-decreasing agent.

hesperidin methyl chalcone—a citrus bioflavonoid. Extracted from the peel of sweet oranges, it has antioxidant properties. Used in eye care preparations for reducing the appearance of dark circles.

hesperitin laurate—antioxidant and skin conditioning.

hexadecanol—*see* cetyl alcohol.

N-hexadecyl-n, n, n-trimethylammonium-trans-retinoate—has some effect in inhibiting the *P. acnes* bacteria associated with acne formation.

hexamidine—a preservative.

hexamidine diisethionate—an antimicrobial and preservative targeting fungi and yeast. It also may have some emollient capacities.

hexyl cinnamal—also known as hexyl cinnamic aldehyde. A fragrance that provides a floral, jasmine-like scent.

hexyl laurate—a mild emollient and a vehicle for lipid-soluble active ingredients. Nonirritating and practically odorless. It enhances product spreadability and feel on skin. *See also* lauric acid.

hexyl nicotinate—penetrates rapidly and dilates blood vessels, thereby temporarily activating blood circulation. This increased blood flow results in an enhanced supply of oxygen, nutrients, and moisture to the skin cells, along with a faster elimination of wastes by means of the metabolic process.

hexylene glycol—could be considered a solubilizer. *See also* polyethylene glycol.

hibiscus extract *(Hibiscus sabdariffa)*—moisturizing and refreshing. It provides a tightening effect without stripping the skin of its natural oils. Hibiscus is a botanical recommended for oily skin due to its high degree of astringency and its toning properties. There are about 200 varieties of this plant, whose extract is obtained from the flowers which contain a number of vegetable acids and pigments. Use of hibiscus extract is increasing in popularity, although it is more frequently used in hair care preparations.

A nonirritating form of pyruvic acid is a key constituent of hibiscus extract.

histidine—a skin-conditioning amino acid. *See also* amino acid.

holy thistle—*see* blessed thistle extract.

homomenthyl salicylate—*see* homosalate.

homosalate—a chemical UVB absorber included in the FDA's Category I Sunscreen Chemical list. Its approved usage level is 4 to 15 percent by the FDA and 10 percent by the European Economic Community's Cosmetic Directive.

honey—said to be soothing, softening, and moisturizing. Masks and other cosmetic preparations containing honey create a watertight film on the face and permit the skin to rehydrate itself. Its use in cosmetics is centuries old, and can be traced back at least to ancient Egypt and Cleopatra. Strong antibacterial and immunological properties are attributed to honey. Honey is composed of a variety of sugars, wax, and other substances, including gluconic, citric, malic, formic, and lactic acids; beta-carotene; enzymes; amino acids; and vitamins. It is a saccharic secretion produced enzymatically from flower nectar that is gathered and stored in honeycombs by honey bees. Honey may cause an allergic reaction in people allergic to pollen.

honey extract—an extract obtained from honey. *See also* honey.

honeydew melon (Cucumis melo sp.)—*see* cumumis melo.

honeysuckle extract (Lonicera fragrantissima)—healing, soothing, and anti-inflammatory. Additional uses for external application include cutaneous tonic, protection against sunburn, and overall skin clearing. A dozen or more of the 100 different species of honeysuckle have botanical applications. Apparently, the leaves have more effect than the flowers.

honeysuckle oil—a biological additive with properties similar to those of honeysuckle extract.

hops extract (Humulus lupulus)—general effects attributed to hops include sedative, inflammation reducing, and the promotion of wound healing. Hops are also considered to have preservative value. Their use is claimed effective in acne products. Important constituents include humulone, lupulone, amino acids, chlorogenic acid, rutin, quercatin, flavonoids, and a lupamaric acid. The oil and the bitter principle combine to make hops more useful than chamomile or gentian. Hops extract is made from the cones of the hops vine and can cause allergic reactions.

H

H

horse chestnut extract *(Aesculus hippocastanum)*—antiphlo-
gistic, anti-inflammatory, spasmolytic, and promotes improved circulation. It apparently also has the ability to
help reduce the permeability of capillaries. This would
make it useful in cases of fragile or broken capillaries. Tannic acid provides horse chestnut extract with toning and
astringent properties. Horse chestnut is recommended for
use in products designed to stimulate circulation and normalize circulatory disorders, such as creams for improving
circulation, and bath salts for the stimulation of the whole
organism. Some suppliers cite a recommended dosage of
2 to 5 percent for use in creams and emulsions, and others
cite 1 to 10 percent for bath and hair products. Detected
constituents include starch, sugar, protein, tannin, oil, vitamins, phytosterol, and an Aesculus Saponine content.
The extract is usually obtained from the seed (fruit).

horseheal—*see* elecampane.

horseradish extract *(Armoracia lapathifolia)*—traditionally
used against sunburns and superficial and other nonextensive burns, and to give the skin clarity and freshness. Its
antiseptic and skin-clearing properties are linked to its
ascorbic acid content. The extract is made primarily from
the plant's roots.

horsetail extract *(Equisetum arvense)* **(shave grass)**—stimulating,
astringent, soothing, healing, and softening. Horsetail is
also described as able to increase the skin's defense mechanism, regulate the skin due to the plant's rich mineral
content, and even strengthen connective tissue due to the
presence of silicic acid. Some product manufacturers
state that when mixed with lady's mantle and eyebright
extracts, horsetail extract works to prevent and counteract
wrinkles in the eye area. This is an extract of the sterile
caules of *Equisetum arvense*, a fern plant whose sprouts
have high silicic acid content as well as flavone glycosides and saponine. Amino acids such as citruline, valine,
asparaginic acid, lucine, and serine have also been detected as constituents of this extract. The recommended
usage level is 1 to 10 percent of a formulation's total composition. Can be beneficial in both antiaging and acne
products.

hortensis extract—*see* savory.

huang qin extract—a plant extract said to have soothing
properties.

hyaluronic acid—a glycosaminoglycan component. Hyaluronic acid occurs naturally in the dermis. It is thought to play a critical role in healthy skin by controlling the physical and biochemical characteristics of epidermal cells. It also regulates general skin activity, such as water content, elasticity, and the distribution of nutrients. Its water-absorption abilities and large molecular structure allow the epidermis to achieve greater suppleness, proper plasticity, and turgor. Hyaluronic acid is a natural moisturizer with excellent water-binding capabilities. In a solution of 2 percent hyaluronic acid and 98 percent water, the hyaluronic acid holds the water so tightly that it appears to create a gel. However, it is a true liquid in that it can be diluted and will exhibit a liquid's normal viscous flow properties. When applied to the skin, hyaluronic acid forms a viscoelastic film in a manner similar to the way it holds water in the intercellular matrix of dermal connective tissues. This performance and behavior suggests that hyaluronic acid makes an ideal moisturizer base, allowing for the delivery of other agents to the skin. Manufacturers claim that the use of hyaluronic acid in cosmetics results in the need for much lower levels of lubricants and emollients in a formulation, thereby providing an essentially greaseless product. Furthermore, its ability to retain water gives immediate smoothness to rough skin surfaces and significantly improves skin appearance.

hyaluronidase—an enzyme with moisturizing properties, it is credited with improving skin elasticity, reducing skin dryness, and increasing the skin's moisture content by 33 percent. It is reported to have a greater moisturizing effect when used in conjunction with hydrolyzed protein than when used alone. In the skin, hyaluronidase is an important glycosaminoglycan component.

hydrocotyl asiatica—*see* gotu kola extract.

hydrocotyl extract—*see* gotu kola extract.

hydrogen peroxide—a bleaching and oxidizing agent, detergent, and antiseptic. Generally recognized as a safe preservative, germ killer, and skin bleacher in cosmetics. If used undiluted, it can cause burns of the skin and mucous membranes.

hydrogenated coco glyceride—an emulsifier and emollient, it also has skin-conditioning and water-binding capacities.

hydrogenated tallow octyl dimonium chloride—a conditioner used in clear or emulsion systems. It provides a soft feel and is lubricating in skin care products.

H

hydrolyzed albumen—*see* hydrolyzed egg.

hydrolyzed animal protein—refers to processed collagen and other animal proteins. The primary function of these proteins is to form a glossy film on the skin. However, depending on the degree of hydrolysis, and thus the size of the final molecule, the action can range from film-forming, in order to reduce moisture loss, to that of individual amino acids, which can penetrate the top layers of the corneum layer. The process of hydrolysis, commonly produced by means of enzyme hydrolysis, breaks the bonds of the larger molecules, making them smaller and smaller until finally one gets the amino acids themselves. Manufacturers hydrolyze the proteins in controlled environments to obtain the desired chain length appropriate for the properties of their formulations. The name listed as such does not indicate any specified level of hydrolysis. *See also* animal protein; collagen; collagen hydrolysates; elastin.

hydrolyzed collagen—*see* collagen hydrolysates.

hydrolyzed corn protein—forms a film on the skin's surface. It is used to reduce loss of the skin's natural moisture. *See also* hydrolyzed vegetable protein.

hydrolyzed egg—a skin conditioning agent that can aid in skin moisturization and improve skin texture and feel. It is also used in cosmetics as a natural viscosity controller. *See also* egg protein and egg extract.

hydrolyzed elastin—forms a film on the skin's surface. A processed form of elastin that facilitates its use in skin care formulations. *See also* elastin (hydrolyzed).

hydrolyzed fibronectin—a humectant and moisturizing agent for skin creams and lotions. It is a processed form of fibronectin that facilitates its use in skin care formulations. *See also* fibronectin.

hydrolyzed glycosaminoglycans—has hygroscopic properties and a small molecular structure that favors penetration into the outer epidermal layers. This ingredient contains low molecular weight oligosaccharides and can be found in hydrating cosmetics. Recommended for stressed and aging skin. *See also* glycosaminoglycans.

hydrolyzed golden pea protein—forms a film on the skin's surface. This is a water-soluble liquid protein derivative and a vegetable protein of interest because of its high soluble tyrosine content. Tyrosine is considered to play an important role in stimulating cell growth, and is an integral component of tyrosinase, which is responsible for the formation of melanin. Considered by some as the best replacement for hydrolyzed animal protein. *See also* hydrolyzed vegetable protein.

hydrolyzed keratin—a processed form of keratin that facilitates its use in skin care formulations. *See also* hydrolyzed animal protein; keratin.

hydrolyzed lupine protein—may help promote the synthesis of epidermal proteins and lipids. It is also said to limit transepidermal water loss and strengthen the barrier function of the skin. Rich in glutamine peptides and oligosaccharides, it is generally incorporated into repairing, regenerating, and hydrating products. *See also* lupine extract.

hydrolyzed milk protein—forms a film on the skin's surface that allows the skin to retain moisture. This is a processed form of milk protein that facilitates and improves performance in skin care formulations. *See also* milk protein.

hydrolyzed mucopolysaccharides—a skin hydrator due to its strong water-binding properties that helps decrease transepidermal water loss. This is a mixture of polysaccharides derived from the hydrolysis of animal connective tissue. *See also* mucopolysaccharides.

hydrolyzed oat protein—an anti-itching skin protectant with a soothing effect on sensitive skin, its lipid content provides improved lubricating and emollient properties. This is a very smooth vegetable protein, derived by acid, enzyme, or other method of hydrolysis. *See also* hydrolyzed vegetable protein; oat; oat protein.

hydrolyzed potato protein—a vegetable protein that serves as a moisturizing agent. Reported to have a unique amino acid profile, with reasonable levels of the sulfur-containing amino acids cystine and methionine. This is the hydrolysate of potato protein derived by acid, enzyme, or other method of hydrolysis. *See also* hydrolyzed vegetable protein.

hydrolyzed rice protein—a vegetable protein that serves as a good moisturizing agent. This is the hydrolysate of rice protein derived by acid, enzyme, or other method of hydrolysis. *See also* hydrolyzed vegetable protein.

hydrolyzed rice bran protein and glycine soja protein and oxido reductases—a mixture of ingredients that is said to reduce puffiness and dark circles around the eyes. This is a manufactured combination of rice bran protein, soybean

H

protein, and a yeast and enzyme mixture (oxido reductases). *See also* rice bran; soybean protein.

hydrolyzed serum proteins—a film-former and skin-conditioning substance that reduces transepidermal water loss and has anti-irritant properties. It is also nourishing to the cells. *See also* hydrolyzed animal protein; serum protein.

hydrolyzed vegetable protein—forms a protein-lipid film on the skin, giving products a moisture-retention capacity. These proteins are obtained from wheat, soybean, corn, peas, or other vegetable source. They are made by the hydrolysate of vegetable protein derived by acid, enzyme, or other method of hydrolysis. Some vegetable proteins have, at least theoretically, a composition that can make them appealing as a replacement for animal protein. However, vegetable proteins generally exhibit a different behavior from animal proteins, which affects the chemical reaction, additive, requirements, and cosmetic product stability.

hydrolyzed wheat protein—offers conditioning, moisturizing, and film-forming properties. It is an effective moisturizer in skin care products, where it helps retain moisture in the skin. It is almost always used as a replacement for hydrolyzed animal protein. It is produced by an enzymatic hydrolysis of wheat gluten. *See also* hydrolyzed vegetable protein.

hydrolyzed wheat protein (AMP isostearoyl)—a skin-conditioning ingredient. This is a neutralized alcohol-soluble wheat protein/fatty acid condensate. It can be found in skin tonics. *See also* hydrolyzed vegetable protein; hydrolyzed wheat protein.

hydrolyzed wheat protein polysiloxane copolymer—upon drying, it forms a protective conditioning film on the skin that reduces water loss. This is a wheat protein attached to silicone, which enhances the effects of protein and silicone on the skin. *See also* hydrolyzed wheat protein.

hydrolyzed whole wheat protein—a modified form of wheat protein to facilitate its performance and incorporation in skin care formulations. *See also* hydrolyzed wheat protein.

hydrolyzed yeast—the hydrolysate of yeast derived by acid, enzyme, or other method of hydrolysis. *See also* protein; yeast.

hydrotriticum wheat amino acids—an ingredient with good moisture-retention properties. It is reportedly able to penetrate the corneum layers and moisturize from within.

hydroquinone—a pigment-lightening agent used in bleaching creams. Hydroquinone combines with oxygen very rapidly and becomes brown when exposed to air. Although it occurs naturally, the synthetic version is the one commonly used in cosmetics. Application to the skin may cause allergic reaction and increase skin sun sensitivity. Hydroquinone is potentially carcinogenic and is associated with causing ochronosis, a discoloration of the skin. The U.S. FDA allows a maximum of 2 percent concentration in a cosmetic formulation. Its use in cosmetics is prohibited in some European countries.

Hydroviton—a trade name for a natural moisturizer derived from rose water, plant sugars, and plant-sourced amino acids. It contains glycerin, sodium lactate, TEA-lactate, serine, lactic acid, urea, sorbitol, lauryl diethylenedi-aminoglycine, lauryl aminopropylglycinel, and allantoin.

2-hydroxy-p-methoxycinnamate—*see* cinoxate.

5-hydroxy-2-hydroxymethyl-gamma-pyridone—a skin-lightening agent apparently 32 times more effective than kojic acid.

hydroxyacetic acid—*see* glycolic acid.

hydroxyacetone—*see* dihydroxyacetone.

hydroxycitronellal—used to mask odor.

hydroxydecyl ubiquinone—a potent antioxidant. *See* idebenone.

hydroxyethyl cellulose—suggested as a thickener, protective colloid, binder, stabilizer, and suspending agent. It is obtained from wood pulp or chemical cotton by treatment with an alkali. *See also* ethyl cellulose.

hydroxyisohexyl 3-cyclohexene carboxaldehyde—fragrance with a light floral scent. May cause skin irritation.

hydroxylated lanolin—a modified form of lanolin. It increases the tackiness, stickiness, and emulsifying capacity of lanolin. A good suspending agent. It is obtained by the controlled hydroxylation of lanolin. *See also* lanolin.

6-hydroxy-5-methoxyindole—a skin pigmenter said to promote melanine synthesis. Thus it is incorporated into cosmetics to create a tanned look, as with dihydroxyacetone. Claimed to yield a pigmentation quality that would be obtained from natural tanning.

hydroxyoctacosanyl hydroxystearate—a consistency regulating agent for water-in-oil emulsions used to improve the body of an emulsion. Used in creams, liquid makeup, and lipsticks. This is a synthetic beeswax substitute.

H

hydroxyproline—a skin-conditioning amino acid. It is a component of collagen.

hydroxypropyl methylcellulose—improves foaming properties, lubricity, and formula stabilization. It can help formulators reduce active surfactant concentrations in a product without the loss of the desirable lathering properties, thereby resulting in a milder product. Mild to the skin and eyes. *See also* cellulose gum.

hydroxypropyltrimonium hydrolyzed wheat protein—enhances skin moisturization. This is considered an upgraded version of hydrolyzed wheat protein, particularly with respect to moisturizing properties. It is also a mildness agent for surfactants.

hydroxyproylated y-cyclodextrin—helps prevent skin roughness.

8-hydroxy stilbenes—a skin-lightening compound. It inhibits melanin formation by inhibiting tyrosinase activity. Not known to cause skin irritation.

6-hydroxy-2,5,7,8-tetramethylchroman-2-carboxyic acid—a free-radical inhibitor. Studies indicate it penetrates the skin more effectively than vitamin E. Can be used in moisturizing lotions.

hypericum extract (Hypericum perforatum)—see St. John's wort extract.

hyssop oil (Hyssopus officinalis)—attributed properties include healing, tonic, and stimulating. It can also be used as a fragrance. Hyssop oil is indicated for dermatitis, eczema, and wounds because of its cicatrizant properties. An infusion of the leaves is reportedly used externally for the relief of muscular rheumatism, bruises, and discolored contusions. The oil is obtained from the distillation of the whole plant in flower.

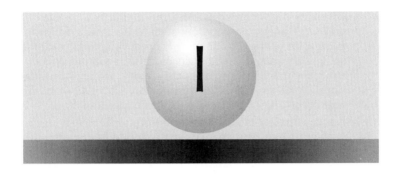

I

Iceland moss extract (Cetraria islandica)—used in cosmetics for its tonic properties, it can also be incorporated for its cleansing, emollient, skin-smoothing and skin-soothing capacities. Despite its name, this plant is not a moss but rather a lichen containing about 70 percent lichen starch, plus fumaric acid, oxalic acid cetrarin, and licheno-stearic acid.

ichthammol—*see* sodium shale oil sulfonate.

ichthyol—*see* sodium shale oil sulfonate.

idebenone—an antioxidant capable of protecting the skin from a variety of free-radical attacks, including the formation of secondary chemicals that negatively affect skin physiology. Its claimed properties include the improvement of intrinsic as well as extrinsic skin damage caused by free-radical formation. Idebenone is a synthetically manufactured form of coenzyme Q10 and has a smaller molecular structure. This allows it to penetrate the skin and apparently the cellular membrane, as well. It demonstrates an ability to produce clinically visible improvement in photodamaged skin, reducing skin roughness and dryness, decreasing fine lines and wrinkles, and increasing skin hydration. In addition, idebenone helps improve hyperpigmentation as its molecular structure is similar to that of hydroquinone. While most of the associated improvements are seen primarily in the epidermis, some increase in dermal collagen has also been confirmed. Idebenone has been used for such health-related problems as Alzheimer's and heart disease.

illipe butter—also known as *Shorea stenoptera* seed butter. Emollient and moisturizing, it can promote skin suppleness.

Given its high melting point, illipe butter can be used to make a cosmetic preparation, such as lipstick or bar soap, more solid or rigid. Its chemical composition and cosmetic activity are similar to that of cocoa butter. Found in skin and sun care preparations, massage creams, makeup foundations, lipsticks, and hair conditioners. Obtained from the nuts of the *Shorea stenoptera* tree, native to Borneo.

illite—a clay similar in structure to montmorillonite. It can be used as an exfoliant and skin softener and to draw impurities and oil to the skin's surface. Red and yellow illite clay may also be used as a color additive. Green illite is particularly appropriate in oily skin products. Illite is generally found in masks, body wraps, exfoliators, and cleansers, and can also be incorporated as a bulking agent. *See also* montmorillonite.

ilomastat—helps prevent the formation of matrix metalloproteinases. Matrix metalloproteinases are a category of enzymes that contribute to the degradation of the extracellular matrix and its proteins, including collagen. Ilomastat therefore helps prevent the formation of this family of enzymes. It also inhibits certain strains of bacteria.

imidazolidinyl urea—one of the most commonly used antibacterial preservatives, given its low sensitizing potential. In 2005, it was the sixth most frequently used preservative in the United States (parabens were in first to fourth place). Generally, imidazolidinyl urea is not used alone but as a copreservative, with parabens for broad-spectrum activity. Although it may yield low levels of formaldehyde when subjected to destructive methods—such as exposure to high temperatures—under normal use conditions, there is no detection of free formaldehyde release. Of all the formaldehyde-releasing preservatives, imidazolidinyl urea is the one least likely to cause skin sensitization and allergic reactions. *See also* urea.

imidurea—an abbreviated annotation for imidazolidinyl urea. *See* imidazolidinyl urea.

immunoglobulins—an ingredient being tested for use in antiacne cosmetic preparations given its potential ability to decrease the *P. acnes* count by about half after one week of use. Obtained from cow's milk.

Indian chestnut extract—*see* chestnut extract.

inositol—used in emollients for its ability to hold and retain moisture. Belongs to the vitamin B family. While found naturally in plant and animal tissue, for commercial use it is isolated from corn.

iodopropynyl butylcarbamate—a preservative with broad fungicidal activity used in skin care products. It is recommended for use in difficult formulation systems.

iris extract (Iris sp.)—the juice of fresh iris root has been employed as a cosmetic and freckle remover. Depending on the part of the plant used—flower, root, or leaf—the activity in a cosmetic product can include tonic, perfuming, masking odor and improving skin condition. There are many varieties of iris, many of which have a considerable reputation for their medicinal virtues. The *Iris versicolor* variety, for example, produces an official drug in the *U.S. Pharmacopoeia* and is used in cosmetics for its emollient, masking, and tonic activity.

Irish moss—*see* carrageen extract.

iron oxide (iron oxide black, red, or yellow)—an inorganic compound frequently used to add color to cosmetics. It may have some slight sunscreening ability. Iron oxide can vary in color from red to brown, black to orange or yellow, depending on the purity and amount of water added.

isoamyl p-methoxycinnamate—also known as isopentyl-4-methoxycinnamate. An organic UV filter and absorber with an approved usage level of up to 10 percent in the European Union.

isoarachidyl neopentanoate—an emollient with SPF-enhancing ability. It is generally used in sunscreen preparations. Considered noncomedogenic.

isobutyl paraben—a preservative.

isocetyl alcohol—a skin conditioner with emollient properties, it may also be used as a viscosity builder within a formulation.

isocetyl stearate—an emollient.

isocream—an emollient. This is a mixture of mineral oil, lanolin, petrolatum, and lanolin alcohol.

isocreme—*see* isocream.

isodecyl citrate—a chemical compound used to inhibit the peroxidation of skin lipids. It is also used in cosmetics as an emollient and to facilitate the incorporation of other, hard to work with, ingredients. Often used in such items as antiaging creams and lotions, sunscreen preparations, and other skin care cosmetics.

I

isodecyl isononanoate—an emollient with a very low irritancy level that gives the skin a light, dry feel. Considered non-comedogenic.

isodecyl oleate—an emollient and moisturizer with wetting and pigment-binding properties.

isodecyl paraben—a preservative.

isododecane—a solvent.

isoeugenol—a volatile oil fraction derived from eugenol, it is also found in ylang-ylang and nutmeg oils. Used in cosmetics as a fragrance or to mask odor.

isoflavones—a family of phytoestrogens related to flavonoids. Clinical studies also indicate an antiaging application, given its ability to inhibit the chemical process leading to collagen degradation in the skin. Some sources cite antioxidant and anti-inflammatory properties as well. Among commonly used isoflavones are genistein, genistin, glycitein, glycitin, orobol, and prunetin. Generally isolated from soy, isoflavones used commercially are also obtained from red clover.

isoflavonoids—a family of ingredients derived from isoflavones. Isoflavonoids have demonstrated antioxidant properties through UV protection and some might also be immunoprotective. *See also* isoflavones.

isohexadecane—an excellent, nongreasy emollient.

isononyl isononanoate—an emollient and skin conditioner, it improves skin smoothness and softness.

isoparaffin—a solvent and dilutent.

isoparaffin, C$_{12-14}$—see paraffin.

isoparaffin, C$_{13-14}$—see paraffin.

isoprene glycol—a possible substitute for propylene glycol. It has good humectant properties, rubs nicely on the skin, and does not leave a greasy feeling. Isoprene glycol is also compatible with a variety of other organic chemicals commonly used by cosmetic formulators. Tests show good tolerance with respect to toxicity and irritation.

isopropanol—see isopropyl alcohol.

isopropyl alcohol—a carrier, antibacterial, and solvent for skin care lotions. Isopropyl alcohol is made from propylene, a petroleum derivative.

isopropyl hydroxycetyl ether—an emollient and skin-conditioning ingredient.

isopropyl lauroyl sarcosinate—a neutral amino-acid ester that functions as a skin conditioner.

isopropyl isostearate—an emollient that leaves the skin surface with a smooth and supple finish. It also acts as a binder. Isopropyl isostearate is a derivative of isostearic acid. *See also* stearic acid.

isopropyl lanolate—a skin softener and binder, it aids in the proper spreading of a product. It can also assist in extract penetration, and improve skin feel and texture. A lanolin derivative. *See also* lanolin.

isopropyl methoxycinnamate—a sunscreen chemical that acts as a UV absorber.

isopropyl myristate—an emollient, moisturizer, binder, and skin softener that also assists in product penetration. It is an ester of myristic acid, naturally occurring in coconut oil and nutmeg. Although isopropyl myristate is generally considered comedogenic, some ingredient manufacturers clearly specify noncomedogenicity on their data sheets.

isopropyl palmitate—an emollient and moisturizer, it also acts as a binder and solvent. Similar to isopropyl myristate, it is produced from the combination of palmitic acid (coconut or palm oil) and isopropyl alcohol. Enzymes are able to metabolize this ingredient and studies do not show allergic reactions or toxicity. Some sources indicate a comedogenicity potential.

isopropylbenzyl salicylate—a UV absorber, it is also credited with antioxidant properties that serve to prevent lipid peroxidation. It is found often in moisturizers and antiaging products.

isopropylparaben—a preservative. *See also* propylparaben and parabens.

isopropyl stearate—a binder, emollient, and moisturizer. It leaves the skin with a smooth and supple finish. *See also* stearic acid.

isosorbide monolaurate—lends greaseless emollience to creams, lotions, and stock preparations.

isostearamidopropyl PG dimonium chloride—an emulsifier that leaves the skin with a soft smooth feeling. It is not subject to oxidation or rancidity, and has a very mild toxicological profile.

isostearic acid—an emollient that forms a lipid film on the skin permeable to water vapor, oxygen, and carbon dioxide.

I

Isostearic acid is recommended for use in moisturizing cosmetics. This fatty acid is similar to waxes secreted by birds for feather maintenance.

isostearyl alcohol—an emollient and viscosity builder derived from isostearic acid. It gives the skin a silky feel after product application.

isostearyl isostearate—an emollient resembling jojoba oil. It leaves an almost imperceptible afterfeel. Some sources cite it as comedogenic with a slight irritancy potential. This is a derivative of isostearic acid.

isostearyl neopentanoate—an emollient, binder, and skin-conditioning agent with a moisturizing and softening effect. It has minimal allergenicity potential.

isostearyl stearoyl stearate—an occlusive skin-conditioning agent able to increase the viscosity of a formulation.

isothiazolin 3 one—a mixture that acts as a preservative against bacteria, fungi, and yeast. It is nontoxic at use levels of 0.02 to 0.1 percent although it is severely irritating at concentrations of 1.5 percent.

isotretinoin—a retinoid derivative with improved bioavailability and percutaneous absorption for acne treatment products.

ivy extract (Hedera helix)—said to have a slimming and anti-cellulite effect due to its ability to prevent water accumulation in the skin tissue. Ivy extract is considered antibacterial, astringent, tonic, and soothing, particularly in burn cases. Apparently, ivy also has detergent, antiparasitic, decongestant, and analgesic properties. In addition, ivy is indicated as vasoconstrictive and antiexudative given its vitamin P content and ability to reduce capillary wall permeability. This extract seems to improve massage tolerance of sensitive skin areas as well. It lowers tissue sensitivity, activates circulation, and helps reduce local inflammation. Ivy extract contains saponines, foaming emulsion stabilizers, and surface active agents that assist in ingredient penetration and the emulsification of fats. Ivy is effective as a circulation stimulant in shower gels and in bath salts for "orange peeled" and bloated skin. In herbal medicine, a decoction of ivy leaves was traditionally used to treat various skin eruptions and skin ulcers. Fresh ivy leaves were used to dress wounds and pus-exuding sores.

I

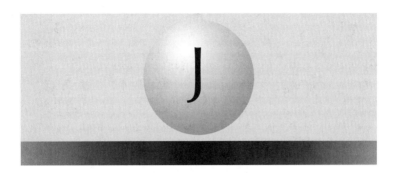

jasmine extract *(Jasminum officinale)*—a fragrance, it is also moisturizing, soothing, and skin conditioning. Some ill-defined and unclear medicinal properties have been attributed to the root extract of several varieties of the 150 jasmine species. These properties include the difficult-to-prove benefit of stimulating the fibroblast with an increase in epidermal cell turnover. Jasmine may cause allergic reactions such as swelling. *See also* jasmine oil.

jasmine oil—fragrance. Credited with moisturizing, soothing, and healing properties. Given these properties, it is indicated for dry and sensitive skins, and also for skin with dermatitis. In truth, there is no essential oil of jasmine. The essence is extracted through a very time-consuming and costly process, making jasmine oil one of the most expensive oils available. This can lead to the use of adulterated versions. Its sweet odor is so delicate and unique that until recently, artificial or synthetic production was believed impossible. Today, synthetic otto of jasmine exists. However, a portion of the natural oil must be added to the synthetic mixture for a satisfactory product. The oil is extracted by a process known as enfleurage. The freshly gathered flowers are sprinkled over oiled glass trays and the flowers are renewed every morning while the plant is in bloom. Finally, the pomade is scraped off the glass, melted at as low a temperature as possible, and then strained. When olive oil is used, the flower petals are placed on coarse cotton cloths previously saturated with the olive oil. The cloths are squeezed under a press, yielding what is termed *huile antique au jasmin*. The oil of jasmine is

J

later separated from the olive oil. Jasmine oil may cause allergic reactions such as swelling—which can last several days.

Job's tears extract—emollient, with anti-inflammatory, tonic, cooling, and calming properties. As a traditional botanical remedy, Job's tears were often used in cases of acne.

jojoba oil *(Simmondsia chinensis)*—a moisturizer and emollient. Jojoba oil was traditionally held in high regard by Native Americans of the Sonora Desert for its cosmetic properties. Mystical properties have been attributed to it for its apparent ability to heal the skin. Jojoba oil reduces transepidermal water loss without completely blocking the transportation of water vapor and gases, providing the skin with suppleness and softness. In addition, it gives cosmetic products excellent spreadability and lubricity. Studies indicate a rapid penetration ability by means of absorption by the pores and hair follicles. From these areas, it seems to diffuse into the stratum corneum layer and acts with intercellular lipids to further reduce water loss. Ingredient manufacturers claim that the chemical composition, functionality, blending ability, appearance, and feel of synthetically produced jojoba oil is the same as the natural oil. Jojoba oil is not a primary skin irritant and does not promote sensitization. Although it is generally considered noncomedogenic, laboratory studies indicate slight-to-moderate comedogenicity depending on the potency of the oil. Jojoba oil is derived from the plant seeds.

jojoba esters—an emollient and skin-conditioning agent made from jojoba oil and jojoba wax. *See also* jojoba oil.

jojoba wax—employed as a natural scrub bead in scrub gels, scrub soaps, and exfoliating products. It is also emollient, used to control product viscosity, and helps improve the skin's look and feel. Jojoba wax is a waxy substance obtained from the jojoba seed.

jonquil—*see* narcissus flower extract.

juniper extract *(Juniperus communis)*—a fragrance, it is also considered a mild skin stimulant. It is believed to help increase epidermal cell turnover. There are some indications that it could also be beneficial for cellulite treatment.

juniper oil—antiseptic, astringent, cleansing, and toning, if used properly. Also credited with good penetration capabilities. Juniper oil is considered helpful in treating acne and good for use with oily skin. It is also indicated for dermatitis and eczema. Obtained from the distillation of the plant's small branches, juniper oil can be irritating in improper amounts. *juniper berry oil*—effective for treating acne. Juniper berry oil has the same properties as those of juniper oil, but it is extracted from the plant's berry rather than its small branches. A distillation of the berries yields the best quality oil.

J

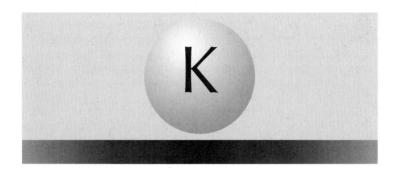

kaolin (China clay)—a mixture of various aluminum silicates. It is often used in powders and masks, given its absorbent, abrasive, bulking, and opacifying properties. This white, soft powder has good coverage and absorption abilities for both water and oil, making it an appropriate absorber of the oil and sweat secreted by the skin. It adheres well to the skin's surface, yet is easily removed with normal cleansing procedures. Kaolin is considered a noncomedogenic raw material.

kaolin China clay—*see* kaolin.

karite (unsaponifiable)—also known as butyrospermum parkii; shea butter. One of a group of vegetable oils with a small molecular structure that is capable of penetrating and possibly becoming involved in the biochemical process of the dermis. It is considered a biological precursor in ceramide synthesis. Karite contains steroidal and triterpenic structures. It is believed that the unsaponifiable fraction of karite can stimulate the dermal fibroblast to synthesize collagen, elastin, proteoglycans, and glycoproteins. *See also* shea butter.

karite butter—*see* shea butter.

kelp—a marine product derived from the giant Pacific kelp. *See* seaweed extract.

keratin—a surface protective agent with film-forming and moisturizing action. Keratin is often used in cosmetics for its moisture retention and protective effect. *See also* protein.

keratin amino acids—a mixture of amino acids obtained from the complete hydrolysis of keratin. *See also* amino acids; keratin.

K

khus-khus—*see* vetiver oil.

kiwi powder—used in scrubs for its abrasive properties. Obtained from ground kiwi seeds.

kojic acid—a skin-lightening agent. Kojic acid is a tyrosinase inhibitor, although it is not as effective as licorice extract. When combined with allantoin and other proper ingredients in sunscreen preparations, the mixture can inhibit UV-caused erythema and accelerate wound healing. It is also found to be skin sensitizing and can be irritating.

kojic acid dipalmitate—preparations containing kojic acid dipalmitate are said to inhibit UV-induced erythema. *See also* kojic acid.

kojic acid monostearate—a kojic acid derivative said to inhibit tyrosinase, and thus the formation of melanin. Kojic acid monostearate is used in skin-lightening preparations. *See also* kojic acid.

kola extract (*Cola acuminata*)—largely known for its stimulating, astringent, and healing properties, research has also established anti-inflammatory and anti-irritant properties. This extract may be used for dressing wounds. Kola extract is also somewhat effective for preventing viable epidermal penetration of certain substances. It has a high content of caffeine and other stimulants. The extract is obtained from the kola nut.

krameria triandra root extract—manufacturers note an ability to modulate stress-related hormone production in the epidermis. Therapeutic benefits include anti-inflammatory, free-radical scavenging, antiaging and an ability to protect against lipid peroxidation. Beneficial for red, chapped, and stressed skin. The plant is native to Peru.

kukui nut oil (*Aleurites moluccana*) (candlenut)—the kukui nut tree was used by early Hawaiians to soothe cuts and burns and to help protect the skin from damage due to sun and surf. Kukui nut oil is reported to have excellent penetration properties, to aid in soothing and moisturizing the skin, and relieve chapped skin and irritations. This oil does not leave the skin with a greasy afterfeel. Kukui nut oil is apparently an excellent treatment for psoriasis and eczema, and is also beneficial for acne and other common skin disorders. In addition, it is a sunscreen solubilizer that reduces the greasy feel often associated with sun products. Studies indicate possible natural sunscreen capabilities of its own, and when

K

used with other sunscreens, may enhance a formulation's efficacy. Native to Hawaii, the nuts and kernels are roasted and then pressed for their clear oil, which has a high linoleic and linoleic acid content. It is usually supplemented and stabilized with vitamins A, C, and E.

K

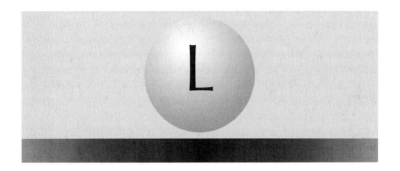

lactamide MEA—a surfactant that can also act as a thickener, foam booster, and stabilizer.

lactic acid (sodium lactate)—a multipurpose ingredient used as a preservative, exfoliant, and moisturizer, and to provide acidity to a formulation. In the body, lactic acid is found in the blood and muscle tissue as a product of the metabolism of glucose and glycogen. It is also a component of the skin's natural moisturizing factor. Lactic acid is an alpha hydroxyacid occurring in sour milk and other lesser-known sources, such as beer, pickles, and other foods made through a process of bacterial fermentation. Lactic acid has better water intake than glycerin. Studies indicate an ability to increase the water-retention capacity of the stratum corneum. They also show that the pliability of the corneum layer is closely related to the absorption of lactic acid; that is, the greater the amount of absorbed lactic acid, the more pliable the corneum layer. Investigations report that continuous use of preparations formulated with lactic acid in concentrations ranging between 5 and 12 percent provided a mild to moderate improvement in fine wrinkling and promote softer, smoother skin. Lactic acid is caustic when applied to the skin in highly concentrated solutions. *See also* alpha hydroxy acid.

lactobacillus/papaya fruit ferment extract—a papaya extract obtained through a fermentation process using lactobacillus as the fermenting agent. Lactobacillus is a "friendly bacteria" that is naturally occurring in the body and that is used in the fermentation process for certain foods, such as yogurt and sour milk. *See* papaya enzyme.

L

197

lactobacillus/solanum lycopersicum (tomato) fruit ferment extract—considered antioxidant, antiaging, and able to provide long-term skin conditioning activity. This is a filtrate obtained through a fermentation process using lactobacillus as the fermenting agent. Lactobacillus is a "friendly bacteria" that is naturally occurring in the body, and used in the fermentation process for certain foods, such as yogurt and sour milk. *See also* tomato.

lactobacillus/Theobroma cacao fruit ferment filtrate—helps reduce inflammation.

lady's mantle extract (Alchemilla vulgaris) (alchemilla)—said to have UV-absorption ability for both the UVA and UVB spectrums. Other properties include anti–free radical, healing, and anti-inflammatory. It is effective in acne treatment products. Herbalists considered lady's mantle extract to be one of the best wound-healing herbs, and credit it with an ability to dry wounds, reduce inflammation, and promote quicker healing. Though the root was seldom used, an extract of fresh root was considered valuable to stop all bleedings. The active constituents of this perennial plant include tannins, rendering it effective against irritation, itching, and skin burns. Lady's mantle extract contains silicon/silicic acid, and it is reported that when combined with eyebright and horsetail, they all work synergistically to strengthen connective tissue.

lady's thistle extract—*see* milk thistle.

Laminaria saccharina extract—a member of the kelp family. *See* seaweed extract.

laneth-10—an emulsifier that is particularly effective when working with lanolin, it is also used as a surfactant for improving product spreadability and to control product viscosity. This is the polyethylene glycol ether of lanolin alcohol.

laneth-10-acetate—an emulsifier with emollient properties. This is the acetylated ester of an ethoxylated ether of lanolin alcohol.

lanolide—a vegetable-derived substitute for lanolin. It is believed to be a good replacement because of its absence of pesticides, antiparasitic constituents, and heavy metals. These can be present in lanolin and have caused quite a few problems in the cosmetic industry.

lanolin—an emollient with moisturizing properties and an emulsifier with high water-absorption capabilities. It has

L

been found to form a network on the skin's surface rather than a film, as is the case with petrolatum (Vaseline). While long-term studies associate a low incidence of allergic reactions to lanolin, it remains a controversial ingredient based on a potential pesticide content and potential comedogenicity. There is a move among high-quality lanolin manufacturers to produce low-pesticide lanolin and among high-quality cosmetic formulators and manufacturers to use the purist form available. With respect to comedogenicity, this ascribed property is increasingly debated as some researchers believe it to be inaccurate, especially when lanolin is used in an emulsion. Lanolin is a sheep's wool derivative formed by a fat-like viscous secretion of the sheep's sebaceous glands. Some consider it a natural wax.

lanolin (hydrogenated)—a lanolin derivative. *See also* lanolin.

lanolin USP (modified)—an emollient and an emulsifier. This is a highly purified lanolin meeting USP monograph specifications that require analysis for trace contaminants. *See also* lanolin.

lanolin acetate—a lanolin derivative. *See also* lanolin.

lanolin alcohol—widely used as an emulsifier and emollient in water-in-oil systems. It absorbs a considerable amount of water that is then slowly released for moisturization purposes. Lanolin alcohol is a mixture of organic alcohols obtained from the hydrolysis of lanolin. It may cause skin sensitivity and allergic reactions.

lanolin oil—a lanolin derivative. This is the liquid fraction of lanolin obtained by physical means from whole lanolin. *See also* lanolin.

lanolin wax—a lanolin derivative. This is the semisolid fraction of lanolin obtained by physical means from whole lanolin. *See also* lanolin.

lanolin derivatives—a mixture of unspecified lanolin-derived products. *See also* lanolin.

lappa extract—*see* burdock extract.

Lapsana cummunis extract (hawk's bread; crepin)—skin protective and antioxidant properties are attributed to extracts from the whole *Lapsana* family, and particularly to the *cummunis* species. Formulations with this extract are said to have antiaging and antiwrinkle activity. It has also demonstrated an ability to protect the skin against free-radical damage. Other properties include antiseptic and disinfectant.

L

lasilium—*see* sodium lacate methylsilanol.

lauramide DEA (lauric acid diethanolamide)—a thickener, foam stabilizer, and viscosity builder in cosmetic formulations. It is added to liquid detergents and cleansers of the lauryl sulfate-type to help stabilize the lather and improve foam formation.

laurel (Laurus nobilis) (bay laurel)—when used in oil form, it is said to have antiseptic and astringent properties. This would make it effective for healing and skin problems. The oil is pressed from the berries and leaves.

laureth-2—a surfactant and emulsifying ingredient. It is the polyethylene glycol ether of lauryl alcohol. Increasing the number of moles (laureth-3, laureth-7, and so on) usually makes the product milder. *See also* lauryl alcohol.

laureth-3—a surfactant, detergent, and emulsifier used in cosmetic preparations. *See also* lauryl alcohol.

laureth-7—a wetting agent also used as an emulsifier, surfactant, detergent, and solubilizer for active substances. *See also* lauryl alcohol.

laureth-12—a surfactant, detergent, and emulsifier in cosmetic formulations. *See also* lauryl alcohol.

laureth-23—an emulsifier used with more frequency in oil-in-water than water-in-oil emulsions, though it is effective in both. It is also an emulsion stabilizer and can act as a surfactant. Laureth-23 may cause very minor irritation to skin and eyes. *See also* lauryl alcohol.

lauric acid (n-dodecanoic acid)—due to its foaming properties, its derivatives are widely used as a base in the manufacture of soaps, detergents, and lauryl alcohol. Lauric acid is a common constituent of vegetable fats, especially coconut oil and laurel oil. It is a mild irritant but not a sensitizer, and some sources cite it as comedogenic.

lauric acid diethanolamide—*see* lauramide DEA.

lauroamphocarboxyglycinate—an organic cleansing agent that removes oil and dirt, but that can be slightly irritating to the skin.

lauroamphodiacetate—a mild cleansing agent.

lauroyl methionine lysinate—a free-radical scavenger used in antiaging skin care cosmetics.

lauroyl lysine—an amino acid that also serves as a skin-conditioning agent. *See also* lysine.

L

lauryl alcohol—used in chemical formulations for a variety of purposes, including as an emulsion stabilizer, a skin-conditioning emollient, and a viscosity-increasing agent.

lauryl aminopropylglycine—a skin-conditioning agent.

lauryl betaine—a skin-conditioning agent. In hair care, it is used as an antistatic conditioning agent and a foam booster.

lauryl diethylenediaminoglycine—a skin-conditioning ingredient that appears to have greater application in hair formulations, where it is reported to work as an antistatic agent.

lauryl glucoside—a mild surfactant.

lauryl lactate—an emollient, detergent/emulsifier, and surfactant used in cosmetic formulations.

lauryl methyl gluceth-10 hydroxypropyl dimonium chloride—benefits include anti-irritancy, conditioning, humectancy, and moisturization.

laurylmethicone copolyol—an emulsifier with excellent waterproof properties when used in the proper concentration and with other emulsifiers.

lauryl PCA—an emulsifier that has good affinity with skin lipids. It can increase a product's moisturizing action by decreasing transepidermal water loss. Lauryl PCA is a lipophilic moisturizer with a delayed and remnant effect. Also used as a thickener or viscosity-control agent, it is derived from natural raw materials. This is the lauric ester of PCA.

lauryl sarcosine—a surfactant for cosmetic formulations.

lavender flower oil—the principal constituent of lavender is the volatile oil, of which the dried flowers contain 1.5 to 3 percent; fresh flowers yield about 0.5 percent. Lavender flower oil is pale yellow, yellowish-green, or nearly colorless. Oil distilled from the earliest flowers is pale and contains a higher proportion of the more valuable esters. The oil distilled from later flowers has a preponderance of the less valuable ester and is darker in color. Lavender oil owes its delicate perfume primarily to its esters. In the oil, there are two esters that practically control the scent. Of these, the principal one is linalyl acetate; the second is linalyl butyrate. Other esters present include geraniol, linalool, and limonene. *See also* lavender oil.

lavender green oil—see lavender flower oil; lavender oil.

lavender oil (Lavandula officinalis)—a fragrance. Lavender oil is considered an all-purpose oil credited with many therapeutic

L

properties. These include antiallergenic, anti-inflammatory, antiseptic, antibacterial, antispasmodic, balancing, energizing, soothing, healing, tonic, and stimulating. In addition, it is said to help clean small wounds after washing and regulate skin functions. It may also have insect repellent properties. Lavender oil works well on all skin types and produces excellent results when used for oily skin as well as in the treatment of acne, burns (sunburns as well as other superficial and nonextensive types), dermatitis, eczema, and psoriasis. Its benefit to the dermis is immediate since it is easily and rapidly absorbed by the skin. Lavender oil is said to normalize any skin type and to stimulate cellular growth and regeneration. When added to other oils, lavender can enhance and balance their effect. Lavender is also claimed to help relieve stress, and as such, is believed to be useful in treating skin problems caused or aggravated by stress. The known use of this oil extends at least to the Roman era, when it was a popular additive to baths. It derived its name from this practice and from the Roman word *lavare,* meaning to wash. The oil's main component is linalool acetate; other actives include geraniol, borneol, ocimene, and pinene. Lavender oil is distilled by using the flower tops and stalks. It is generally considered nontoxic, nonsensitizing, and nonirritating.

lawsone with dihydroxyacetone—one of the 21 FDA-approved sunscreen chemicals and listed as a Category I UVB-absorber. Its approved usage level is 3 percent. Dihydroxyacetone (DHA) alone is used as a self-tanning agent in self-tanning products. DHA and lawsone together act as a sunscreen.

lecithin—a natural emollient, emulsifier, antioxidant, and spreading agent, lecithin is a hydrophilic ingredient that attracts water and acts as a moisturizer. Generally obtained for cosmetic products from eggs and soybeans, it is found in all living organisms.

lecithin (hydrogenated)—an emulsifier.

lemon balm—*see* balm mint oil.

lemon bioflavonoids extract—obtained by extraction of oil rind. *See also* bioflavonoids; lemon extract.

lemon extract (Citrus limonum)—its botanical properties are described as antibacterial, antiseptic, astringent, and toning. It is also perfuming. Lemon extract is suggested for treating sunburn, acne problems, and oily skin. This extract contains citric acid and vitamins B and C. It can cause irritation and allergic reactions.

L

lemon oil—as one of the most versatile essential oils in aromatherapy, it is considered a counterirritant, antiseptic, blood purifier, and lymphatic stimulant. The volatile oil is obtained from the fresh peel of *Citrus limon* (citrus lemon) that contains an essential oil and a bitter principle. Crystals of the glucoside hesperidin are deposited by the evaporation of the white, pulpy portion when boiled in water. Diluted acids decompose it into hesperidin and glucose. The oil is more fragrant and valuable if obtained by expression rather than distillation. Lemon oil can cause an allergic reaction.

lemon peel—*see* lemon oil.

lemongrass oil *(Cymbopogon citratus)*—considered astringent and tonic, it has also exhibited antifungal properties. It is widely used in the perfume and soap industries. Lemongrass oil is the volatile oil distilled from the leaves of the lemon grasses.

lettuce extract *(Lactuca virosa)*—said to have emollient properties in its fresh state, but after processing for use in cosmetics, this property is unlikely to be retained. Herbologists attribute a sedative, narcotic property to lettuce extract. It is obtained from wild lettuce (not the garden and salad variety), a plant growing to a maximum height of six feet. The whole pant is rich in milky juice that flows freely from any cut made to it.

lichen extract—a preservative that can be used against certain types of bacteria, fungi, and yeast. It also contributes to the activity of other preservatives. Lichen extract is a water-free, natural, active agent extracted from alpine lichen. Nontoxic and nonirritating to skin.

licorice extract *(Glycyrrhiza glabra)*—considered an anti-irritant, studies indicate an ability to absorb UVA and UVB rays. Studies also conclude that licorice extract has a depigmenting effect as well as an inhibitory effect on melanin synthesis due to its ability to act as a tyrosinase inhibitor. As a depigmenting agent, licorice extract is described as more effective than kojic acid and 75 times more effective than ascorbic acid. The chief constituent of licorice root is glycyrrhizin, present in concentrations that range from 5 to 24 percent depending on the variety of licorice used. A member of the bean family, licorice's pharmacological properties are found in the plant's roots and stem.

licorice root extract—*see* licorice extract.

L

lily extract—there are almost 100 different known varieties of lilies to which antiseptic and skin-clearing properties are generally ascribed. Herbalists have also credited the Madonna lily variety with demulcent (soothing) and astringent properties. The extract, obtained from the bulbs of this variety, is used primarily for its emollient, healing, soothing, and anti-inflammatory action. The extract from leaves and roots of the white pond lily variety has been described as astringent, healing, and anti-inflammatory.

lime blossom extract—perfuming. It is also an emollient with soothing and antiseptic properties. Lime blossom extract is a source of vitamin C. It can cause adverse reactions when the skin is exposed to sunlight.

lime oil (Citrus acida, Citrus aurantifolia)—has similar properties and uses as lemon oil. Lime oil is extracted from lime skin by cold pressure or distillation. *See also* lemon oil.

lime tree extract—the main extract from the lime tree is the one obtained from the blossoms. Some extract may also be obtained from leaves and sap. Lime tree extract is sometimes referred to as linden. *See also* linden extract.

d-limonene—used for perfuming and to mask odor, it is a chemical constituent of citrus oil. *See* lemon oil.

linalool—a fragrant component of both lavender and coriander. It can be incorporated into cosmetics for perfuming, deodorant, or odor-masking activity.

linden extract (Tilia sp.)—extract from the bark can be used to help problem or blemished skin, and is considered refreshing and soothing to the skin. Linden extract can also be obtained from linden blossoms and is credited with antiseptic, skin-clearing, soothing, sedative, circulation-stimulating, hydrating, and astringent properties. Linden extract may be used effectively in creams and emulsions for irritated skin, as well as in bath salts for the relaxation of muscle tension and cold. In oil form, linden may be used for its odor-masking properties as well as a skin conditioner.

linoleamide DEA—a highly effective thickener. It enhances product slip and feel, and is also a conditioner, stabilizer, and viscosity builder. *See also* linoleic acid.

linoleamidopropyl PG-dimonium chloride phosphate—a vegetable-derived emulsifier. It leaves the skin with a smooth afterfeel. It is nonirritating.

linoleic acid (vitamin F)—also known as omega-6. An emulsifier, it is also cleansing, emollient, and skin conditioning. Some

L

formulations incorporate it as a surfactant. Linoleic acid prevents dryness and roughness. A deficiency of linoleic acid in the skin is associated with symptoms similar to those characterizing eczema, psoriasis, and a generally poor skin condition. In numerous laboratory studies where a linoleic acid deficiency was induced, a topical application of linoleic acid in its free or esterified form quickly reversed this condition. In addition, linoleic acid is being found to inhibit melanin production in laboratory tests by decreasing tyrosinase activity and suppressing melanin polymer formation within melanosomes. Linoleic acid is an essential fatty acid found in a variety of plant oils, including soybean and sunflower.

linoleic acid ethylester—*see* ethyl linoleate.

linoleic acid triglyceride—an emollient and good penetrating agent, it is not widely used because its unsaturated nature creates rancidity problems.

linolenic acid—also known as alpha-linolenic acid; omega-3. An essential fatty acid found in most drying oils. It is slightly irritating to the mucous membranes. It may be used in a cosmetic preparation for any of the following broad uses: antistatic, cleansing, emollient, skin conditioning and surfactant properties.

linolenic acid triglyceride—an emollient of limited use due to potential rancidity problems. It is a good penetrating agent.

linseed oil—its botanical properties are listed as emollient, antiinflammatory, and healing. Derived from the flax plant seed, the oil is obtained by expression with little or no heat.

lipid concentrate—a vague description, as it does not refer to the lipid's origin or source. Lipids, when added to the skin, are considered moisturizers. They renew the skin's barrier function and reduce moisture loss.

lipohydroxy acid—also known as LHA. *See* beta-lipohydroxy acid.

liposomes—extremely small, double layer, hollow, spherical, phospholipid membrane vesicles able to encapsulate water-soluble as well as oil-soluble substances. Their compatibility and affinity with cellular membranes allows them to be easily accepted and metabolized by the skin, and provide the skin with "actives" that would not be so readily accepted otherwise. Liposome effectiveness is measured by their ability to deliver encapsulated actives ingredients to target sites. By varying the type of phospholipids used to

L

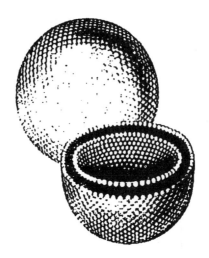

Liposomes

make liposomes and/or by attaching certain molecules to the surface of liposomes, they can be engineered to have many useful properties, which include: releasing their active content upon reaching the target site; protecting ingredients from acidic and enzymatic degradation before reaching the target site; protecting compounds from premature oxidation; targeting certain tissues or cell types; acting as time releasers of valuable actives. In addition to their carrier abilities and penetration properties, liposomes provide the upper stratum corneum with a pleasant and smooth feeling. Liposomes are predominantly formed by phospholipids of natural, semisynthetic, and/or synthetic origin. Liposomes have brought to the cosmetic field widespread interest in the concepts of microencapsulation and targeted substance delivery.

liquid paraffin—*see* paraffin.

liquorice extract—*see* licorice extract.

liquorice root extract—*see* licorice extract.

live yeast cell derivative—*see* tissue respiratory factor.

lovage oil (Levisticum officinale)—ascribed properties include cleansing, depurative, and draining. Lovage oil is appropriate for use on oily skin. In addition, the roots and fruit have aromatic and stimulant activity. This oil is produced by distillation of the roots, though the leaves and seeds are also used for therapeutic purposes.

L

lupine amino acids—reported to have excellent hydrating capabilities, lupine amino acids are often found in moisturizers, cleansers, and washes. Derived from the seeds of *Lupinus albus*. *See also* lupine extract.

lupine extract (Lupinus albus)—research attributes a number of physiological benefits to lupine extract, impacting both the stratum corneum and the epidermis. Generally, lupine extract appears to enhance cellular activity (evidence indicates that it may penetrate down to the basal layer) and thicken the epidermis and stratum corneum. It strengthens the epidermal structure by stimulating the production of epidermal proteins, notably filaggrin (which promotes keratin synthesis) and epidermal lipids, including ceramides, cholesterol, and di- and triglycerides. Studies also indicate an improvement and/or restoration of the stratum corneum's barrier function, resulting in reduced transepidermal water loss. This might be attributed to lupine's ability to promote protein and lipid production. Lupine extract is rich in oligosaccharides and low molecular-weight peptides that are high in glutamic acid. It may be particularly beneficial when used in combination with such moisturizing ingredients as lactic acid. Lupine extract is most likely to be found in skin restructuring, repairing, and hydrating preparations. *See also* lupine amino acids.

lysine—a skin conditioning amino acid. *See also* amino acid.

lysine PCA—increases cellular oxygen intake and improves moisturization. Lysine PCA is also used as a neutralizing agent and pH buffer in skin care formulations.

lysine carboxymethyl cysteinate—a water-soluble amino acid complex with the ability to regulate oil secretion.

lysine lauroyl methionate—an amino acid that acts to improve the skin's look, feel, and overall condition.

L

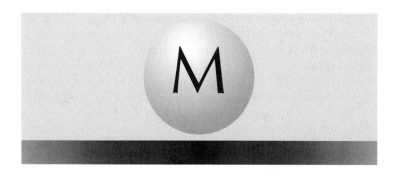

MI/MCI (methylchloroisothiazolinone)—a preservative that works against bacteria and fungi. In 2005, it was the tenth most commonly used preservative. However, it is associated with a sensitizing potential, including allergic reactions, in products intended to stay on the skin (for example, night creams). Its recommended concentration levels range from 7.5 ppm (parts per million) for leave-on products to 15 ppm for rinse-off preparations such as soaps and cleansers. However, MI/MCI in concentrations as low as 7 ppm may induce sensitization.

macadamia nut oil (Macadamia integrifolia)—a carrier and an emollient with excellent spreadability, lubrication, and penetration properties. It is moisturizing, leaves a good, smooth, nongreasy afterfeel, and is very gentle to the skin. Its fatty acid composition is similar to the major fatty acid composition of skin sebum, including some of the acids that are crucial to maintaining the skin's water-barrier functions. Macadamia nut oil is beneficial in skin softening and nourishing preparations. It is also useful in products for mature and/or dry skin due to its palmitoleic acid content (up to 20 percent). Palmitoleic acid is a naturally occurring fatty acid produced by the sebaceous glands, the production of which decreases with age. The nut's weight is 70 to 80 percent oil, specifically triglyceride oil and palmitoleic oil. It is very cosmetically stable with low rancidity, and naturally contains tocopherols. The macadamia (nut) tree is grown primarily in Australia and the Hawaiian Islands.

Macrocystis pyrifera extract—also known as bladder kelp. *See* kelp; seaweed extract.

Madonna lily—*see* white lily bulb extract.

magnesium—plays an important role in various processes within the skin, including amino acid synthesis, the synthesis of proteins (e.g., collagen), and in the metabolism of calcium, sodium, and phosphorus.

magnesium aluminum silicate—a thickener with texture-modification and emulsion-stabilizing abilities, as well as astringent properties. This is a refined and purified smectite clay. It is noncomedogenic and nontoxic.

magnesium ascorbyl phosphate (magnesium-1-ascorbyl-2-phosphate)—a stabilized, synthetically derived version of vitamin C. It is reported to be equally as effective as vitamin C in regulating collagen biosynthesis, and as an antioxidant. *See also* vitamin C.

magnesium aspartate—used in a cosmetic to improve skin condition, look, and feel. Some manufacturers note an ability to promote the adhesion of basal layer cells to the dermal–epidermal junction and in particular to the collagen found there. It would be used in antiaging and antiwrinkle cosmetics.

magnesium laureth sulfate—a mild surfactant and cleansing agent.

magnesium silicate—*see* talc.

magnesium sulfate—an inorganic salt used as a bulking agent in cosmetic preparations.

maize germ oil—*see* corn oil.

maize gluten amino acids—*see* corn amino acids.

maleated soya bean oil—*see* soybean oil.

malic acid—the third smallest alpha hydroxyacid in terms of molecular size. While it is used in numerous cosmetic products, particularly those indicating a "fruit acid" content and generally designed for antiaging, unlike glycolic and lactic acids, its skin benefits have not been extensively studied. Some formulators consider it difficult to work with, particularly when compared to other AHAs, and it can be somewhat irritating. It is rarely used as the only AHA in a product. Found naturally occurring in apples. *See also* alpha hydroxyacid.

mallow extract (Malva sylvestris)—anti-inflammatory, soothing, refreshing, emollient, and wound-healing properties are attributed to this ingredient. Mallow extract has a high mucilage content that, when in contact with water, swells and forms a soft, soothing, protective gel. It is beneficial in eye treatment preparations. The extract is often derived from the leaves and flowers of *Malva sylvestris*, generally known as blue, common, or high mallow, although it can be obtained from other types of mallow such as marsh, musk, dwarf, and tree-sea.

M

malpighia glabra fruit extract—*see* acerola.

malt extract—has rubefacient properties in cosmetics due to the presence of yeast. It is used in face masks and toning lotions as a nutrient and texturizer. Malt extract is a dark syrup obtained by evaporating an aqueous extract of partially germinated and dried barley seeds.

maltodextrin—a polysaccharide obtained most often from corn, potato, or rice starch. It is considered absorbent, and skin conditioning. It can also be employed as an emulsion stabilizer and/or a film former. Maltodextrin is incorporated into a variety of cosmetic preparations, including face powders, makeup, creams, lotions, gels, and soaps.

malva—a traditional emollient and moisturizer. Malva is part of the mallow family. *See also* mallow extract.

mandarin extract—has similar properties to those of orange extract. Obtained from mandarin orange peel. *See also* orange extract.

mandarin oil—its botanical properties are very close to those of orange, with mandarin's sedative and antispasmodic properties being more pronounced. Expressed from the peel of mandarin oranges.

manganese—as an oligoelement, manganese plays a role in collagen synthesis and skin moisturizing. Patents have been assigned on the use of manganese, zinc, and copper in the treatment of acne and sunburns. It can also be used as a colorant, providing a violet color to a product.

manganese aspartate—a skin conditioner, this is the combination of L-aspartic acid and manganese salt.

manganese gluconate—a skin conditioner used to improve or maintain the skin's texture and feel.

mango (Mangifera indica)—associated with various benefits, including antioxidant properties and skin softening and smoothing thanks to natural enzymatic activity. When listed simply as mango, it is difficult to identify which

M

part of the plant is used. This limits a full understanding of why the plant was selected for a cosmetic formula. While mango fruit is considered astringent in a cosmetic, the extract of both the fruit and leaf are skin conditioning. Mango seed is abrasive and hence used in scrubs, while the seed oil is emollient. Thus, more specific information as to the form or portion of the plant used is necessary to determine function in the cosmetic formulation.

mango butter—emollient, moisturizing, and anti-inflammatory. It could also promote cellular rejuvenation. Mango butter demonstrates some ability to protect against UV rays and appears to release salicylic acid. Constituents include tocopherol, phytosterols, olein, and fatty acids (including stearic and oleic acids). Mango butter is very stable when exposed to oxygen, and can replace paraffin-based emollients. Studies have indicated overall consumer preference for lotions containing mango butter over those using avocado butter or apricot kernel oil. Obtained from the kernel within the mango stone. Used in skin care cosmetics, sun and post-sun products, hair conditioners, and shampoos.

mannuronate methylsilanol—see methylsilanol mannuronate.

margosa oil—considered a healing oil for its antiseptic and sebum-regulating properties.

marigold extract (Calendula officinalis)—the general effects attributed to marigold extract include antiseptic, healing, and soothing. It is useful in eye treatment cosmetics. In addition, it may be used against sunburns and other superficial burns due to some emollient capabilities. Traditionally, marigold extract was used to heal skin rashes and to clean minor wounds after washing. Marigold extract's constituents include flavonoids, glycosides of oleanoic acid, carotenoids, and phenolic acid. Marigold is also a source of carotenoids, particularly lutein and zeaxanthin. The recommended usage level for this extract is 1 to 10 percent. The extract is obtained from the flowers. See also xanthophylls.

marine plasma extract—may help in organizing the structure of connective tissue. It is considered healing due to its iodine content, which is present in a natural form complexed with algal peptides and polysaccharides. This makes it a more active and gentler product when applied to the skin. This extract contains plasma (the fluid part of the tissue from which suspended matter such as cells has been removed), vitamins, polysaccharides, essential sea minerals, and some cellular reagents. Trace minerals also include calcium, iron, magnesium, potassium, sodium, and silicon. Vitamin A, water-soluble vitamin B, vitamin C, pantothenic acid, and niacinamide are also present. Marine plasma extract is a trade name for a mixture that combines brown algae and marine animals. It is obtained by extracting the liquid from the cellular mass of marine organisms. Not known to cause skin irritation.

M

marine seaweed extract—*see* algae extract; seaweed extract.

marine sediments—an all-encompassing name for an unspecified marine-based compound. *See also* algae extract; marine plasma extract; seaweed extract.

marjoram (Origanum vulgare)—described as tonic and antifungal. Although there are numerous species of marjoram, sweet marjoram and wild marjoram are the most popular for botanical applications. Similar properties are reported for both. *See also* marjoram oil.

marjoram oil—its ascribed botanical properties include antispasmodic, calming, and sedative—indicating applications for sensitive or irritated skin. The oil is obtained through distillation. It may cause allergic reactions expressed as skin redness and itching.

marshmallow extract (Althea officinalis)—emollient and soothing. It can be pain relieving, especially in the case of burns, sunburns, or scrapes. In traditional medicine, marshmallow extract was used as a local adjunct soothing and anti-itching agent for dermatological treatments. In folklore, it has been used for rough skin, scruff, dry scabs, burns, scalds, and swelling. *See also* althea extract; mallow extract.

marshmallow root extract—*see* althea extract; marshmallow extract.

matricaria extract—an extract of the flowerheads of Matricaria chamomilla. *See also* chamomile extract.

matrimony vine (Lycium barbarum)—also known as goji berry, wolfberry. Credited with astringent, skin conditioning, antioxidant, tonic, and antibacterial properties. Constituents include vitamins A, C, and E, and essential fatty acids. In cosmetic preparations, it is either the fruit extract or the seed oil which is used.

Mauritia flexuosa fruit oil—*see* buriti pulp oil.

meadowfoam oil (Lamnanthes alba)—a rich emollient. This mild, stable oil is resistant to oxidation. It is of much interest to

M

cosmetic formulators because of its "dryness" and quick penetration into the skin. When combined with shea butter, the mixture acts as an emollient and emulsifier, and can serve as a lanolin replacement. The oil is extracted from the meadowfoam seeds that contain 20 to 30 percent oil by weight.

meadowsweet extract *(Filipendula ulmaria* **or** *Spirea ulmaria)*—appears to have strong anti-free radical properties, as well as aromatic, astringent, analgesic and topical anti-inflammatory activity. The anti-free radical activity is attributed to its flavonoid and tannin content; the anti-inflammatory and analgesic properties are due to nonvolatile salicylate derivatives, including salicylic acid and methyl salicylate. Gallic acid is another constituent. Its analgesic, anti-inflammatory, and anti-free radical activity make it particularly useful in sun care preparations. The word *aspirin* is derived from this plant's Latin name: *a* from acetyl and *spirin* from *Spireae*. Meadowsweet is a perennial plant that grows abundantly at the edges of rivers and ditches in meadows and damp woods.

medanione—used as a preservative in emollients. This is a synthetic ingredient with the properties of vitamin K. Used medically to prevent blood clotting.

medlar *(Mespilus sp.)*—a fruit-bearing tree that is related to pear and hawthorn. Constituents are said to include carotenes and vitamins A, B, and C. Used in antiaging cosmetics.

melanin—a water-soluble form of melanin that can be formulated into a product as a free-radical scavenger. Melanin can be naturally extracted from cuttlefish ink or synthetically produced. Research indicates that when employed as a sunscreen, melanin provides better UVA protection and requires lower usage concentrations than other available sunscreens. Its safety is supported through studies conducted with radioactive melanin, which showed no penetration through human skin.

melhydran—increases the skin's moisture-binding capacities. This is a concentrated and purified extract of Provence honey from thyme, lavender, and rosemary. It can also be produced synthetically.

melaleuca—*See* cajeput oil.

melilot *(Melilotus officinalis)* **(sweet clover; white clover)**—credited with emollient, bactericidal, sedative, and virustatic properties. Traditionally, it was used on a couperose

M

condition. Coumarin is melilot's only important constituent. Its related compounds are hydrocoumaric (melilotic) acid, orthocoumaric acid, and melilotic anhydride (lactone), which is a fragrant oil. There are several species of this perennial herb. The whole herb is used for botanical purposes.

melissa *(Melissa officinalis)*—*see* balm mint extract.

melissa oil—*see* balm mint oil.

menhaden oil—contains essential fatty acids vital to the metabolism of healthy skin. The oil is obtained from the small North Atlantic menhaden fish, which is a little larger than a herring.

menthol—a fragrance. It is also said to be antiseptic, cooling, refreshing, and a blood-circulation stimulant. Menthol gives the skin a "cool" feeling after use. It constitutes almost 50 percent of peppermint oil but can also be made synthetically by hydrogenation of thymol. It is nontoxic in low doses, but in high concentrations it can be irritating to the skin, especially the mucous membranes. *See also* mint.

menthol extract—*see* menthol.

menthol methyl lactate—cooling and used also as a fragrance.

menthyl anthranilate—the only FDA-approved liquid sunscreen chemical with UVA-absorption capabilities. It has an approved usage level of 3.5 to 5 percent. This is a stable ingredient and can be combined with other sunscreen chemicals to increase SPF while providing UVA protection.

menthyl lactate—a fragrance component. This is the ester of menthol and lactic acid.

mercaptopyridine—used in skin-lightening preparations due to its ability to retard melanin production and provide a skin-lightening effect.

mercurials—a category of preservative with a high sensitizing potential, particularly in products intended to be left on the skin. They are used in minute amounts as a preservative in some eye makeup preparations to inhibit bacterial proliferation.

methicone—a type of silicone used primarily in the formulation of free-flowing cosmetic powders. Methicone can also be found in cosmetic preparations as a skin surface sealant to reduce transepidermal water loss.

methionin—*see* methionine.

methionine—slows down and normalizes oil gland sebum production. Methionine is also used as a texturizer in cosmetic

M

creams. It is an essential amino acid found in a number of proteins and obtained by means of fermentation.

methoxy PEG-22 dodecyl glycol copolymer—an effective water-in-oil emulsifier with a high water-binding capability. This ingredient has good dermatological and toxicological properties, and is very compatible with other skin care ingredients. This facilitates its incorporation into cosmetic preparations.

4-methoxybenzoic acid—*see* anisic acid (p-anisic acid).

3,1-methoxypropane-1,2 diol—provides a cool sensation when used in facial masks.

methoxy propyl gluconamide—an alpha hydroxyacid derivative used as a moisturizer and an emollient. Its minimal acidity favors its use on dry and very dry, scaly skin surfaces, where other alpha hydroxyacid compounds may not be well tolerated.

methyl dihydroxybenzoate—*see* methyl gentisate.

methyl gentisate—also known as methyl dihydroxybenzoate. A skin-lightening ingredient that acts by inhibiting the melanocyte's production of tyrosinase. Can be naturally obtained from gentian root. *See also* gentian.

methyl gluceth-10—a skin humectant and a preservative. This is the polyethylene glycol ether of methyl glucose.

methyl gluceth-20—a humectant skin-conditioning agent.

methyl glucose isostearate—an emulsifier with highly effective moisturizing properties.

methyl glucose sesquistearate—a sucrose-based emulsifier.

methyl hydroxy stearate—an emollient used in moisturizing formulations. This is the ester of methyl alcohol and hydroxystearic acid.

methyl paraben—one of the most frequently used preservatives because of its very low sensitizing potential. It is one of the oldest preservatives in use to combat bacteria and molds. Noncomedogenic.

methylbenzylidene camphor—also known as 4-methylbenzylidene camphor. A UV filter and absorber not known to cause photoallergies.

methylchloroisothiazolinone—a preservative. *See* MI/MCI.

methylisothiazolinone—a preservative. *See* MI/MCI.

methylsilanol elastinate—a protein derivative used as a skin-conditioning agent.

methylsilanol hydroxyprolinate aspartate—classified as a skin-conditioning agent that can perform a number of different functions within a skin care formulation.

methylsilanol mannuronate—tests indicate that as a result of its cutaneous hydration activity, it increases skin suppleness and moisturization and aids in the reduction of cellulite.

M

mica—used as a texturizer and coloring agent in cosmetics, it is employed to provide a "glimmer" or "shimmering" quality in makeup powders. Mica is the group name for a series of ground silicate minerals with similar physical properties but varied chemical composition. Micas range in color from colorless to pale green, brown, or black.

microcrystalline cellulose—provides good slip and softness, and acts as a binder. A cellulose fiber isolated from colloidal crystals. *See also* cellulose.

microcrystalline wax—an emulsifier. This is a beeswax substitute characterized by the fineness of its crystals (in comparison with the larger crystals of paraffin wax). It is derived from petroleum.

micronutrients—*see* trace elements.

milfoil extract (Achillea millefolium)—credited with antiseptic and antibiotic properties. *See also* yarrow extract.

milk lipid(s)—emollient and skin conditioning.

milk protein—gives a smooth feel to the skin. Milk protein is primarily casein that is well absorbed by the skin, and gives it a gloss and fine touch by forming a soft film. It has a water-retention ability in the range of 13 percent. Milk protein is obtained from milk. If it is hydrolyzed, it is broken down into smaller pieces and is referred to either as hydrolyzed milk protein, milk amino acids, or casein amino acids. Its constituents include the flavones silybin, silydiamnin, and silychristin.

milk thistle (Carduus marianus)—credited with wound-healing. It is used in toners and aftershave preparations.

milkweed (Asclepias syriaca)—used in traditional medicine for its cicatrizant properties on wounds, and therapeutic value on various skin eruptions, including warts. Constituents include tannins, dextrose (sugar), and such fatty acids as oleic, linoleic, and linolenic.

millepertuis oil (Hypericum perforatum)—emollient and antiinflammatory, it is used for sunburns, burns, and bruises.

M

Millepertuis oil is the fixed oil obtained from St. John's wort flowers.

mimosa bark extract—see mimosa tenuiflora.

mimosa essence—fragrance. Mimosa essence is credited with anti-inflammatory and astringent properties. It may produce allergic skin reactions. *See also* mimosa tenuiflora.

mimosa tenuiflora (mimosa bark extract; tepescohuite [Mexican name])—used in cosmetics for its believed epidermal-tissue regenerating, repairing, and protecting properties, as well as to help reduce moisture loss. It has also been described as a healing oil with antiseptic properties. It can be used effectively in post-sun preparations, baby skin care creams, and protective creams. Mimosa tenuiflora has a high bioflavonoid and tannin content. It also contains zinc, necessary for DNA synthesis and cellular nutrition; iron, vital for oxygen transport and intracellular metabolism; magnesium, for its protective role; copper, for anti-inflammation; and manganese, that is said to stimulate cellular metabolism. The mimosa tenuiflora tree, related to the acacia, is found only in Mexico's southeastern state of Chiapas. The bark is the part that is used. Mayan healers used bark powder on cutaneous lesions, and the Guatemalan inhabitants of the region still use it today. May produce allergic skin reactions.

mineral oil (Russian white oil)—an emollient cleanser and demulsifier of dirt trapped in pores. Although widely used in European skin care products, its use is looked on with distrust in the United States, as many sources have classified it as comedogenic. Mineral oil is excellent for use in cleansers. In leave-on cosmetics, its comedogenicity or lack thereof appears related to the level of raw material refinement; therefore, some suppliers state that their product is noncomedogenic. When used in leave-on preparations, mineral oil's occlusive capability is considered to help improve the epidermal barrier function. This is a clear, odorless oil derived from petroleum and is not known to cause allergic reactions.

mineral pigments—provide UV protection. Mineral pigments refer to ingredients such as titanium dioxide or zinc oxide, which are usually incorporated into sunscreens, makeup bases, and even daytime moisturizers to enhance the product's sunscreening ability.

mineral wax—see ozokerite.

M

mink oil—a gentle and effective emollient with skin-softening abilities. Its occlusive properties give it skin-conditioning qualities as well. Obtained from the subdermal fatty tissues of the mink.

mint oil (Mentha sp.)—cooling, tonic, stimulating, antiseptic, and relaxing properties are attributed to mint. Mint was traditionally used as an adjunct soothing and anti-itching treatment in dermatological disorders. It has also been considered helpful for scratches and insect bites. In addition, this aromatic herb is widely used as a fragrance in beauty products. There are about 20 species in the *Mentha* genus growing around the world, including peppermint and spearmint, the two most widely used in skin care preparations. These serve as cleansers and decongestants indicated for acne and for dermatitis. Mint oil is produced by distillation of the plant.

mireth-3 myristate—an emollient employed as a skin-conditioning agent in cosmetic formulations.

mistletoe extract (Phoradendron flavescens; Viscum album)—antispasmodic, healing, and calming properties are attributed to this ingredient. Mistletoe is an evergreen, parasitic plant growing on tree branches where it forms pendent bushes two to five feet in diameter. The extract is obtained from the plant's berries.

mitracarpus—extracts obtained from plants of the mitracarpus genus (*Rubiaceae* family) are credited with skin-lightening and improving overall complexion. The most common species used include *M. Scaber zucc.*, *M. Villosus*, and *M. verticillatus*. The extract is typically obtained by traditional methods, including maceration. Active components include flavonoid, phenolic, and hydroquinone derivatives.

monoammonium glycyrrhizinate—*see* glycyrrhizinate.

monomethylsilanetril lactate—an alpha hydroxyacid derivative with silicone.

monosodium n-cocoylglutamate—a surfactant.

montmorillonite—used as an abrasive in exfoliants and as a bulking agent in masks. It is also used to increase a formula's viscosity, as an emulsion stabilizer, and as an opacifying agent. Montmorillonite, a complex silicate, is a clay mineral that forms the main ingredient of bentonite and Fuller's earth.

Morus alba—*see* mulberry extract.

M

mucopolysaccharides—their strong moisture-binding capacity enhances a formulation's moisture-binding quality and reduces transepidermal water loss. Studies show that mucopolysaccharides will reduce the amount of moisture lost by the skin and will stimulate its moisture intake. This ingredient exhibits the desirable moisture-binding qualities of healthy skin, giving the skin turgor, increased water content, and elasticity. Mucopolysaccharides are highly effective in skin treatment products. As a natural skin component, mucopolysaccharides fill the spaces between collagen and elastin protein fibers in the dermis, giving them support and providing lubrication and moisture. *See also* glycosaminoglycans.

mucoprotein (soluble)—*see* protein.

mucus of quince—*see* quince.

mud—a mixture of a powder and a liquid. Usually applied wet as a facial mask and allowed to dry. If the powder and/or liquid contain therapeutic ingredients, these will interact with the skin. Identifying its therapeutic action requires knowing the nature of the powder and liquid being used. In a mask, it also acts as an occlusive agent for the time the mask remains on the skin. This favors the interaction of ingredients in a cream or other products applied prior to the mud.

mugwort (Artemisia vulgaris)—improves skin feel and condition, it is also perfuming. Constituents include volatile oil, cineole, linalool, thujone, glycosides, insulin, and tannin. *See also* wormwood.

mulberry extract (Morus sp.)—increasingly used in cosmetics for its skin-lightening properties. Mulberry extract appears to inhibit tyrosinase and oxidation activity. While there are several mulberry varieties, these properties are attributed to white mulberry (*Morus alba*). Studies have indicated that extract obtained from young twigs (ramulus mori) of the white mulberry are particularly potent skin lighteners. White mulberry is the variety originally found in China and used as a food source for silkworms. Mulberry was very highly regarded in ancient times and commonly cultivated throughout Europe for multiple uses, including an expectorant and flavoring agent. It is an official entry in the *British Pharmacopoeia*. Constituents of the berry include glucose, protein, tartaric, and malic acids. *See also* ramulus mori.

mulberry glycolic extract—astringent.

mung bean extract (Phaseolus aureus)—a botanical used in cosmetic preparations since ancient times. It is credited with anti-inflammatory and some antioxidant properties. Its active constituents include vitexin and isovitexin, both flavonoids.

M

musk rose oil (Rosa moscata; Rosa moschata)—see rose hip oil.

myristal myristate—an ester of myristyl alcohol and myristic acid. *See also* myristic acid; myristyl alcohol.

myristic acid—a surfactant and cleansing agent. When combined with potassium, myristic acid soap provides a very good, abundant lather. This is a solid organic acid naturally occurring in butter acids such as nutmeg, oil of lovage, coconut oil, mace oil, and most animal and vegetable fats. Although some sources cite it as having no irritation potential, they do indicate a comedogenicity potential.

myristyl ether propionate—an emollient and skin-conditioning agent used in preshave lotions and moisturizing preparations.

myristyl alcohol—an emollient often used in hand creams, cold creams, and lotions to give them a smooth, velvety feel. Sources indicate it as being mildly comedogenic and potentially irritating.

myristyl lactate—a light emollient and moisturizer with good spreadability. It leaves a smooth, satiny afterfeel. Sources indicate it as being comedogenic and with a slight irritancy potential. *See also* lactic acid; myristyl alcohol.

myristyl myristate—an occlusive skin-conditioning agent that enhances product spreadability and can reduce a product's transparency. It is particularly useful in emulsions that have to "melt" once in contact with the skin. This is an ester formed by the combination of the myristyl alcohol and myristic acid fractions of coconut oil. *See also* myristic acid; myristyl alcohol.

myristyl ocatanoate—a light emollient and moisturizer. It leaves the skin's surface with a smooth and supple finish.

myrrh extract (Commiphora myrrah)—said to have disinfectant, antiseptic, anti-inflammatory, anti-itching, cicatrizant, tonic, stimulant, sedative, and astringent properties. It is also a good fixative. Myrrh extract can be valuable in products designed for acne treatment. Myrrh is a traditional and ancient ingredient for perfumes and incense, and was used by ancient Egyptian women in facial masks

M

and other cosmetic preparations. Myrrh oil is produced by the distillation of the gum.

myrtle—astringent and antiseptic with botanical properties closely resembling those of eucalyptus. Indicated for acne and oily skin. Myrtle is obtained by distillation of the branches.

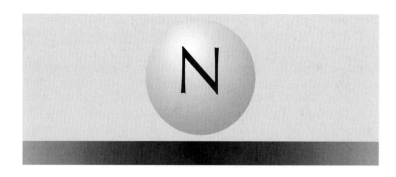

NaAl silicate—*see* sodium aluminum silicate.

nalidone—*see* pyrrolidonic carbon acid.

NaPCA—*see* sodium PCA.

narcissus *(Narcissus poeticus)*—a fragrance, it is also used as an antispasmodic. Recommended for use in very low concentrations as its oil has been shown to impair cellular functions when added to in-vitro cell cultures. In addition, large amounts of the extract may produce headaches. This general name may also include narcissus flower extract and narcissus essential wax. As a wax, it can also help thicken an emulsion.

naseberry *(Manilkara zapotilla)*—also known as sapodilla. Antioxidant and antiaging. Its constituents include tannin, fructose, pectin, ascorbic acid, mineral salts, and bioflavonoids, particularly proanthocyanidins, which have emollient, humectant, and antioxidant activity. The fruit is the part of the plant that is used.

nasturtium extract *(Tropaeolum majus)*—considered to have disinfectant and rubefactant attributes. It is effective in acne treatment products. May produce allergic reactions.

natrium mud extract—*see* mud.

natural moisturizing factor (NMF)—refer to entry in Chapter 4.

neem extract—may have insect-repellent properties.

neopentyl glycol dicaprate—an emollient also used to increase a formulation's viscosity. Primarily used in hand and body preparations.

neopentyl glycol dicaprylate/dicaprate—an emollient and formula viscosity-increasing agent used mostly in the manufacturing of lipsticks.

nerol—a primary alcohol used in perfumes, especially those with rose and orange blossom scents. Nerol is a naturally occurring fraction in oil of lavender, orange leaf, palmarosa, rose, neroli, and petitgrain. It is colorless and has a rose-like scent.

neroli—*see* neroli oil; orange flower oil.

neroli oil—a fragrance. It is used in skin care preparations to stimulate cell regeneration. Given its sedative and soothing properties, it is indicated for sensitive and delicate skin. However, neroli oil appears beneficial for all skin types. True neroli is extracted from bitter orange blossom. This is one of the most expensive oils and, therefore, is widely adulterated with the distillation of other citrus blossoms such as sweet orange, lemon, and mandarin. *See also* orange flower oil.

neroli water—*see* orange flower water.

nettle extract (Urtica dioica)—its botanical properties are listed as anti-inflammatory, astringent, bactericidal, healing, mildly deodorant, and stimulating. Some consider it effective for treating eczema and sunburn. According to some sources, this is the botanical with the highest vitamin E content, and as such, it would have good antioxidant properties. Nettle's important constituents include acetylcholine, amino acids, histamine, carotinoids, and chlorophyll. An analysis of fresh nettle also shows the presence of formic acid, mucilage, mineral salts, ammonia, carbonic acid, and water. The formic acid in nettle, along with the phosphates and a trace of iron, makes it a valuable botanical. There are more than 500 species of nettle growing mainly in tropical countries. The whole herb is employed for therapeutic purposes.

niacin—a conditioning agent, it helps smooth the skin.

niacinamide—used as a skin stimulant and skin smoother, it is a derivative of niacin, and part of the vitamin B family. *See also* vitamin B.

niaouli oil—its therapeutic properties indicate possible improvement in circulation, antibody activity, and healing in cases of infected wounds and burns. Some of its medicinal properties and indications are the same as those for eucalyptus.

Niaouli oil is produced through distillation of the leaves of the *Melaleuca quinqueneriva* plant.

niosomes—nonionic surfactant vesicles that act as a delivery system and are similar to liposomes. According to manufacturers, niosomes interact desirably with human skin when topically applied. They are prepared from suitable nonionic surfactants. *See also* liposomes.

nonfat dry milk—soothing and moisturizing it is often used in facial masks. Nonfat dry milk consists mostly of protein and also contains lactic acid, lactose, vitamins, and minerals. *See also* milk protein.

nonoxynol—*see* polyoxyethylene nonylphenyl ether.

nonoxynol-14—a surfactant and emulsifying agent. It is used as a nonionic surface-active agent and as a dispersing agent in cosmetics.

norvaline—a protein amino acid used as a skin-conditioning agent. *See also* valeric acid.

nutmeg (Myristica fragrans)—studies credit nutmeg extract with a skin-lightening effect based on an ability to inhibit tyrosinase activity. An extract, powder, or oil can be obtained from the nut. However, nutmeg oil, credited with tonic and stimulating properties, is not commonly used in cosmetic preparations as it could cause skin irritation.

Nutrilan (hydrolyzed animal protein)—a trade name for hydrolyzed animal protein. Manufacturers claim that this ingredient creates a smooth, velvety feeling on the skin's surface. It contains amino acids present in the skin. Nutrilan is an example of how cosmetic companies can list their ingredients and create ambiguity with respect to identity or source. *See also* hydrolyzed animal protein.

nylon—a commonly known synthetic material used as a fiber in eyelash lengtheners and mascaras, and as a molding compound to shape cosmetics. Nylon gives bulk to a formulation and, when appropriate, provides opacifying properties. It can cause allergic reactions.

nylon 11—a bulking agent used primarily in makeup preparations and in some moisturizers.

nylon 12—a bulking and opacifying agent that provides good feel and good elasticity to moisturizers and makeup preparations, including foundations. Nylon 12 reduces oiliness. It is a polyamide derivative of acid 12-aminododecanioic.

nylon 66—a bulking agent.

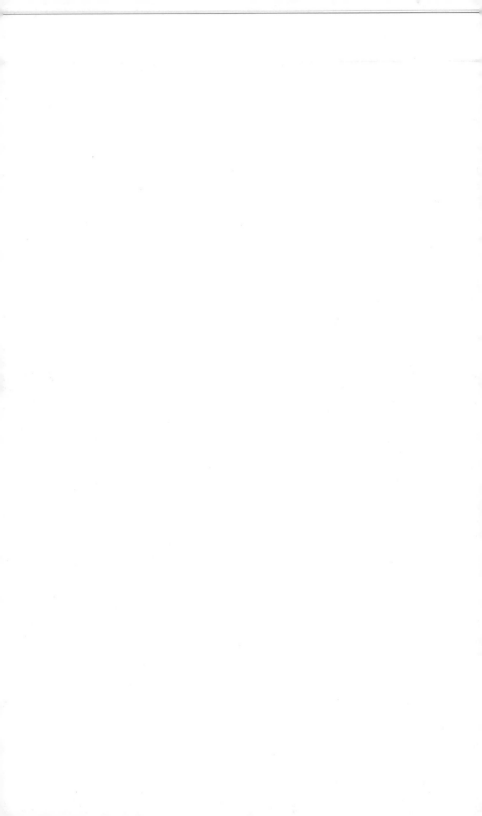

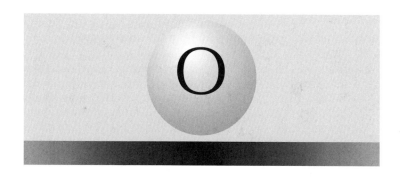

oak bark *(Quercus sp.)*—its botanical properties are described as slightly tonic, strongly astringent, and antiseptic. It also reduces inflammation and prevents infection. Oak bark extract appears to have greater therapeutic effects than oak root.

oak bud extract—*see* aleppo gall.

oak root—exhibits soothing and anti-inflammatory properties. Oak root is recommended for sensitive skin, protecting it against unwanted reactions such as swelling or redness. The extract is generally obtained from the younger part of the plant.

oakmoss empuree *(Evernia prunastri)*—a fragrance component derived from any one of several resin-yielding lichens that grow on oak trees.

oat *(Avena sativa)*—contains a colloid that has soothing properties on the skin. Generally speaking, all oat grades enhance emulsion stability, increase viscosity, leave a smooth after-feel, and provide a source of whole natural vegetable protein. Dermatologists indicate oatmeal-based preparations for irritated skins resulting from sunburn, psoriasis, or allergic dermatitis, as oatmeal seems to reduce irritation and relieve redness and itching. In addition to acting as a soap-free cleanser, oats in the form of bran, flour, or meal provide a gentle base for face masks designed to work with delicate, sensitive skin. Oatmeal masks absorb oil from the skin's surface and reduce the redness of irritated, broken-out skin. Oatmeal soaps are nonirritating and good for people with delicate, sensitive skin.

oat bran—see oat.

*oat extract—*an extract obtained from the seeds of oats. *See also* oat.

*oat flour—*an abrasive, absorbent, bulking, and viscosity-increasing substance obtained by the fine grinding of oat kernels. It is used in a variety of cosmetic preparations including powders, masks, mudpacks, moisturizers, suntan gels, hand and body creams, and soaps. *See also* oat.

*oat meal flour—*used as an abrasive and bulking agent in paste masks and soaps. Obtained by grinding oats from which the husks have been removed. *See also* oat.

octadecanol—see stearic acid.

*octadecene/maleic anhydride copolymer—*an emulsion stabilizer, film former, and viscosity-increasing chemical used in cosmetic formulations. It is also used in sunscreens as a waterproofing agent.

*octadodecyl stearyl stearate—*an emollient.

*octinoxate—*the drug name for the sunscreen chemical generally known as octyl methoxycinnamate and ethylhexyl methoxycinnamate. *See* octyl methoxycinnamate.

*octisalate—*a UVB protector. This is the drug name for ethylhexyl salicylate and octyl salicylate. *See* ethylhexyl salicylate.

*octocrylene—*a UVB sunscreen with strong water-resistant properties and a rather broad-band absorption range. It exhibits good photostability, and is being evaluated by many companies as an effective SPF booster and waterproofing enhancer. This is an expensive ingredient with an approved usage level of 7 to 10 percent in both the U.S. and the European Union. Although gaining in popularity among formulators, its cost and usage level can limit use.

*octyl dimethyl PABA (padimate-O; p-aminobenzoic acid)—*an FDA-approved sunscreen chemical whose INCI name is now listed as ethylhexyl dimethyl PABA. *See* ethylhexyl dimethyl PABA.

*octyldodecanol—*formerly listed as octyl dodecanol. An emollient alcohol with good spreadability and skin-conditioning properties. This is a good vehicle for oil-soluble ingredients. It is also used for perfuming.

*2-octyl-1-dodecanol—*an emollient.

*octyl methoxycinnamate (ethylhexyl methoxycinnamate; ethylhexyl p-methoxycinnamate; 2-ethylhexyl p-methoxycinnamate)—*an FDA-approved sunscreen chemical with an approved usage level of 2 to 7.5 percent in the U.S. and up to 10 percent in the European Union. Currently, this is the most popular sunscreen chemical incorporated worldwide into sun products. It has an excellent UV absorption capability, a good safety profile, broad solubility in oils, insolubility in water, and rarely causes photoallergy. These attributes all add up to make it an almost perfect sunscreen chemical. Considered a noncomedogenic raw material, it is derived from balsam of Peru, cocoa leaves, cinnamon leaves, and storax. *See also* cinnamate.

octyl p-methoxycinnamate—*see* octyl methoxycinnamate.

octyl palmitate—a nongreasy, nonoily moisturizing ester with good spreadability and good solvency properties.

octyl pelargonate—a light emollient that does not leave a greasy feel on the skin.

octyl salicylate (2-ethylhexyl 2-hydroxybenzoate; 2-ethylhexyl salicylate; ethylhexyl salicylate)—*see* ethylhexyl salicylate.

octyl stearate—an emollient with similar properties to those of octyl palmitate. *See also* stearic acid.

octyl triazone—*see* ethylhexyl triazone.

2-octyldodecyl alcohol—*see* octyldodecanol.

octyldodecyl benzoate—an emollient and a solvent with high spreadability. It leaves a pleasant feel on the skin.

octyldodecyl myristate—an emollient.

octyldodecyl neopentanoate—an emollient with skin-conditioning properties.

octyldodecyl stearate—a noncomedogenic emollient.

octyldodecyl stearoyl stearate—a noncomedogenic skin-conditioning agent that provides occlusive properties. It is also used to increase viscosity in cosmetic formulations.

octyl hydroxystearate—an emollient used as a skin-conditioning agent.

old English walnut—*see* walnut.

oleamine—an antistatic agent used in the formulation of cosmetics.

oleate sorbitan—*see* sorbitan oleate.

oleic acid—also known as omega-9. Can improve the skin penetration abilities of a preparation's components. An essential fatty acid, it is obtained from various animal and vegetable fats and oils. Can be mildly irritating to the skin.

oleostearine—a mixture of the fatty acid triglycerides remaining after the physical separation of the low titre oils from beef tallow. It acts as a binder and an emollient in cosmetic preparations.

oleth-2, -5, -10, -20, -30—all are emulsifiers and solubilizers, and all are versions of a polyethylene glycol ether of oleyl alcohol. Cosmetic formulators will often select a specific one depending on the formulation's other requirements. For example, oleth-5 is also a spreading agent; oleth-20 is particularly useful as a fragrance solubilizer and can be successfully employed in some clear gel systems; oleth-30 has additional surfactant and cleansing properties. *See also* oleyl alcohol.

oleyl alcohol—an emollient, solvent, viscosity-increasing agent, and carrier employed in a wide variety of cosmetic formulations including makeup, skin care, and hand and body preparations. Oleyl alcohol is an unsaturated fatty alcohol found in fish oils and can also be produced synthetically. According to some sources, it is comedogenic and has a mild irritancy potential.

oleyl betaine—a mild emollient, conditioning surfactant, and formulation thickener. *See also* betain; oleamine.

oleyl erucate—an all-purpose emollient sometimes used as a jojoba oil substitute.

olibanum—*see* frankincense.

olibanum oil—a fragrance component. It is astringent with slight anti-inflammatory properties. *See also* frankincense.

oligo active liposomes—liposomes encapsulated with oligo elements.

oligoelements—refer to entry in Chapter 4. *See also* trace elements.

olive extract—*see* olive leaf extract.

olive oil (Olea europaea)—a carrier oil with excellent lubricity, pale color, and low odor. Olive oil is considered an especially good carrier for essential oils. Its unsaponifiable fraction is described also as a type of precursor, although not a biological one, with some claims of its targeting epidermal keratinocytes and stimulating the synthesis of such substances as collagen, elastin, proteoglycans, and glycoproteins.

olive leaf extract—astringent and antiseptic, it also has vasodialating capacities. Olive leaf extract has demonstrated some antioxidant and free-radical scavenger activities.

Olive leaves contain both bioflavonoids and polyphenols. Generally found in antiaging products.

omega-3—an essential fatty acid. *See* alpha linolenic acid.

omega-6—an essential fatty acid. *See* linoleic acid.

omega-9—an essential fatty acid. *See* oleic acid.

orange essence—used for fragrance.

orange oil (*Citrus aurantium* ***[bitter orange] and*** *Citrus sinensis* ***[sweet orange])***—primarily used in perfumery. Its botanical properties in skin care are considered anti-inflammatory, antibacterial, antispasmodic, and sedative, making it suitable for sensitive, delicate skin.

orange flower extract—used in folk medicine as a mild sedative. It is considered effective for dry skin.

orange flower oil—a fragrance. Credited with soothing and calming properties when used in skin care preparations. Orange flower oil should not be confused with orange flower extract. The flowers from the bitter orange tree yield, by distillation, an essential oil known as neroli, which forms one of the principal elements of eau de cologne. A pomade and an oil are also obtained from orange flowers through maceration. The oil from sweet orange blossoms is far less fragrant than that from bitter orange. The flowers are distilled immediately after being gathered. The essential oil, which rises to the surface of the distillate, is drawn off while the aqueous portion is sold as orange flower water. One hundred kilograms of flowers will yield 600 grams of oil by volatile solvents, 400 grams by the maceration method, and only 100 grams by enfleurage. Obtained by extraction or pressing of orange skin.

orange flower water—has similar activity to that of orange oil, but its soothing properties appear to be more pronounced.

orange roughy oil—in skin care preparations, it demonstrates superior spreading and skin-softening properties. A fish oil.

orchid extract (*Orchis sp.)*—a restorative and rejuvenator apparently due more to the beauty of the flower than to any specific stimulant properties. However, it is noted as both soothing and skin conditioning. Some sources credit it as good for dry skin. The extract is obtained from the tubers of various orchid species.

orizanol (orysanol)—a protector from UV radiation with an antioxidizing effect on fats and oils. Orizanol is a powder obtained from rice germ oil.

O

orysanol—*see* orizanol.

oxido reductases—a mixture of naturally occurring yeast and enzymes that acts as an antioxidant by reducing or blocking oxygen.

2-oxothiazolidine carboxylic acid—a glutathione precursor, this ingredient is being studied for its antiaging, antiwrinkle properties. *See also* glutathione.

oxybenzone (benzophenone-3)—the drug name for an FDA-approved UV filter and absorber. *See* benzophenone-3.

oxyquinoline sulfate—a disinfectant and a preservative against fungus growth. Made from phenols.

ozokerite (cresin)—a naturally occurring microcrystalline wax. It regulates formulation viscosity, has suspension properties, and gives products stability. Ozokerite is a hydrocarbon wax derived from mineral or petroleum sources that, when refined, yields a hard white microcrystalline wax known as cresin.

O

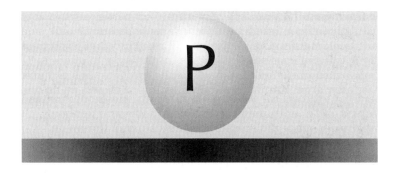

P

PABA—also known as p-aminobenzoic acid. A sunscreen chemical with an approved usage level of 5 to 15 percent. It is found to be irritating to sensitive skin, has the potential to cause sensitization, and is considered too water soluble. Once extremely popular, this ingredient has practically disappeared from sunscreen formulations. PABA is a yellowish or colorless acid found in vitamin B complex.

padimate A—*see* pentyl dimethyl PABA.

padimate O—the drug name for ethylhexyl dimethyl PABA, a sunscreen chemical formerly known as octyl dimethyl PABA. *See* ethylhexyl dimethyl PABA.

palm oil (hydrogenated)—used as a consistency regulator and a formula stabilizer in the manufacture of creams, lotions, makeup, and decorative cosmetics.

palm oil glycerides (hydrogenated)—used as a coemulsifier, dispersing agent, and consistency regulator in the manufacture of cosmetics. It imparts a pleasant skin feel.

palm kernel glycerides (hydrogenated)—an emulsifier and consistency regulator. It is a mixture of mono-, di-, and triglycerides derived from palm kernel oil.

palm kernel oil—used primarily for making soaps and ointments. It is a natural oil obtained from the kernel of *Elaeis guineensis*.

palm kernelamide DEA—used as a nonionic surfactant, thickener, foam booster, and formula stabilizer in cosmetic preparations. It is also able to control the viscosity of a formulation.

palmarosa oil (Cymbopogon martini)—properties attributed to this oil are soothing, moisturizing, antiseptic, tonic, and cell regenerating. Palmarosa oil is said to have immediate calming and refreshing action on the skin. Its use is indicated for acne skin and dermatitis condition as well as for dry skin. This oil is widely used in perfumery and cosmetology, as its fresh, rose-like scent makes it useful for the adulteration of rose oil, one of the most expensive essential oils. It can also be used to mask odors. Palmarosa oil is obtained by distillation of this flowering grass-like plant.

palmitic acid—one of the skin's major fatty acids produced by the sebaceous glands. In cosmetic preparations, it is used as a formula texturizer. This acid is naturally occurring in allspice, anise, calamus oil, cascarilla bark, celery seed, butter acids, coffee, tea, and many animal fats and plant oils. It is obtained from palm oil, Japan wax, or Chinese vegetable tallow.

palmitoyl hydroxypropyltrimonium amylopectin/glycerin crosspolymer—a skin conditioner.

palmitoyl oligopeptide-3—a synthetic peptide used in antiaging products. It is said to help smooth and reduce the appearance of wrinkles as well as repair age-related skin problems by stimulating collagen production.

palmitoyl pentapeptide-4—a synthetic peptide with derivatives of serine, threonine, and hexadecanoyl. It is a skin conditioner. Clinical studies of manufacturers credit it with an ability to promote collagen, elastin, and glycosaminoglycan synthesis. This would result in an ability to restore skin thickness, which diminishes with age, and to reduce the appearance of lines and wrinkles.

palmitoyl tetrapeptide-3—a peptide that appears to improve skin elasticity and firmness. It also hydrates, smoothes, and protects the skin. An additional anti-inflammatory activity is attributed to its ability to control the secretion of specific chemicals responsible for skin aging (i.e., cytokines and specifically interleukin-6), and hence it may function in a manner similar to the antiaging hormone, DHEA.

pansy extract (Viola tricolor)—its botanical properties include soothing, healing, and cleansing. The active constituents of this extract include saponins, salicylic compounds, tannins, and flavonoids (for example, rutin, violantin, scoparin, vitexine, saponaretin, orientin), volatile oils, and the glycosides of the methyl ester of salycilic acid. Pansy extract is recommended for use in dry skin preparations and for skin problems of various types.

P

pantethine—emollient and conditioning, often found in hair care preparations.

pantetheine sulfonate—skin conditioning.

panthenol (vitamin B$_5$)—acts as a penetrating moisturizer. Panthenol appears to stimulate cellular proliferation and aid in tissue repair. Studies indicate that when topically applied, panthenol penetrates the skin and is converted into pantothenic acid, a B complex vitamin. Such action could possibly influence the skin's natural resources of pantothenic acid. It imparts a nonirritant, nonsensitizing, moisturizing, and conditioning feel and promotes normal keratinization and wound-healing. Panthenol protects the skin against sunburn, provides relief for existing sunburn, and enhances the natural tanning process. Panthenol's humectant character enables it to hold water in the product or attract water from the environment, resulting in a moisturizing effect. As a skin softener, it provides suppleness, and claims are that it also acts as an anti-inflammatory agent. Considered a noncomedogenic raw material.

panthenyl triacetate—a panthotenic acid derivative with vitamin B activity. *See also* pantothenic acid.

pantothenic acid—part of the vitamin B complex. It is considered a biological precursor capable of acting as a bioactivator. Pantothenic acid's relatively small molecule facilitates permeation of the epidermis, allowing it to participate in the metabolic process of the dermis. Some studies indicate a benefit when incorporated into products destined for treating eczema, psoriasis, skin inflammation, and skin allergies. It is found naturally occurring in liver, eggs, dried brewer's yeast, and royal jelly.

papain—a papaya enzyme with the ability to dissolve keratin. Papain is used in face masks and peeling lotions as a very gentle exfoliant. Papain can be irritating to the skin but is less so than bromelin, a similar enzyme found in pineapples and also used in cosmetics. Considered a noncomedogenic raw material.

papaya (Carica papaya)—considered a cleanser for skin with acne condition. Its value resides in its papain enzyme content. *See also* papain.

papaya enzyme extract—used as a gentle exfoliant, it also softens the skin and can help smooth the appearance of fine line and wrinkles. *See also* papain.

paprika—used to stimulate blood circulation in the skin.

P

parabens—one of the most commonly used group of preservatives in the cosmetic, pharmaceutical, and food industries.
Parabens provide bacteriostatic and fungistatic activity
against a diverse number of organisms, and are considered
safe for use in cosmetics, particularly in light of their low
sensitizing potential. An evaluation of preservatives for use
in leave-on cosmetic preparations lists parabens among the
least sensitizing. The range of concentrations used in cosmetics varies between 0.03 to 0.30 percent, depending on
the conditions for use and the product to which the
paraben is added. *See also* parabens entry in Chapter 4.

paraffin—used in cosmetics as a beeswax substitute. Paraffin is a
solid mixture of hydrocarbons obtained from petroleum, although it can also be obtained from wood or coal. Pure paraffin is harmless to the skin, but the presence of impurities
may result in irritation, eczemas, and other skin problems.

Parinari curatellifolia seed oil—said to have regenerative, restructuring, and moisturizing capacities, thanks to its eleostearic
acid content.

parsley extract (Petroselinum sativum)—serves as a deodorant.
It is said to have disinfectant, anti-inflammatory, and skin-
conditioning properties.

parsley oil—traditionally used for soothing and anti-itching treatment in dermatological disorders. It may also be used as a
preservative. Parsley oil is extracted from the seeds that
contain an oil called apiol. It may cause allergic reactions in
sensitive skin.

parsley seed—*see* parsley oil.

partially hydrolyzed protein—*see* protein.

passion flower extract (Passiflora sp.)—its botanical properties
are described as antispasmodic and calming. Extract
specifically from the *incarnata* variety is credited with an
ability to protect the skin against harmful external factors
(e.g., climate). Its active principle, passiflorine, appears to
be somewhat similar to morphine.

passion fruit extract—an emollient with moisturizing and refreshing properties. Depending on the varietal, passion
fruit extract can be soothing to the skin as well as act as a
skin conditioner and protector. A listing of "passion fruit"
alone is insufficient to determine the variety used or the associated activity. There are four primary *Passiflora* varieties used in cosmetics: *edulis, incarnata, laurifolia, and*

P

quadrangularis. Depending on the variety and the portion of the plant used (flower, fruit, or seed), therapeutic properties can range from improving skin condition to astringent, soothing, refreshing, and skin protecting, for example. Some of passion fruit's most important constituents include vitamins, polysaccharides, minerals, and amino acids. This extract has an aromatic, fruity, tropical scent.

passion fruit oil—seen most often on suncare product labels, the oil extracted from the plant's seed is considered emollient, and, depending on the plant's varietal, may also offer some skin protecting capacity.

patchouli lite oil—*see* patchouli oil.

patchouli oil (Pogostemon patchouli) (patchouly)—its botanical properties are described as astringent, anti-inflammatory, and decongestive. Other properties are listed as tonic, stimulant in low doses, and sedative at high doses. Its botanical attributes make it useful for acne, aged and chapped skin, and skin redness. In Asia, it was a renowned antidote against insect and snake bites. Also used as a perfume in soaps and cosmetics to impart a long-lasting Oriental aroma. This oil has a strong, sweet, musty, and very persistent fragrance. The patchouli leaves are dried and fermented prior to distillation. May produce an allergic reaction in sensitive individuals.

patchouly—*see* patchouli oil.

PCA (Ajidew; Ajidew A-100; l-2-pyrrolidone-5-carboxylic acid)—a hygroscopic moisturizing ingredient, it serves as a fine humectant. It is frequently used in moisturizing products.

peach extract (Prunus persica)—used for a variety of functions, including as an abrasive, to add bulk and for moisturizing activity. There are differences based on the portion of the plant employed. For example, an extract from peach leaves is considered emollient and moisturizing, and is credited by herbalists with an ability to help stop bleeding and heal wounds. Extract of peach bud is used for its humectant properties, and peach flower extract is moisturizing. Peach extract is recommended for use in products for dry skin.

peach kernel oil—a carrier credited with emollient, calming, and soothing properties. This oil is expressed from the peach kernels.

peach stones (ground)—used in scrubs as exfoliants.

P

peanut fat—used to add consistency to cosmetic products. Peanut fat is hydrogenated peanut oil. *See also* peanut oil.

peanut oil—utilized as a skin softener, emulsifier, and emollient. It can also be used as a substitute for more expensive oils such as almond and olive in cosmetic creams. Peanut oil has a higher vitamin A, vitamin E, and nicotinic acid content than other nut oils. Peanut oil is obtained by pressing the seed kernels.

pectin—used as a thickening agent in cosmetic preparations due to its gelling properties. It is soothing and mildly acidic. Extracted from apples or the inner portion of citrus fruit rind.

PEG, PEG-4, -8, -14, -20, -32, -75, -100, -150, -200—the acronym for polyethylene glycol. PEGs are compatible with a wide range of ingredients and are blended into a formulation to obtain the desired humectancy, viscosity, or melting point. PEGs make excellent solvents, binders, vehicles, humectants, lubricants, and bases. When a number is associated with the PEG entry, it indicates the number of moles present (the PEG's weight). While each fundamentally serves the same purpose, a cosmetic chemist might choose one PEG over the other for formulatory requirements. For example, PEG-4 can improve a product's resistance to moisture and oxidation, and is generally used in hair products. Certain types of PEG-8 can be used as a moisture and consistency regulator in creams, lotions, and shaving preparations, and PEG-32 can improve a product's spreadability and skin feel. When they are listed with another ingredient such as PEG-5 stearate, it means that a polyethylene glycol (PEG) chain has been added to the stearic acid to enhance water solubility. *See also* polyethylene glycol.

PEG-2 ceteareth—an emulsifier.

PEG-2 stearate—an emulsifier for creams and lotions. This tan-colored wax is derived from stearic acid. *See also* PEG stearate.

PEG-3 sorbitan oleate, -6 sorbitan oleate—an emulsifying agent. Commonly used in cosmetic, toiletry, and fragrance preparations and in suntan gels.

PEG-3 sorbitan stearate, -6 sorbitan stearate, -60 sorbitan stearate—an emulsifying agent and a popular PEG among cosmetic formulators for use in all cosmetic, toiletry, and fragrance preparations, including suntan gels.

PEG-4 dilaurate—an emulsifier.

P

PEG-4 laurate—used in cosmetic preparations as an emulsifier and a surfactant.

PEG-5 glyceryl stearate—a surfactant-emulsifying agent used in moisturizing and cleansing products.

PEG-5 soy stearol—an emollient, emulsifier, and emulsion stabilizer used in a wide variety of skin and hair care products. PEG-10 soy stearol also has viscosity-modifying properties. These are derived from the sterols found in soybean oil, and are considered noncomedogenic raw materials.

PEG-5 stearate—listed as particularly applicable for hand and body lotions and creams. *See also* PEG stearate.

PEG-6 beeswax, -8 beeswax, -12 beeswax, -20 beeswax—a surfactant-emulsifying agent that can gelate lipids.

PEG-6 caprylic/capric glycerides—an emollient and emulsifying agent that helps preserve the skin's lipid content and keep the skin soft. Studies indicate good effectiveness in psoriasis treatment due to its ability to soften the scaling skin and improve the action of the active ingredient being applied. Manufacturer test results indicate no primary toxic or allergic reactions and good skin tolerance.

PEG-6 dioleate—a surfactant-emulsifying agent derived from oleic acid. Used as a carrier or base in lotions and other cosmetic preparations.

PEG-6 isostearat—an emulsifier.

PEG-6 lauramide—an emulsifier.

P

PEG-6 stearate—used primarily as an emulsifier in the formulation of cleansing products. *See also* PEG stearate.

PEG-7 glyceryl cocoate—a self-emulsifying emollient especially suitable for aqueous formulations.

PEG-7M—a binder, emulsion stabilizer, and viscosity-increasing agent used primarily in soaps and cleansing products.

PEG-8 stearate—an emulsifier and thickening agent generally incorporated into hair care products, hand and body creams, and moisturizing preparations. Also a superfattening agent for shaving preparations and foam baths. *See also* PEG stearate.

PEG-10 sorbitan laurate, -40 sorbitan laurate, -44 sorbitan laurate, -75 sorbitan laurate, -80 sorbitan laurate—cleansing and solubilizing agents. These are among the most popularly used PEGs because of their mildness. They are incorporated into a variety of preparations including skin care cosmetics, suntan products, toiletries, and fragrances. As a group, they are considered noncomedogenic raw materials.

PEG-10 soy stearol—*see* PEG-5 soy sterol.

PEG-16 macadamia glycerides—emollient. Derived from macadamia nut oil glycerides.

PEG-18 castor oil dioleate—an emulsifier for creams and lotions, and a viscosity-increasing agent. It is particularly suitable when animal and vegetable oils are used.

PEG-20 oleate—an emulsifier derived from oleic acid.

PEG-25 PABA—an ultraviolet-light absorber and filter derived from PABA. It is approved for use up to 10 percent in the European Union.

PEG-30 castor oil, -30 castor oil (hydrogenated)—an emollient, detergent, emulsifier, and oil-in-water solubilizer recommended for fragrance oils, and for other oils that may be difficult to solubilize.

PEG-30 dipolyhydroxystearate—an emulsifier for oil-in-water preparations.

PEG-30 stearate—a cleansing and solubilizing agent often suitable for moisturizing preparations. *See also* PEG stearate.

PEG-32 stearate—a cleansing and solubilizing agent often used in face and neck preparations as well as moisturizers. *See also* PEG stearate.

PEG-40 castor oil, -40 castor oil (hydrogenated)—an emulsifier, surfactant and powerful solubilizer used for solubilizing essential oils and perfumes in oil-in-water creams and lotions. It is similar to PEG-30 castor oil but more dense; it is a soft paste rather than a liquid. The hydrogenated version is particularly used as a nonionic emulsifier for essential oils and perfumes.

PEG-40 ricinoleyl ether—*see* ricinoleth 40.

PEG-40 stearate—a hydrophilic emulsifier, stabilizer, antigellant, and lubricant for a variety of skin care products, some hair care preparations, toiletries, and perfumes. *See also* PEG stearate.

PEG-45 palm kernel glycerides—an emollient and emulsifying agent derived from palm kernel glycerides.

PEG-50 lanolin—a surfactant used as a cleansing and solubilizing agent primarily in hair straighteners. A lanolin derivative.

PEG-60 glycerylisostearate—a surfactant-emulsifying agent.

PEG-75 lanolin—an emollient, emulsifier, dispersant, plasticizer, and foam stabilizer. A polyethylene glycol derivative of lanolin.

PEG-85 lanolin—a surfactant.

PEG-100 stearate—a stabilizer and emulsifier for creams and lotions. Technically, it is the polyethylene glycol ester of stearic acid containing 100 moles of PEG. It is also a cleansing agent and surfactant utilized in skin care products, some hair care preparations, toiletries, and some perfumes. *See also* PEG stearate.

PEG-120 methyl glucose dioleate—a cleansing agent used in soaps, cleansers, and shampoos.

PEG-150 distearate—a surfactant used as a cleansing and solubilizing agent.

PEG-180/laureth-50/TMMG copolymer—a thickener with emulsifying and film-forming properties. Can also add lubricity and humectancy to a product.

PEG-180/octoxynol-40/TMMG copolymer—*see* PEG-180/laureth-50/TMMG copolymer.

PEG-200 hydrogenated glyceryl palmate—a polymer with cleansing, emulsifying, and solvent action. It is often found in cleansing products for face, body, and hair.

PEG-octanoate—all PEG octanoates are listed as emulsifying agents regardless of the number of PEGs in the formulation.

PEG stearate—all PEG stearates are emulsifying agents. Some are more frequently used or are more suitable for use in particular types of preparations, such as body creams and lotions versus cleansers.

pentaerythrityl stearate/caprate/caprylic adipate—an extremely emollient compound with moisturizing and protective properties. It is also a viscosity-building agent.

pentaerythrityl tetraoctanoate—an emollient.

pentasodium ethylenediamine tetramethylene phosphate—a chelating agent similar to EDTA.

pentasodium pentate—an inorganic salt used as a water softener, emulsifier, and sequestering and dispersing agent in cleansing creams and lotions. Prepared from the dehydration of mono- and disodium phosphates. It is moderately irritating to the skin and mucous membranes.

pentyl dimethyl PABA (Amydimethyl PABA)—a chemical UVB absorber infrequently used due to the PABA component.

P

pentylene glycol—an alcohol with humectant and antibacterial properties.

peony extract (Paeonia sp.)—credited with immunostimulant, anti-inflammatory, antispasmodic, and antibiotic properties. It is also said to be a circulation stimulant and have general skin beautifying properties. Clinical studies show peony extract to help improve the acne condition and some skin diseases.

pepper (Capsicum annuum)—depending on the form in which it is used (i.e., extract of the whole plant versus extract of just the fruit, or as juice, powder or resin) a wide range of therapeutic properties are attributed to pepper. Extract from the whole plant can help mask odor, is tonic, and also serves to improve skin condition. In a skin care formulation, extract from the fruit can be used for such properties as antimicrobial, antioxidant, astringent, and skin protecting. In hair care products, it could be used as an antidandruff and hair-conditioning ingredient. The juice, powder, and resin forms are all considered skin conditioning. Among pepper's constituents are carotenoids, capsaicin, volatile oil, organic acids, vitamin C, flavonoids (e.g. rutin), and mineral salts.

peppermint (Mentha piperita)—in extract form, it helps relieve skin irritation and itching. It reduces skin redness due to inflammation or acne, cools by constricting capillaries, and has refreshing and tonic properties.

peppermint oil—credited with refreshing, cooling, bactericidal, and anti-irritant properties. It is also used as a fragrance. Peppermint oil can produce allergic reactions such as hay fever, skin rashes, and irritation, especially if a dressing is applied over the oil. Extracted from the leaves of the peppermint plant, menthol accounts for more than 50 percent of its content. *See also* mint oil.

peptide—*see* peptides entry in Chapter 4.

peptide CLB-253, -CL-2572, -CLF-5—trade names for a series of different peptides found in the products of a particular cosmetic product manufacturer. *See* peptide.

peptones—a protein derivative. *See* protein.

PERA—*see* polyethoxylated retinamide.

perfluoropolyether—a liquid polymer able to form a protective and lubricating film on the skin. Recommended as a skin protectant against aggressive chemicals such as surfactants, alkalis, and organic solvents, as it might also help prevent irritant contact dermatitis. It is suitable for dry and oily skins due to its lipo and hydrophobic properties. This ingredient also enhances product stability and improves product feel on the skin.

perfluoropolymethylisopropylether—used in formulations to stabilize emulsions, reduce skin moisture loss, and provide a product with a silky texture.

perhydroxysqualene (squalane)—an emollient that can be obtained from a variety of sources, including wheat germ, olive and bran oils, and shark liver oil. When obtained from shark liver oil, it must be converted from squalene through a process of hydrogenization.

petit grain biguarade—*see* petit grain oil.

petit grain extract—credited with tonic and antiseptic properties. *See also* petit grain oil.

petit grain oil (petitgrain)—widely used in pharmacy and perfumery for its therapeutic and tonic effect. Its fragrance is fresh, invigorating, and slightly floral with a bitter note. Like neroli, real petitgrain (or petitgrain biguarade) is obtained by distilling the leaves of the bitter orange tree. Petitgrain bergamot, petitgrain lemon, and petitgrain mandarin are also produced. May be irritating to the skin.

petitgrain—*see* petit grain oil.

petrolatum (petroleum jelly; Vaseline)—softens and smoothes the skin. It forms a film on the skin's surface, preventing moisture loss due to evaporation, and protecting against irritation. Its disadvantage lies in the difficulty of effectively and properly removing it from the skin. Studies indicate that petrolatum accelerates the recovery of skin surface lipids and neither forms nor acts as an impermeable membrane. Rather, it permeates throughout the corneum layer, allowing normal barrier recovery despite its occlusive properties. Petrolatum imparts a greasier feeling than other emollients and also has the potential for clogging pores and causing comedogenicity. It is a purified mixture of semi-solid hydrocarbons from petroleum. Although it can cause allergic skin rashes, petrolatum is nontoxic to the skin when properly purified and of high grade.

petroleum jelly—*see* petrolatum.

phenethyl alcohol—*see* phenylethyl alcohol.

phenol—frequently used for medical chemical face peels. It may trap free radicals and can act as a preservative. Phenol,

P

however, is an extremely caustic chemical with a toxicity potential. It is considered undesirable for use in cosmetics. Even at low concentrations, it frequently causes skin irritation, swelling, and rashes.

L-phenylalanine—an amino acid used as a skin-conditioning agent. It has greater use in hair care than in skin care products.

phenoxyethanol—a broad-range preservative with fungicidal, bactericidal, insecticidal, and germicidal properties. It has a relatively low sensitizing factor in leave-on cosmetics. Phenoxyethanol can be used in concentrations of 0.5 to 2.0 percent, and in combination with other preservatives such as sorbic acid or parabens. In addition, it is used as a solvent for aftershaves, face and hair lotions, shampoos, and skin creams of all types. It can be obtained from phenol.

phenoxyethylparaben—a preservative considered a noncomedogenic raw material.

2-phenyl-5-benzimidazolesulfonic acid—*see* phenylbenzimidazole sulfonic acid.

phenyl dimethicone—an antifoaming agent and an occlusive skin-conditioning agent. This mixture of linear siloxane polymers is a silicone-derived material. *See also* dimethicone.

phenyl trimethicone—serves as a barrier protecting the skin from excessive water loss. It leaves the skin feeling soft and smooth, adds emolliency to a formulation, and reduces any feeling of tackiness. It can also be used to control or prevent a cosmetic preparation from foaming. It is a form of silcone, which is similar to dimethicone but has a broader range of compatibility with organic oils and waxes.

phenylalanine—a conditioning agent with greater application in hair care than in skin care preparations. It is also used in suntan products.

phenylbenzimidazole sulfonic acid (2-phenyl-5-benzimidazolesulfonic acid; 2-phenylbenzimidazole-5-sulfonic acid)—one of 21 FDA-approved sunscreen chemicals for UVB absorption. It has an approved usage level of up to 4 percent in the U.S. and up to 8 percent in the European Union. When combined with a proper base, it becomes a water-soluble sunscreen. It exhibits a very effective use level versus SPF relationship when compared to other sunscreen chemicals. In addition, when combined with other UVB absorbers, it seems to significantly boost SPF. Also excellent for use in clear sunscreen gels.

P

2-phenylbenzimidazole-5-sulfonic acid (2-penyl-5-benzimidazolesulfonic acid)—*see* phenylbenzimidazole sulfonic acid.

phenylethyl alcohol (phenethyl alcohol)—used as a disinfectant, a preservative, and for its fragrance properties. It is a primary component of rose oil, and is also found in oranges, raspberries, and tea.

phosphatides—*see* phospholipids.

phospholipids (phosphatides)—used topically as a moisture/ emollient because of their inherent compatibility with skin lipids. In general, natural phospholipids have a short-lived effect when topically applied, and are a primary material in the manufacture of liposomes. Phospholipids are complex fat substances that, together with protein, form the membrane of all living cells. *See also* liposomes.

phosphatidic acid—one of several minor components of cosmetic and pharmaceutical liposomal membranes.

phosphatidylcholine—a major component of most cosmetic and pharmaceutical liposome structures, derived from commercially available egg yolk or soybean lecithin.

phosphatidyl ethanolamine—a minor component of cosmetic and pharmaceutical liposomal membranes.

phosphatidylinositol—a minor component of cosmetic and pharmaceutical liposomal membranes.

phosphatidylserine—used in the manufacturing of large quantities of liposomes.

phosphoenolpyruvic acid—skin care preparations containing this ingredient are said to improve dry skin due to its moisturizing properties and its ability to accelerate cell turnover.

P

phosphoric acid—a preservative and an antioxidant. It is irritating to the skin in concentrated solutions.

phytic acid—used to help maintain product stability, its therapeutic activities are said to include skin-lightening, antiinflammatory and antioxidant properties. Naturally occurring in grains, seeds, and beans.

phytosterol oleate—the prefix phyto- means plant. *See also* sterols.

phytosterols—*see* plant sterols.

pine bark extract—used as a solvent. It is also an antiseptic and stimulant. Pine bark extract can cause skin irritation.

pine cone extract—said to be a skin stimulant. This extract is obtained from pine cones. *See also* pine extract.

pine extract (Pinus sp.)—the different varieties of pine yield resin in greater or smaller quantities, of which a very small amount is employed for therapeutic purposes, primarily as ointments. Pine's therapeutic properties are described as bactericidal and stimulating to blood circulation. Manufacturers usually specify if the extract is from the pine's bark, cone, or needle. Can be irritating to the skin and cause red splotches.

pine needle extract—recommended for use as a skin stimulant. It is the extract of the needles of various pine species.

pine oil—originally used as a solvent and a disinfectant. Studies are now showing that pine oil may stimulate the growth of fibroblasts, which would mean an increase in the turnover of epidermal cells. Pine oil is produced by distillation of small pine branches. It may be irritating to the skin and mucous membranes.

pineapple enzyme—used in folkloric medicine as an anti-inflammatory. It is currently used in face masks and peeling lotions to remove the top layers of cells. Pineapple's activity is based on bromelin, an enzyme that dissolves keratin. Its important constituents include mucins, amino acids, polysaccharides, minerals, flavonoids, and enzymes. It can be irritating to the skin.

piscine oil, C_{30}-C_{46}—a fish oil used as an emollient.

plant extracts—an all-encompassing and vague term usually used for marketing effect. Its lack of specificity does not allow for the identification of potential benefits, botanical properties, or irritating effects.

plant sterols—active principles that can perform a variety of functions, including moisturizing. Used by cosmetic formulators to add a lipophilic property to a formulation. Often derived from plants associated with oils such as soy and canola seed.

plantain extract (Plantago sp.)—credited with cooling, soothing, antiseptic, astringent, and bacteriostatic botanical properties. It is a banana-like fruit.

plantain fruit—see banana oil.

pollen extract—an extract of flower pollen.

poloxamer 188—a liquid surfactant polymer.

poloxamer 788—a surfactant polymer. A change in number (for example, poloxamer 188 versus poloxamer 788) indicates the consistency of the ingredient, generally from liquid to

P

paste to solid. The higher the number, the more solid the consistency.

polyacrylamide—a binder, film former, and fixative with greater use in hair and nail than in skin care preparations. It is used in some hand and body lotions and cleansing creams.

polyacrylamidomethyl benzylidene camphor—a sunscreen chemical that works as a UV filter and absorber. It has an approved usage level of up to 6 percent in the European Union.

polyacrylic acid salt—a binder, emulsion stabilizer, film former, and viscosity-increasing agent primarily used in shampoos.

polyalkoxy ester—a thickener, auxiliary emulsifier, and body agent in cosmetic formulations.

polybutene—a binder and viscosity-increasing agent used more in makeup than skin care preparations. Polybutene is a polymer of one or more butylenes obtained from petroleum oils.

polybutylene terephthalate—a film former and viscosity-increasing agent.

polycaprolactone—a synthetic polymer that acts as a suspending agent.

polydecene—an emollient and skin conditioner.

polydimethyl cyclosiloxane—*see* cyclomethicone.

polyether-1—a thickener with emulsifying properties. Can also provide humectancy and lubricity.

polyethoxylated retinamide (PERA)—has characteristics similar to retinoic acid and retinol, improving collagen synthesis and promoting wrinkle reduction. The penetration potential of PERA is said to be three times greater than that of retinol and six times greater than that of retinyl palmitate. PERA is a combination of retinoic acid with polyethylene glycol, and is designed for enhanced stability and skin permeability. *See also* retinoids entry in Chapter 4.

polyethylene—used to regulate viscosity, suspension properties, and general stability in cosmetic formulations. It is derived from petroleum gas or dehydration of alcohol.

polyethylene beads—used in scrubs as replacement for almond particles. Some companies prefer it as they consider it less abrasive for delicate skins.

polyethylene glycol (PEG)—a binder, solvent, plasticizing agent, and softener widely used for cosmetic cream bases and pharmaceutical ointments. PEGs are quite humectant

P

up to a molecular weight of 500. Beyond this weight, their water uptake diminishes.

polyethylene glycol monostearate—an emulsifier. *See also* PEG.

polyethylene particles—*see* polyethylene beads.

polyethylene terephthalate—a film former and viscosity-increasing agent. This is a synthetic polymer.

polyglucadyne—a trade name for polyglucan. *See* polyglucan.

polyglucan (beta-glucan; polyglucadyne)—reported to enhance the skin's natural defense mechanism, which becomes less effective with age and exposure to UV light. It is also credited with wound-healing properties and it promotes cellular activity; serves as a topical moisturizer with long-lasting moisturizing effects; reduces wrinkles; helps protect the skin from infection; and protects the skin from invasion by toxic agents caused by pollution and injuries due to abrasions, exposure to UV light, and extremes in climatic conditions. In addition to this impressive list, polyglucans are also credited with immunostimulatory properties. A polyglucan is a hydrophilic ingredient, able to absorb more than 10 times its weight in water. It can be absorbed into the outer layers of the epidermis due to its extremely small size, thereby facilitating penetration into the pores and follicular openings of the skin. Once applied on the skin, it forms a protective, hydrated film with superior adhesive properties that do not appear to interfere with normal skin respiration. These film-forming and protective properties are particularly valuable for aging skin suffering from diminished collagen and elastin, as well as impaired hydration and elasticity. Derived from yeast cell walls, polyglucans are compatible for formulation with all normally used skin care and other cosmetic ingredients. *See also* glucans; betaglucan.

polyglyceryl-3-dioleate—an emulsifier for water-in-oil emulsions. Listed as being very suitable for use in baby care products, water-resistant sun-protection products, skin creams, and dry skin treatment products. It is an ester of oleic acid with polyglycerol.

polyglyceryl-3 distearate—an emulsifier used in oil-in-water emulsions.

polyglyceryl-3 methylglucose distearate—an emulsifier and skin conditioner.

polyglyceryl-4-oleate—used as an emulsifier in cosmetic formulations. It may also be used as a lubricant, plasticizer,

P

gelling agent, and dispersant. It is prepared by adding alcohol to coconut oil or other triglycerides.

polyglyceryl-10 dipalmitate—also known as decaglyceryl dipalmitate. An emollient and emulsifier.

polyglyceryl-6 distearate—an emulsifier. Can be found in products for sensitive skin, baby products, and sun care products.

polyglyceryl methacrylate—a film former used in moisturizers, skin care products, and fragrance preparations. It is a synthetic polymer.

polyisobutene (hydrogenated)—an emollient.

polymethylacrylate—a film former. It is a synthetic polymer used in suntan gels, creams, and liquids as well as a variety of makeup preparations such as blushes, foundations, and powders.

polymethoxy bicyclic oxazolidine—a preservative active against yeast, bacteria, and mold. It can be used alone or with parabens, in which case it contributes to the preservative activity. This ingredient can be used in rinse-off and leave-on cosmetics, with manufacturers reporting a good toxicological profile at recommended use levels.

polyols stearate—an emulsifier and a thickening agent.

polyoxyethylene cetyl ether—*see* polyoxyethylene compounds.

polyoxyethylene compounds—emulsifiers used in cosmetic formulations.

polyoxyethylene monooleate—an emulsifier. *See also* PEG 20-oleate.

polyoxyethylene nonylphenyl ether (nonoxynol)—an emulsifier.

polyoxyethylene stearyl alcohol—an emulsifier. *See also* PEG stearol.

polyoxyethylene-(21)-steryl alcohol—an emulsifier. *See also* PEG-21 stearol.

polyoxyethyleneglycol monostearate—an emulsifier.

polypentaerythritol tetralaurate—an emulsifier. Considered a noncomedogenic raw material.

polypeptides—*see* hydrolyzed animal protein; protein.

polyphenol—the coloring agent in phenolic compounds. It is also considered a natural antiseptic. Polyphenol is rather irritating and sensitizing.

polyquaternium-10—a cellulose polymer and conditioning agent used in skin-conditioning formulations.

P

polyquaternium-24—suggested by some companies to be used as an SPF enhancer in sunscreen formulations. This is a film former similar to polyquaternium-10, but it gives better skin feel and has a lipophilic character that enables it to act as a secondary emulsifier and help form a thicker, more uniform sunscreen film.

polyquaternium-51—used as a film former and for skin conditioning properties including to improve skin feel.

polysaccharide xanthan—see xanthan gum.

polysorbate 20—a solubilizer, emulsifier, viscosity-modifier, and stabilizer of essential oils in water.

polysorbate 40—an emulsifier and stabilizer of essential oils in water. It is also a detergent. Employed in a variety of cleansing and moisturizing preparations.

polysorbate 60—an emulsifier, wetting agent, and detergent emulsifier for mineral oil, fats, and waxes. It is also a stabilizer of essential oils in water. Widely used in cosmetic and toiletry preparations.

polysorbate 60 NF—an oil-in-water emulsifier and a fragrance solubilizer used in cosmetic and pharmaceutical creams and lotions. *See also* polysorbate 60.

polysorbate 80—an oil-in-water emulsifier.

polysorbate 80 NF—a hydrophilic emulsifier, pigment dispersant, and solubilizer for oils and fragrances. Used in creams, lotions, and makeup bases.

polysorbate 120—a fragrance solubilizer and an emulsifier used in sunscreen preparations and moisturizing creams and lotions.

polytetrafluoroethylene—see PTFE.

polyvinyl acetate emulsion—a binder, emulsion stabilizer, and film-forming substance. *See also* polyvinylpyrrolidone.

polyvinyl alcohol—a binder, film former, and viscosity-increasing agent used primarily in makeup and nail polish preparations.

polyvinylpyrrolidone (PVP)—a chemical ingredient that, depending on the formulatory requirement, can act as a binder, viscosity controller, emulsion stabilizer, or film former. Its benefits include water and wear resistance, pigment dispersion, a nongreasy feel, and improved stick integrity. PVP is commonly found in waterproof sunscreens, mascaras, and lipsticks in order to improve their wear.

pomegranate extract (Punica granatum)—has cleansing, astringent, tonic, and purifying properties. It also is a

P

strong natural antioxidant with skin-protecting and anti-inflammatory properties. Its constituents include polyphenols and anthocyanidins. In addition to pomegranate extract, and depending on a formula's requirements, cosmetic formulators can use bark extract, the fruit juice, the seed, and the seed oil. The juice is the part that is used.

poplar bud extract—said to be antibacterial and support wound-healing. It may also be used topically for treating superficially broken skin as well as sunburn.

Portulaca oleracea—commonly known as purslane. Its therapeutic activities are considered to include antimicrobial, antifungal, anti-inflammatory, and analgesic (pain-relieving). Used in extract form, its constituents include alkaloids, coumarins, glycosides, omega-3 fatty acids, proteins, and flavonoids.

potassium PCA—a humectant that improves skin moisturization.

potassium alginate—*see* algin.

potassium alum (alum)—a cosmetic astringent.

potassium carbomer 941—*see* carbomer entry in Chapter 4.

potassium chloride—a laboratory reagent used as a viscosity-increasing agent in cosmetic and pharmaceutical preparations.

potassium hydroxide—used as an emulsifier in lotions and as an alkali in liquid soaps, protective creams, and shaving preparations. Depending on the concentration used, it can be highly irritating to the skin and/or cause a burning sensation.

potassium myristate—a cleansing and emulsifying agent.

potassium phosphate—a humectant and pH adjuster used in cosmetic formulations. Potassium phosphate is an inorganic salt.

potassium sorbate—a preservative primarily against mold and yeast, and used in concentrations of 0.025 to 0.2 percent. It is nontoxic but may cause mild skin irritation.

potassium stearate—a cleansing and emulsifying agent.

potassium sulfate—a reagent in cosmetics. Potassium sulfate is an inorganic salt with a primary function as a viscosity-increasing agent.

potato extract (Psoralea coryfolia)—studies indicate value in products for the treatment of severe dry skin conditions such as psoriasis. Psoralen, the relevant fraction of potato extract, appears to prevent keratinocyte proliferation, and is known to inhibit DNA synthesis.

P

potato starch (modified)—a thickener that works well in acidic formulations. *See also* potato extract.

PPG-2 isoceteth-20 acetate—an emulsifier.

PPG-2 methyl ether acetate—a solvent, it is also used as a formula stabilizer and to improve skin penetration in topically applied acne preparations containing erythromycin.

PPG-2 ceteareth-9—a surfactant and emulsifying agent.

PPG-2-PEG 20 isocetyl acetate—a fragrance solubilizer and oil-in-water emulsifier.

PPG-3 benzyl ether myristate—an emollient that provides silicone-like characteristics to a formulation. Used to give shine in hair products and gloss to lip products. It can also be found in sun care preparations to improve SPF values.

PPG-4 myristyl ether propionate—an emollient.

PPG-5-ceteth 20—a surfactant and emulsifying agent.

PPG-15 stearyl ether—an emollient and skin conditioning agent.

PPG-20 methyl glucose ether—an emollient.

PPG-30 cetyl ester, -50 cetyl ester—both are emollients.

pregnenolone hemisuccinate—used topically as an anti-inflammatory and anti-itch agent. A corticosteroid. *See also* primula extract.

primrose—*see* primula extract.

primula extract (Primula officinalis or Primula vulagris) (primrose)—traditionally used as adjunct soothing and anti-itching treatment. It is useful in dry skin preparations. The leaves of some species are known to cause skin irritation sometimes resulting in a form of eczema.

procollagen—water-binding and moisturizing. Procollagen is a triple helical molecule of collagen, and is fully soluble and membrane permeable. It is hygroscopic and, as such, is able to bind many times its weight in water. Procollagen is found naturally in the skin as a first stage in the production of collagen. With age, there is a decrease in the skin's procollagen content that may have some correlation to the increased dryness and reduction in elasticity often associated with mature skin.

proline—a skin-conditioning agent. An amino acid found in the collagen molecule. *See also* amino acid.

propanetriol—*see* glycerin.

propolis—once considered a mystical cure for such problems as infections and troubled skin. Chemists now recognize propolis as having a sun protective function, and many

P

preparations for acne problems also contain propolis as an active substance for its healing, cleansing and antiseborrhoeic properties. It is also moisturizing and can help smooth the skin. Propolis is made up of resins, balsam, various waxes, essential oils, pollen, flavonoids, amino acids, vitamins, and minerals. This is a component of beeswax, often referred to by beekeepers as "bee glue." It is collected from trees, shrubs, flowers, and other types of plants visited by bees.

propolis extract HD 10%—*see* propolis.

propyl gallate—an antioxidant with preservative properties.

propyl paraben—one of the most frequently used preservatives against bacteria and mold. It has a low sensitizing and low toxicity factor, and is reputed to be very safe. Considered a noncomedogenic raw material. *See also* parabens entry in Chapter 4.

propylene carbonate—used in chemical reactions as a solvent, plasticizer, solubilizer, or dilutent.

propylene glycol—next to water, this is the most common moisture-carrying vehicle used in cosmetic formulations. It has better skin permeation than glycerin, and it also gives a pleasant feel with less greasiness than glycerin. Propylene glycol is used as a humectant since it absorbs water from the air. It also serves as a solvent for antioxidants and preservatives. In addition, it has preservative properties against bacteria and fungi when used in concentrations of 16 percent or higher. There is a concern that propylene glycol is an irritant at high concentrations, though it appears to be quite safe at usage levels under 5 percent. *See also* glycerin.

propylene glycol ceteth-3 acetate—an emollient used in moisturizing preparations.

propylene glycol dicaprylate/dicaprate—has very good emollient properties. It also provides a product with good skin coverage, and spreadability and absorption promotion properties. It does not cause skin irritation.

propylene glycol di-isostearate—considered an excellent emollient. Similar to jojoba oil.

propylene glycol di-pelargonate—an emollient ester with good skin penetrating and spreadability properties. Does not leave a greasy feel.

propylene glycol mono-isostearate (propylene glycol isostearate)—an emollient.

P

propylene glycol monomethyl ether—a stabilizer and skin penetration enhancer often found in topical acne preparations in which erythromycin is the active substance.

propylene glycol myristyl ether acetate—a skin conditioning agent and emollient; also used in lipstick.

protein (partially hydrolyzed protein; peptide; peptone; polypeptide)—its main function in skin care preparations is to produce a good film on the skin, thus helping reduce the loss of natural moisture. The films formed by animal proteins, such as collagen and elastin, are not occlusive as may be the case with mineral oil. Rather, they lie on the skin and have an affinity for it. All proteins, whether animal, vegetable, or silk derived, are built up from amino acids linked together to form a polymer. Depending on its source, the molecular weight of naturally occurring proteins may range from several thousands to millions, and the amino acid composition, which also influences the protein's properties, may vary widely. In the case of collagen-derived proteins, attributes include the ability to form clear solutions, contribute viscosity, stabilize oil-in-water emulsions, bind moisture, and form glossy films. The benefits claimed are soft and silky skin feel, increased moisture retention with a related improvement of elasticity, and a decrease in chapping and irritation conditions. Adding protein to skin cleansing surfactants reduces skin irritation and dryness. Animal-derived collagen protein has been the preferred protein because of performance, ease of availability, and cost. However, due to consumer preferences to move away from animal products, vegetal proteins have been perfected for use in skin care cosmetics. The most popular appears to be wheat-based hydrolyzed protein. Proteins are usually hydrolyzed to achieve lower molecular values, which enhances moisture-binding properties.

pseudoalteromonas ferment extract—a humectant derived from marine bacteria, it can help reduce skin roughness.

pseudocollagen—acts in much the same way as collagen, leaving the skin feeling soft and supple. Pseudocollagen forms a moisture-retentive film on the skin in a similar way to soluble collagen. It represents the pseudocollagenous extract of yeast cells. It is plant derived.

PTFE (polytetrafluoroethylene)—a bulking agent, it is also used in cosmetic preparations to improve the formulation's feel and spreadability. PTFE may also have some waterproofing potential.

P

pumice powder—usually employed in cosmetics for removing rough skin. Used in hand cleansing preparations, skin cleansing grains, powders, and soaps for acne. Because of its abrasive action, daily use is not recommended. If used continuously on dry, sensitive skin, it will most likely cause irritation. It can also be an irritant when used in soapless detergents. Pumice is of volcanic origin and consists primarily of complex silicates of aluminum and alkali metals.

pumpkin (Curcubita pepo)—credited with purative properties. Cosmetic applications include use in acne products and as an antiseborrheic. While the seeds have medicinal value, it is often the root that is used for obtaining the extract.

pumpkin enzyme—exfoliating and softening, it can help smooth the appearance of fine line and wrinkles.

purcellin oil (nonanimal) (cetearyl octanoate)—used as a fixative in perfumes. This is a synthetic mixture of fatty esters designed to simulate the natural oil obtained from the preen glands of waterfowl.

PVP—*see* polyvinylpyrrolidone.

PVP/eicosene copolymer—a waterproofing polymer with sunscreen absorption properties. *See also* polyvinylpyrrolidone.

PVP/hexdecene copolymer—designed for use in formulations where unique delivery systems are desired. *See also* polyvinylpyrrolidone.

PVP/triacontene copolymer—a PVP with greater waterproofing abilities and significantly improved retention of UV absorbers in sunscreen products than PVP/eicosene. *See also* polyvinylpyrrolidone.

pyridoxine dipalmitate—a skin-conditioning agent used in moisturizing formulations.

pyridoxine hydrochloride—*see* pyridoxine HCL.

pyridoxine HCL—a skin-conditioning agent that is also widely used in hair products.

pyridoxine tripalmitate—soothing to the skin. This is a stable, oil-soluble form of vitamin B_6. It prevents scaling and skin dryness, and is also used as a product texturizer.

pyrrolidonic carbon acid (nalidone)—a natural moisturizing factor that protects the skin from dehydration and increases its moisture-retention capabilities.

pyrrolidone-carboxylic acid—a moisturizing agent. *See also* PCA.

P

pyruvic acid—an alpha hydroxyacid that can be irritating and is considered difficult to work with. It has a larger molecular size than the most commonly used AHAs. Sodium pyruvate is more commonly used, and is an organic salt. *See also* alpha hydroxyacid.

P

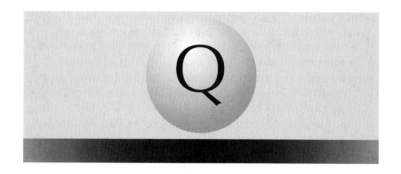

quassia *(Picraena excelsa)*—an antibacterial. Quassia yields quassin, a bitter alkaloid obtained from the wood of *Quassia amara*. Quassia is primarily a denaturant for ethyl alcohol.

quaternium-15—an all-purpose preservative, it is active against bacteria, mold, and yeast, and used in concentrations of 0.02 to 0.3 percent. Though not a primary skin irritant, quaternium-15 is considered a highly sensitizing preservative when used in leave-on cosmetic preparations. Dermatologists find it to be the most frequent sensitizer among preservatives in the United States. It is probably the greatest formaldehyde releaser among cosmetic preservatives, causing dermatitis in people who are allergic to formaldehyde and even in those who are not. The technical data of some manufacturers indicates, however, that quaternium-15 does not contain or release free gaseous formaldehyde. These would most likely be versions of quaternium-15 that have been specially formulated and adjusted to avoid formaldehyde release.

quaternium-18—a surfactant.

quaternium-18 bentonite—a thickener and conditioning agent, it helps control product viscosity.

quaternium-18 hectorite—used as a thickener and suspending agent, it helps control product viscosity. Produced by a reaction of hectorite and the quaternary salt. Used in concentrations of 1.5 percent. *See also* hectorite.

quercus extract *(English oak extract)*—*see* oak.

quinaquina—*see* cinchona extract.

Q

quince extract *(Pyrus cydonia)*—when obtained from the juice of the fruit, it is astringent and tonic and mentioned as appropriate for dry skin and in eye treatment preparations. See also quince seed.

quince seed—an emollient, emulsifier, and thickening agent, it can also be used as an abrasive. Quince seed extract can also help mask odor. It may cause allergic reactions.

quinine extract—an alkaloid from the bark of *Cinchona officinalis.* *See* cinchona extract.

Q

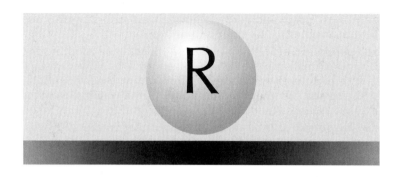

ramulus mori extract—credited with strong skin-lightening abilities due to tyrosinase inhibition activities. Even at low concentrations, ramulus mori has demonstrated more efficacious tyrosinase inhibition capacities than kojic acid and arbutin. Studies indicate little to no irritation caused by this extract. Ramulus mori extract is derived specifically from the young twigs of the white mulberry tree (*Morus alba*). These properties would make ramulus mori beneficial in products designed to even skin tone. *See also* mulberry extract.

raspberry concentrate (*Rubus idaeus*)—botanical properties are described as astringent and tonic. Raspberry concentrate is added to cosmetics to give them the fruit's fresh smell. Some sources claim that there is no evidence of raspberries having any external value for the skin, and that they may increase allergenicity.

raspberry seed oil—made up of a very high percentage of essential fatty acids (including omega-3 and omega-6), as well as vitamin E, which gives it antioxidant capacities. It is emollient, skin conditioning, and anti-inflammatory. It also exhibits UVB absorption capacities.

red algae extracts—*see* seaweed extract.

red clover—described as beneficial for acne and eczema. *See also* clover; isoflavones.

red currant (*Ribes rubrum*)—the fruit has astringent properties, while the fruit extract is considered tonic and refreshing. When used in cosmetic preparations, red currant juice can help improve the skin's general condition. Constituents of

R

red current include vitamin C, fruit acids, pectin, and flavonoids.

red poppy extract *(Papaver rhoeas)*—considered soothing and emollient, this extract is obtained from the flower's petals. When the extract is derived from poppy seeds it is soothing and skin conditioning. Poppy flower water is known to be astringent and able to mask odor.

red raspberry extract—considered astringent. *See also* raspberry concentrate.

red vine extract—anti-inflammatory and anti-itching. Traditionally used for broken or fragile capillaries.

red wine—contains tartaric acid, a member of the alpha hydroxyacid family. Red wine can be used in cosmetics, given its anti-inflammatory and polyphenol-based antioxidant properties. Red wine's therapeutic benefits are more closely linked to its botanical constituents, rather than a topical application of red wine on the skin. *See also* alpha hydroxyacid; grape.

resin—used to give gloss, flow, adhesion, and water resistance to cosmetics. This is a brittle substance, usually translucent or transparent, that can be either naturally derived or synthetically obtained. Among the natural resins are dammar, elemi, and sandarac, which are formed from the hardened secretions of these plants. Toxicity and allergenicity depend on source used.

resorcinol—in very mild solutions, used as an antiseptic and soothing preparation for itchy skin. In slightly higher concentrations, resorcinol removes the top layer of the stratum corneum and is used particularly in cases of acne. In still higher concentrations, it can act as an aggressive surface skin exfoliant. Resorcinol can also be used as a preservative. While it is a beneficial skin care ingredient when used in low concentrations, it causes irritation in higher concentrations with a strong burning sensation and a reddening of the skin. Used in high concentrations as a peel, resorcinol may cause a variety of problems, including swelling. Resorcinol is obtained from various resins.

restharrow extract *(Ononis arvensis **and** Ononis spinosa)*—an emollient that provides relief for skin itching. Traditionally used for relieving the problems of eczema. The extract is obtained from the plant's roots.

R

reticulin (soluble)—a protein that, when on the skin's surface, acts as a protective agent against water loss. It helps increase the water content of the skin's outer layers, plumping up the epidermis and leaving the skin softer and smoother. Unlike proteins of a similar molecular weight, when reticulin dries, it leaves the skin feeling pleasant and without tackiness.

retinaldehyde—a mild retinoid credited with increasing epidermal thickness without producing erythema.

retinoic acid (tretinoin)—a vitamin A derivative. Has demonstrated an ability to alter collagen synthesis, increase dermal hyaluronic acid levels, and stimulate the growth of fibroblasts and the extracellular matrix. It is used for keratinization disorders and for treating acne. Retinoic acid's antiaging effect has been convincingly documented, and it is often used for treating the visible signs of aging. It is associated with a number of adverse effects, including irritation, photosensitivity, skin dryness, redness, and peeling. *See also* retinoids in Chapter 4.

retinol—a retinoid considered to be a skin revitalizer, retinol is reported to enhance skin radiance and treat conditions associated with chronological aging, such as wrinkles and fine lines, as well as dermatological disorders, including acne, follicular and lesion papules, actinic keratosis, oily skin, and rosacea. According to clinical dermatologists, retinol is one of the few substances with a demonstrated ability to reduce and prevent fine lines and wrinkles. It is able to alter the behavior of aged cells so they act in a more youthful manner. It is considered necessary for normal epidermal cell growth and differentiation and stimulates the production of new blood vessels in the skin, improving skin tone. In addition, retinol has antioxidant capacities and protects dermal fibers by counteracting the increased activity of enzymes that degrade collagen and elastin when the skin is exposed to UV rays. Retinol can be drying to the skin when used for a prolonged period of time or in concentrations that are too high. A weaker retinoid than retinoic acid, retinol converts to retinoic acid once on the skin. When compared to retinoic acid, retinol has an increased penetration potential and is less irritating, making it an effective cosmetic antiaging ingredient. The antiaging benefits of topically treating skin with retinol are believed to be based on its penetration ability, which allows it to reach the sites in the skin requiring treatment. When used on sensitive skin for a prolonged period of time or in concentrations that are too high, retinol can cause dermatitis. *See also* retinoids in Chapter 4.

R

retinyl esters—precursors of retinoic acid. Common retinyl esters include acetate, propionate, and palmitate. When compared to retinol, they have a more difficult time penetrating the skin and they demonstrate a lower clinical effectiveness. However, they are more stable than retinol and hence considered easier to incorporate into a formulation. Given the improvements in delivery technology for retinol, and depending on the formulatory needs, manufacturers are increasingly using retinol rather than the retinyl esters, given retinol's greater activity. *See also* retinoids in Chapter 4.

retinyl linoleate—a conditioning agent, this is an ester of retinol and linoleic acid. *See also* retinol; linoleic acid.

retinyl palmitate—a skin conditioner, this retinoid is considered a milder version of retinoic acid, given its conversion properties. Once on the skin, it converts to retinol which, in turn, converts to retinoic acid. Physiologically, it is credited with increasing epidermal thickness, stimulating the production of more epidermal protein, and increasing skin elasticity. Cosmetically, retinyl palmitate is used to reduce the number and depth of fine lines and wrinkles, and prevent skin roughness resulting from UV exposure. Secondary reactions such as erythema, dryness, or irritation are not associated with retinyl palmitate. It is even more effective when used in combination with glycolic acid because it achieves greater penetration. In the United States, its maximum usage level in cosmetic formulations is 2 percent. Retinyl palmitate is the ester of retinol and palmitic acid. *See also* retinoids; vitamin A palmitate. *See also* retinoids in Chapter 4.

retinyl palmitate polypeptide—allows for the delivery of vitamin A as a water-dispersable substance.

rhubarb extract (Rheum palmatum)—astringent and tonic, rhubarb is said to act as a tyrosinase inhibitor and have skin-lightening properties, as well. Constituents include gallic acid, emodin, glucosides, tannoids, and resins. The root is used for obtaining extract, powder, tinctures, syrups, and infusions.

riboflavin (Vitamin B_2)—used in skin care preparations as an emollient. It can be found in sun care products as a suntan enhancer. Medicinally, it is used for the treatment of skin lesions.

riboflavin tetraacetate—a skin-conditioning agent, it is a vitamin B_2 derivative. *See also* vitamin B.

R

ribonucleic acid (RNA)—a surface film-forming agent with moisturizing action. This is the polyribonucleotide found in both the nucleus and the cytoplasm of cells.

rice amino acids—humectant and conditioning. This is an amino acid complex. Some chemical manufacturers note that it is all natural and vegetable-derived.

rice bran—soothing. It is credited with promoting collagen formation and inhibiting lipid peroxidation in the skin. Recommended for treatment of dry, mature skin. Rice bran is employed in various forms, including extract, oil, and wax. The oil functions as a carrier and an emollient. The germ and bran of unpolished rice contains linolic acid or vitamin F, oleic acid, palmitic acid, vitamin E, and oryzanol.

rice flour—*see* rice starch.

rice oil (Oryza sativa)—emollient, it is recommended for combination skin products where the ingredients must not be too aggressive for the dry skin area, and yet should be helpful for the oily T-zone.

rice germ oil—used in cosmetics for its emollient properties.

rice starch—emollient and able to form a soothing, protective film when applied to the skin. In addition, rice starch is employed in cosmetic formulations for its absorbent, binding and viscosity-controlling action. Rice starch also adds bulk. It is used in baby and face powders. Rice starch is a crystalline polymeric compound obtained from grains of rice.

ricinoleamide DEA—an emulsifier with lubricity, and good wetting and softening properties. It can also serve as a foam booster and formula stabilizer when blended with anionic surfactants such as lauryl sulfates.

ricinoleth—a surfactant used as a cleansing, emulsifying, and solubilizing agent.

RNA—*see* ribonucleic acid.

roe extract (Acipenser stellatus) (caviar)—used in products for oily and mature dehydrated skins in need of revitalization. It has a high and wide-ranging vitamin content that includes vitamins A, B_1, B_2, and B_6, D, and E. Roe extract contains an array of other constituents including cobalt, copper, fluorine, iodine, iron, magnesium, manganese, phosphorus, silicium, and zinc. The amino acids present are glutamic acid, glycine, methionine, lysine, arginine, histidine, and aspartic acid. In addition, roe has essential and sulfured amino acids and unsaturated fatty acids. Usage levels range from 1 to 5 percent depending on the preparation. Prepared from sturgeon roe.

R

Roman chamomile oil *(Anthemis nobilis)*—the most popular variety of chamomile, it is different from German chamomile (matricaria). Considered tonic and healing. *See* chamomile.

rose extract *(Rosa sp.)*—credited with astringent, tonic, and deodorant properties. It is also used as a fragrance.

rose hip *(Rosa canina)*—the seedpod that remains once the rose petals fall from the flower. Rich in vitamin C, the flower is also used to mask odor, while the rose hip fruit is considered astringent. *See also* rose hip oil.

rose hip oil—also known as rosa mosqueta oil. Emollient, it is also wound-healing and antiseptic. Studies indicate an ability to improve skin hydration, and aid in cases of pruritis and xerosis. It also helps regulate oil gland secretion. Rose hip oil is nourishing and rejuvenating and exhibits strong moisture-retention abilities. Its constituents include very high levels of essential fatty acids, and it is a natural source of retinoic acid. It is beneficial for use in sun care products, given its apparent UV-protection abilities. It is also increasingly incorporated into antiaging and antioxidant products.

rose hip powder—incorporated into formulations as a natural abrasive and for its ability to help remove dead surface cells (keratolytic action). Thus, it helps improve the skin's look, feel, and texture.

rose oil—has been credited with antiseptic, disinfectant, slightly tonic, and soothing properties. Some sources also cite moisturizing and moisture-retention abilities. It is found helpful in cases of skin redness or inflammation, and where moisturization and regeneration is needed. Rose oil may be beneficial to all skin types, particularly mature, dry, or sensitive skins. As one of the most expensive essential oils, true rose oil is only used in very high-grade perfumes. Rose oil is almost always adulterated with substances like geranium, lemongrass, palmarosa, and terpene alcohols. However, the process of adulteration has become so refined that it is almost impossible to discover frauds. To produce rose oil, rose buds are picked for only a few hours in the morning, right after the dew, and are immediately distilled. According to some sources, 30 roses are required to make one drop of oil. It is considered the least toxic of all essences. Given the cost and potential of adulteration, rosewater is widely used as a replacement for rose oil in cosmetics and perfumery.

rose petal extract—has mild astringency and tonic value. *See also* rose extract.

R

rose wax—floral waxes such as rose and jasmine complement the skin's natural lipids and give a formulation wear- and smudge-resistant properties. Rose wax is an almost odorless residue left after the extraction of the oily fractions.

rosemary extract (Rosmarinus officinalis)—a general effect attributed to this herb is the promotion of wound-healing, in addition to its astringent, toning, tonic, refreshing, stimulating, deodorant, antiseptic, reactivating, antibacterial, antimicrobial, softening, and invigorating properties. Rosemary also helps improve blood circulation, thereby aiding in skin regeneration. An alcohol fraction of rosemary extract had demonstrated strong antioxidant activity by hindering free-radical induced reactions. Rosemary adds fragrance to a formulation. Some constituents of rosemary extract include a variety of amino acids, caffeic acid, rosemary acid, and apigenin. The leaf is the part of the plant that is used.

rosemary oil—credited with antiseptic properties, it is also used for masking odor and providing fragrance. Rosemary oil is considered beneficial for acne, dermatitis, and eczema. Some reports indicate that rosemary oil may stimulate fibroblast growth with a possible increase in epidermal cell turnover. This would make it useful in products for aging and mature skin. Rosemary oil, obtained through distillation of the herb's flowering tops, is superior to that which is obtained through distillation of the stems and leaves. The latter process, however, is more common among the commercial oils.

rosewater—credited with soothing, astringent, and cleansing properties. In addition, it can be used as a vehicle for other ingredients and as an eye lotion. Ointment of rosewater is said to have soothing and cooling properties when applied to abrasions and other superficial skin lesions. Rosewater is often mixed with glycerin, which provides moisturization and lubricity. *See also* rose oil.

rosewood oil—one of the major perfumery oils used as a middle note. Until recently, it was little used in aromatherapy. Although it does not have major curative power, rosewood oil appears useful as a cellular stimulant and tissue regenerator. As such, it would be applicable to sensitive and aged skin, wrinkles, and general skin care. It is very mild, safe to use, and is obtained by means of distillation of the chopped wood.

R

rowan *(Sorbus aucuparia)*—also known as mountain ash. The extract, which aids in maintaining good skin condition, is obtained from the tree's fruit. Constituents include vitamins B and C, sorbite, tannin, carotene, flavonoids, fruit acids (e.g. malic acid), mineral salt, and glucose.

royal jelly—the therapeutic value associated with royal jelly when used in skin care products includes favoring the regeneration of dermal tissue, stimulating cell metabolism, improving the skin's look and feel, photoprotection, normalizing sebum secretion, and moisturizing, antiseptic, and anti-inflammatory activities. These characteristics are attributed to royal jelly's complex composition. Royal jelly is produced by bees (for the nutrition of the queen bee), and is a mixture of proteins, fats, carbohydrates, water, growth factors, and various trace elements. It has a high amino acid content (including aspartic acid, glutamic acid, glycine, and lysine), a high vitamin content (particularly the B family, but also A, C, and D), and is also made up of such minerals as potassium, calcium, and iron. Manufacturers cite royal jelly as particularly appropriate for use in antiaging products, as well as those for oily skin.

royal jelly extract HD—an extract of royal jelly. *See also* royal jelly.

Russian white oil—*see* mineral oil.

rutin—described as having tightening and strengthening properties for skin capillaries, thus helping to prevent a couperose condition. It also demonstrates antioxidant properties. Rutin is found in rue leaves, buckwheat, and other plants.

R

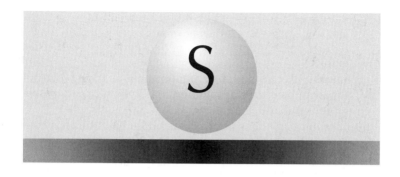

S

saccharide isomerate—a humectant and skin-conditioning agent.

Saccharomyces cerevisiae extract (living yeast)—healing and protecting. This extract is also credited with the ability to protect against infection and boost immunodefenses. Constituents include the polysaccharides d-mannan and d-glucan. *Saccharomyces cerevisiae* is a yeast traditionally used to help raise bread. *Saccharomyces* ferment also acts as a stabilizer for other compounds, particularly enzymes and metals. Given its ease of use and stabilizing activity, it is increasingly incorporated in skin care products.

Saccharomyces/copper ferment—obtained through the fermentation of Saccharomyces in the presence of copper ions. It is used to promote and maintain a good skin condition. It is found in a wide range of cosmetic products, including facial moisturizers, antiaging preparations, acne preparations, and sun care products. *See also Saccharomyces cerevisiae* extract.

Saccharomyces lysate extract powder—a yeast extract in powder form. Manufacturers note a variety of activity, including an ability to stimulate cellular consumption of oxygen, promote cellular proliferation, and stimulate collagen production. It could be incorporated into a number of product types, including antiaging, sun and post-sun products, makeup, and hair care products.

Saccharomyces/manganese ferment—obtained through the fermentation of *Saccharomyces* in the presence of manganese ions. It is found in such cosmetic preparations as eye creams, sun protection products, bronzers, moisturizers, facial powders, antiaging creams, and formulations for reducing skin redness. *See also Saccharomyces cerevisiae* extract.

Saccharomyces/xylinum/black tea ferment—a skin conditioning ingredient that is found in a variety of skin care preparations, including eye creams.

Saccharomyces/zinc ferment—obtained through the fermentation of *Saccharomyces* in the presence of zinc ions. *See also Saccharomyces cerevisiae* extract.

saccharum officinarum—moisturizing and helps keep the skin feeling smooth and supple. It is a sugarcane derivative. Manufacturers claim it to be beneficial for acne.

sacred bark—*see* cascara sagrada extract.

safflower oil *(Carthamus tinctorius)*—a carrier oil also considered hydrating to the skin. It consists primarily of linoleic acid triglycerides. Safflower oil is a noncomedogenic raw material obtained from the plant's seeds.

sage extract *(Salvia officinalis)*—considered to have astringent, antibacterial, antiseptic, anti-inflammatory, stimulating, softening, invigorating, and healing properties. Sage extract was traditionally used as a remedy for every type of inflammation. The extract is obtained from the herb's leaves.

sage oil—credited with depurative and healing properties, and indicated for acne and oily skin. Sage oil is obtained by distillation of sage leaves and flowers. *See also* sage extract.

St. John's wort extract *(Hypericum perforatum)* **(hypericum extract)**—said to have astringent, anti-inflammatory, and possibly soothing properties. St. John's wort offers general skin protection, especially for sensitive skin and areas with burns. This is an herbaceous perennial plant with hypericine as its important constituent.

St. John's wort oil—considered anti-inflammatory. It is beneficial for sensitive and/or rough, chapped skin as well as acne skin or skin suffering from irritation and inflammation. It is also considered effective for improving capillary circulation. In addition, St. John's wort oil is an antibiotic and can act as a natural preservative. This is a deep red oil. *See also* St. John's wort extract.

salicylamide—an analgesic, fungicide, and anti-inflammatory ingredient used to soothe the skin. Salicylamide is an aromatic amide.

salicylic acid—a beta-hydroxyacid with keratolytic and anti-inflammatory activity. It helps dissolve the top layer of corneum cells, improving the look and feel of the skin. Salicylic acid is an effective ingredient in acne products and as such is widely used in acne soaps and lotions. Because it is lipid soluble, it can more easily reduce sebaceous follicle blockage by penetrating the pores and exfoliating the cellular buildup. It is antimicrobial, antiseptic, and enhances the activity of preservatives. For the treatment of aging skin, it appears to help improve skin wrinkles, roughness, and tone. In addition, it is a useful ingredient for products formulated to treat psoriasis, callouses, corns, warts—cases where there is a buildup of dead skin cells. When applied topically, it is reported to penetrate 3 to 4 mm into the epidermis. A small amount of salicylic acid can convert to copper salicylate, a powerful anti-inflammatory. Used at high concentrations, salicylic acid may cause skin redness and rashes. This is a naturally occurring organic acid, related to aspirin. It is found in some plants, particularly the leaves of wintergreen and the bark of sweet birch. Salicylic acid is also synthetically manufactured.

salicyloxy-carboxy acid—a general term for a variety of salicyloxy-based compositions (salicyloxy-propionic acid, among them) acting as a skin-conditioning agent. They may also aid in controlling sebum secretion and improve skin feel. Additional properties are noted as antiaging (the reduction of wrinkles and benefit to photoaging skin); improved skin tone, radiance, and clarity; and promotion of generally healthier, younger looking skin. It can also reduce or help prevent stickiness and shine within a formulation.

salt—*see* sodium chloride.

sambucus extract—*see* elder extract.

sandalwood oil (Santalum album) (santal; santalum)—credited with astringent, anti-inflammatory, antibacterial, tonic, stimulant, cooling, and soothing properties. It is also considered a good antiseptic in cases of acne and an astringent for oily skin. There are indications that sandalwood oil may promote epidermal cell turnover as some report it stimulates fibroblast growth. Sandalwood could help prevent the skin dryness associated with seborrheic dermatitis, psoriasis, and eczema. In addition, some manufacturers utilize it as a natural colorant to give products a light red or rose tone. Sandalwood oil might produce a rash in hypersensitive people, especially if it is present in high concentrations. Produced by distillation of the inner wood.

santal oil—*see* sandalwood oil.

santalum oil—*see* sandalwood oil.

saponaria extract—*see* soapwort extract.

sarcosine—a naturally occurring amino acid that is used in cosmetic formulations as a skin conditioner. Its chemical name is n-methyl glycine.

sarriette oil—a fragrance with healing, tonic, antiseptic, and anti-inflammatory properties. This oil is derived from an herb native to the Mediterranean basin.

sarsaparilla (Smilax officinalis)—among its therapeutic botanical claims for skin care are healing, antiseptic, and beneficial for chronic skin disease, including psoriasis. Its primary constituents include saponins (sarsaponin and parallin) and sterols (sitosterol and stigmasterol). Independent of the variety of sarsaparilla, in every case the sarsaparilla's root is the part that is used.

sassafras oil (Sassafras albidum)—credited with antiseptic, astringent, and stimulant properties. Its main active ingredient is saprol, constituting about 80 percent. Sassafras oil is obtained from the plant's bark and root through a process of steam distillation. It may produce dermatitis in hypersensitive individuals.

savory (Satureia hortensis) (hortensis extract)—considered antiseptic and antibiotic. It is indicated for acne skin. A hardy herb.

saw palmetto fruit extract (Serenoa serrulata)—attributed with anti-inflammatory properties.

scabwort—*see* elecampane.

sclary sage oil—*see* clary sage oil.

sclerotium gum—can be used as a thickener and stabilizer as well as to improve a formulation's skin feel and spreadability.

scurvy grass extract (Cochlearia officinalis)—considered tonic. It is a source of vitamin C.

SD alcohol-40—*see* alcohol SD-40.

SD alcohol-40A—*see* alcohol SDA-40.

SD alcohol-40B—the B denotes a specific denaturing method. *See also* alcohol SD-40.

sea clay—*see* clay.

sea lettuce extract (Ulva lactuca)—anti-inflammatory and antioxidant. *See also* seaweed extract.

sea minerals yeast derivative—described as supplying essential minerals for cosmetic applications. Marine elements have been used for centuries for their beneficial effects on all epidermal structures. The mixture of sea elements with low-molecular-weight yeast glycoproteins apparently results in a degree of biocompatability with the skin and acceptance by the epidermal cells.

S

sea salt—a mild abrasive used in scrubs. Its water solubility allows it to self-dissolve during product use. It is also employed as a dilutant. As sea salt does not seem to form secondary reactions, it is considered a stable ingredient in cosmetic formulations. In large grains, it is colored and perfumed, and utilized in bath salts. Sea salt may cause dryness.

sea wave—*see* seaweed extract.

sea wrack—*see* seaweed extract.

seawater—healing powers have long been attributed to the sea. Salt water can have an antiseptic and stimulating effect when used to treat wounds. Used primarily in oligotherapy and thalassotherapy, its cosmetic benefits have yet to be proven.

seaweed (fresh)—has gelatinous properties. It is the major ingredient in the thin, clear masks that peel off in one piece when applied on the skin. This type of mask allows the skin to build up a supply of water, giving it a moist, supple look. Seaweed is also used in face creams and lotions, providing body and substance to products. Considered good for oily skin.

seaweed extract (Fucus vesiculosus) (algae extract; black tang; bladderwrack; fucus; kelp; laminaria digitata, sea wave; sea wrack)—seaweed has been used by the Chinese for curing burns and rashes; by the Polynesians for treating wounds, bruises, and swelling; and by mariners who recognized its healing properties. Seaweed is found to be stimulating, revitalizing, and nourishing to the skin due to its iodine and sulfur amino acid content, which also give it anti-inflammatory and disinfectant abilities. Seaweed's moisturizing properties are attributed to its ability to react with protein and form a protective gel on the skin's surface, reducing moisture loss due to evaporation. It has potential tissue renewal action and positive effects on facial wrinkles, probably because of its silicon content. It protects sensitive

S

skin against irritation, making it particularly effective in shaving creams. It is also beneficial for treating mature and drier skins due to its smoothing and softening actions. Seaweed extract seems to be effective in treating acne based on its presumed antibiotic properties, which offer the skin protection against infection. Evidence indicates seaweed may help accelerate wound-healing, and improve the healing of burns (including sunburns) and other wounds when in the presence of calcium alginate. It can be utilized as a regenerator in cases of suntanned or "orange peeled" skin. It reportedly improves blood circulation in the skin. Due to its alginates, seaweed is also used by formulators as a thickener for gellants and emulsions. In cosmetic products, its total percentage of use varies between 2 and 7 percent. The benefits of seaweed and seaweed extracts can be attributed to the plant's wealth of components that include water, mineral matters, lipids, protids, glucids, and sulfuric esters. It is rich in vitamins including vitamins A, B_1, B_2, B_3, B_5, B_{12}, C, D, E, and K. Among its mineral constituents are iodine, calcium, iron, phosphorus, sodium, potassium, zinc, nitrogen, copper, chlorine, magnesium, and manganese. It has trace amounts of various other minerals such as silver, lithium, silicon, bromine, titanium, cobalt, and arsenic. The amino acid content of seaweed is extremely high compared to other plants, and its polysaccharides include fructose, galactose, glucose, mannose, and xylose. Additional constituents include folic acid, choline, alginic acid, uronic acid, alginates, carrageenan, cellulose, proteins, agar-agar, algin, and iodine-protein complexes. There are more than 17,000 seaweed species that are classified according to color: green, blue, red, and brown. The red and brown varieties, the ones most commonly used in cosmetic preparations and generally referred to as seaweed or algae extract, are green when fresh and olive-brown when dry. The thallus is the part that is used for cosmetic purposes.

selenium—a trace mineral used for years in topical preparations for its antifungal properties. Selenium has been shown to have other protective effects such as repairing DNA, reducing the DNA-binding of carcinogens, and suppressing gene mutations. In laboratory studies, skin lotions containing selenium compounds have been shown to decrease UV induced skin damage such as inflammation, blistering, and pigmentation.

senna (Cassia angustifolia) (Indian senna, meca senna, tinnevelly senna)—used in traditional medicine as a stimulant.

S

Researchers have isolated a beta-glycan fraction, galactomannan, from the plant's seeds. The cosmetic properties ascribed to this fraction are similar to those of hyaluronic acid. These include skin softening and smoothing; a long-term moisturizing effect with an improvement in the stratum corneum's capacity to hold water; film-forming properties demonstrated by a reduction in transepidermal water loss; and a corrective and repairing ability for dry or rough skin. Senna also acts as an emollient without associated oiliness or leaving an occlusive layer. Due to its galactomannan concentration, senna is recommended for skin care preparations designed to relieve or repair dry, rough skin, and antiaging cosmetics and moisturizers.

sericin—a silk protein that can act as a film former in moisturizers, it also helps maintain skin that is smooth and in good overall condition. *See also* silk protein.

serine—a hydrophilic amino acid. Serine helps retain the skin's moisture balance. *See also* amino acid; protein.

serum protein—contains all essential amino acids. By varying the process, it is possible to concentrate fractions that have high specific essential amino acid contents such as methionine and lysine. Made by a selected fractionation process to isolate the plasma serum proteins present. *See also* amino acid; protein.

sesame amino acids—provides moisturizing properties and has some natural sugars associated with it. This amino acid complex is produced from sesame seed flour.

sesame oil—a commonly used carrier oil for cosmetic products, it has the same emollient properties as other nut and vegetable oils. Sesame oil is useful in suntan lotions as it blocks 30 percent of the sun's burning UV rays. Derived from sesame seeds.

shaddock extract—an extract obtained from the fruit of *Citrus grandis,* it is astringent and tonic. It is an unusual pear-shaped citrus fruit similar to a grapefruit.

shave grass—*see* horsetail extract.

shea butter—protects the skin from dehydration and external aggressions due to harsh climate, and is attributed with anti-inflammatory activity. It restores skin suppleness, increases moisturization, and can improve the appearance of irritated dry skin. Shea butter is a natural fat obtained from the fruit of the karate tree. *See also* shea butter (hydrodispersable).

S

shea butter (hydrodispersible)—an excellent emollient for use in creams, lotions, and makeup preparations. It alleviates skin dryness, and has sun-protection and high skin-penetration properties. Obtained by the hydroxylation of shea butter.

shepherd's purse (Capsella bursa pastoris)—attributed traditionally with wound-healing properties. It is also astringent and anti-inflammatory, making it particularly effective in acne preparations. Its constituents include flavonoids (e.g., diosmin), amines, cholene, acetyl cholene, potassium salt, tannin, resin, and silica.

shinleaf extract (Pyrola elliptica)—a botanical reported to help maintain the balance of normal skin.

shiitake mushroom extract (Lentinus edodes)—a skin conditioner that may also have antimicrobial and antibacterial properties. There is some evidence that it can cause skin irritation.

Shorea stenoptera seed butter—see illipe butter.

silica—also known as silicone dioxide. A carrier for emollients, it is also used to control a product's viscosity, add bulk, and reduce a formulation's transparency. In addition, it may be used to improve a formulation's skin feel. Spherical silica is porous and highly absorbent, with absorption capabilities roughly 1.5 times its weight. A typical claim associated with silica is oil control. It is also found in sunscreens. Tests show it has been successfully used in hypoallergenic and allergy tested formulations.

silicon glyconucleopeptides—a conditioning agent. This is protein attached to a silicone.

silicon oil—a generic description usually referring to dimethicone.

silicone (volatile)—used in face creams to increase the product's protection capabilities against water evaporation from the skin. Silicone polyethers are mainly used in water-based skin care formulations and give improved softness, gloss, and feel. Silicones have been used in cosmetics for more than 30 years. As they are minerals able to repel water, silicones present formulation problems because of poor compatibility with cosmetic oils and emollients. Silicones are not irritating.

silicone wax—gives the formulation improved glide on the skin.

silicum—used in scrubbing preparations for its roughness and texture.

silk amino acids—a silk-derived protein resulting from the complete hydrolysis of silk. *See also* amino acids; silk protein.

silk powder—recommended primarily for use in powder make-ups to improve humectancy, oil absorption, and anticracking properties. However, a large amount of silk powder may be needed to obtain the desired results. Silk powder is a micronized powder of natural silk protein and is not compatible with all inorganic pigments used in color cosmetics. Obtained from the secretion of the silkworm. Silk powder may cause allergic skin reactions.

silk proteins—protect the skin from dehydration and leave it with a smooth feel. Described as very effective for use in eye wrinkle creams. It is being claimed that their low molecular weight allows for penetration in the top layers of the corneum layer.

siloxanetriol alginate—often used in combination with caffeine for use in ant-cellulite products, the siloxanetriol aginate portion provides with skin-conditioning properties.

silverweed—*see* cinquefoil extract.

slippery elm extract (Ulmus fulva)—said to be soothing and emollient. It is found to be beneficial in aftershave preparations and for treating sunburn. *See also* slippery elm bark extract.

slippery elm bark extract—considered to have soothing, antiseptic, anti-inflammatory, and healing action. The inner bark is considered to have important medicinal value. Microscopic examination of the bark's tissue shows round starch grains and very characteristic twin crystals of calcium oxalate.

soap bark—a natural surfactant used for its cleansing properties. Some sources indicate a high allergenicity potential.

soapwart extract (Saponaria offinalis)—credited with cleansing properties due to its saponin content. It is also said to be soothing to the skin and to relieve itching. In traditional medicine, it has been used for treating acne, psoriasis, and eczema. Its constituents include flavonoids and vitamin C. The extract is made primarily from the roots of this herbaceous perennial, though the leaves and stem may be used as well.

sodium acrylate/sodium acryloyldimethyl taurate copolymer—a thickener, gelling agent, and formulation stabilizer.

sodium alginate—*see* algin.

SOD—*see* superoxide dimutase.

sodium aluminosilicate—*see* sodium aluminum silicate.

sodium aluminuschlorohydroxylactate—a cosmetic astringent. This is an inorganic salt.

sodium aluminum silicate (sodium aluminosilicate; sodium silicoaluminate)—abrasive. It is a viscosity-increasing agent.

sodium benzoate—a nontoxic, organic salt preservative that is particularly effective against yeast, with some activity against molds and bacteria. Generally used in concentrations of 0.1 to 0.2 percent.

sodium bicarbonate (baking soda)—an inorganic salt used as a buffering agent and a pH adjuster. Used in skin-smoothing powders. It also serves as a neutralizer.

sodium bisulfate—an inorganic salt used as an antiseptic and a pH adjuster in cosmetic creams. Concentrated solutions can produce strong irritation.

sodium bisulfite—a preservative and antioxidant, it is most frequently used as a pH adjuster.

sodium borate—a preservative and emulsifier with astringent and antiseptic properties. It is also used as a pH adjuster. Sodium borate is the sodium salt of boric acid. It may cause skin dryness and irritation.

sodium carboxymethyl betaglucan—used as a binder and to control the viscosity of a cosmetic formulation.

sodium cetearyl sulfate—a surfactant used as a cleansing agent. Also an oil-in-water emulsifier for creams.

sodium chloride (table salt)—used as a preservative, astringent, and antiseptic to treat inflamed lesions. Diluted solutions are not considered irritating.

sodium chondroitin sulfate—described as a skin-conditioning agent for use in moisturizers and night skin care preparations. A derivative of natural mucopolysaccharides. *See also* mucopolysaccharides.

sodium citrate—may be used in cosmetic formulations as an alkalizer and to bind trace metals in solutions (by means of a chelating action). It is the sodium salt of citric acid.

sodium cocoate—a surfactant used as an emulsifying and cleansing agent primarily in bath soaps and cleansers. This sodium salt of coconut acid may also be listed as coconut oil. *See also* coconut oil.

sodium coco hydrolyzed collagen—a surfactant that is nonirritating to the skin or mucous membranes.

sodium cocoyl glutamate—a very mild cleansing agent that lathers slightly. It is derived from coconut fatty acid and glutamic acid, an amino acid. Can be found in cleansers, acne products, body gels, and shampoos.

sodium cocoyl isethionate—a mild, high-foaming surfactant. Leaves the skin with a soft afterfeel.

sodium cocoylsarcosinate—a surfactant used as a cleansing agent.

sodium dehydroacetate—a preservative against bacteria and fungi that is used at concentration levels of 1.0 percent or less. It is useful in combination with parabens. May cause skin irritation.

sodium dihydroxycetyl phosphate—a surfactant used as a cleansing agent.

sodium hexametaphosphate—a chelating agent and a corrosion inhibitor. This is an inorganic salt.

sodium hyaluronate—used as a moisturizing agent, viscosifier, and emulsifier, sodium hyaluronate is capable of binding 1,800 times its own weight in water. It is the sodium salt of hyaluronic acid. *See also* hyaluronic acid.

sodium hydroxide—commonly referred to as caustic soda. It is a chemical reagent used in making soap. If too concentrated it may cause severe skin irritation.

sodium hydroxymethyl glycinate—an antimicrobial. It is derived from glycine, a naturally occurring amino acid, and is used as a preservative in cosmetics.

sodium isostearoyl lactylate—an ester of lactic acid with moisture retention properties.

sodium lactate—keeps a product's pH from becoming too acidic. Sodium lactate is naturally occurring in the skin, and is moisturizing and moisture-binding. It is also used as a substitute for glycerin.

sodium lactate methylsilanol—an additive used in self-tanning preparations. It helps in obtaining a more uniform color.

sodium laureth-5 carboxylate—a very mild surfactant. It substantially improves the skin's tolerance to cleansers. It also has good emulsifying properties and is not affected by water hardness.

sodium laureth-11 carboxylate—a surfactant. *See also* sodium laureth-5 carboxylate; sodium laureth-13 carboxylate.

sodium laureth-13 carboxylate—an extremely mild surfactant that substantially improves the skin's tolerance of cleansers. It is particularly suitable for high-quality formulations, baby shampoos, and products designed for sensitive skin. This

S

ingredient has good emulsifying properties and is insensitive to water hardness.

sodium laureth sulfate—an emulsifier and versatile surfactant used in personal care products, especially for its cleansing and foaming properties. It enjoys good skin compatibility and is very often found in shower foams, foam bath products, and liquid soaps. It exhibits a mild-to-moderate skin irritation index in irritation tests, and has been found to be less irritating than sodium lauryl sulfate.

sodium lauroamphoacetate—a mild surfactant that is especially suitable for use in products where skin tolerance is important (for example, baby and child care products).

sodium lauroyl glutamate—a surfactant with some moisturizing capacities, it can be derived from vegetal raw materials, and therefore may often be found in "natural" or plant based cosmetics.

sodium lauroyl oat amino acids—a surfactant with skin cleansing and conditioning properties, it is derived from oat amino acids.

sodium lauryl sarcosinate—a foaming agent used primarily in hair products.

sodium lauryl sulfate—serves as a base surfactant, foaming agent with good foaming properties, dispersant, and wetting agent. Formulators have found it ideal for cleansers and soaps intended to be packaged with pump dispensers. However, it is considered among the most irritating surfactants associated with causing skin dryness and redness. Often, it is either replaced by less irritating but related surfactants such as sodium laureth sulfate, or anti-irritant ingredients are incorporated into the formulation together with the sodium lauryl sulfate in order to reduce sensitivity potential.

sodium magnesium silicate—a binder and bulking agent used primarily in makeup products.

sodium mannuronate methylsilanol—a skin-conditioning agent.

sodium metabisulfite—an antioxidant and reducing agent.

sodium methylcocoyl taurate—an emulsifier and mild cleansing agent. Used in cleansing creams, lotions, shampoos, and bath soaps. Derived from coconut oil.

sodium methyloleoyl taurate—an emulsifier and a mild cleansing and foaming agent derived from oleic acid.

sodium oleate—a mild cleansing and foaming agent generally used in soaps. Derived from natural fats and oils.

sodium C$_{12-16}$ olefin sulfonate—a cleansing agent.

sodium PCA (Ajidew NaPCA)—a high-performance humectant due to its moisture-binding ability, sodium PCA also exists naturally in the skin as a component of the natural moisturizing factor. For cosmetic use, it is derived from amino acids. It is considered a noncomedogenic, nonallergenic raw material recommended for dry, delicate, and sensitive skins.

sodium PCS (Ajidew N-50)—a humectant. *See also* PCA; sodium PCA.

sodium phosphate—helps maintain product pH.

sodium polyacrylate—a suspending agent, stabilizer, and emulsifier.

sodium polyacrylate starch—a thickener and gellant with good pH stability.

sodium polyphosphate—a preservative against bacteria, molds, and yeasts. Used at high concentrations it can cause skin irritation.

sodium polystyrene sulfonate—a film former. It holds the actives on site and gives the feeling of skin tightening. It is synthetically manufactured.

sodium ricinolate—an emulsifying agent used in certain soaps and medicines. It is a sodium salt of the fatty acids from castor oil.

sodium shale oil sulfonate—found to be anti-inflammatory, antibacterial, fungicidal, antiseptic, and have analgesic properties. It is also a surfactant. A naturally occurring, water- and glycerin-soluble substance that is distilled from oil-shale, it is used in products for acne, eczema, and psoriasis. Sulfur is among its constituents.

sodium silicoaluminate—*see* sodium aluminum silicate.

sodium stearate—a fatty acid used as a waterproofing agent. One of the least allergy-causing sodium salts of fatty acids. Nonirritating to the skin. *See also* stearic acid.

sodium sulfate—a filler in the manufacturing of synthetic detergents and soaps. A laboratory reagent. It may enhance the irritant action of certain detergents.

sodium sulfite—has antiseptic, preservative, and antioxidant properties. Sodium sulfite is also a topical antifungal.

sodium tallowate (tallow)—a defoamer, emollient, and intermediate and surface active agent. *See also* tallow.

sodium/TEA lauryl—a moderately irritating surfactant.

S

sodium tetraborate—*see* sodium borate.

sodium triceth sulfate—a surfactant.

sodium trideceth sulfate—a surfactant used as a cleansing and emulsifying agent. Its activity and level of irritation depends on the formulation's pH.

soluble elastin—*see* tropoelastin.

sorbic acid—a broad-spectrum, nontoxic preservative against molds and yeasts with moderate sensitizing potential in leave-on cosmetics. It is used in concentrations of 0.1 to 0.3 percent, and its activity is dependant on the formulation's pH. Sorbic acid is used as a replacement for glycerin in emulsions, ointments, and various cosmetic creams. Obtained from the berries of the tree commonly known as mountain ash and rowan. It can also be produced synthetically. Sorbic acid can be irritating.

sorbitan isostearate—an emulsifier used in the preparation of sunscreens, moisturizing creams, and lotions.

sorbitan laurate—an emulsifier in cosmetic creams and lotions as well as a stabilizer of essential oils in water.

sorbitan monostearate—*see* sorbitan stearate.

sorbitan oleate—a mild emulsifier derived from sugar.

sorbitan olivate—an emulsifier.

sorbitan palmitate—an emulsifier with moisture-binding abilities. It also serves as a solubilizer of essential oils in water. Derived from sorbitol.

sorbitan sesquioleate—a surfactant used as an emulsifying agent. *See also* sorbitol.

sorbitan stearate—an emulsifier for water-in-oil creams and lotions, and a solubilizer of essential oils in water. It results from the reaction of stearic acid with sorbitol and is, therefore, synthetically produced from naturally derived materials.

sorbitan trioleate—an emulsifier. *See also* sorbitol.

sorbitan tristearate—an emulsifier and alternate for sorbitan stearate.

sorbitate stearate—a secondary emulsifier that helps formulate glossy emulsions.

sorbitol—absorbs moisture from the air to prevent skin dryness, and leaves the skin feeling smooth and velvety. However, if the skin's moisture content is greater than that of the atmosphere, it will draw moisture out of the skin, thereby increasing the feeling of dryness. Sorbitol is used by formulators as a replacement for glycerin in emulsions, ointments, and various cosmetic creams. Obtained from the leaves and in some cases the berries of mountain ash. Sorbitol also occurs in other berries, cherries, plums, pears, apples, seaweed, and algae.

sorrel extract *(Rumex acetosa)*—an astringent. Although there are many varieties of sorrel including wood sorrel, French sorrel, and garden sorrel, similar properties are attributed to all. The extract is obtained from the whole herb or just from the leaves.

sour cherry *(Prunus cerasus)*—overall beneficial for maintaining a healthy skin condition, a variety of other therapeutic values are attributed to sour cherry, some of which depend on the portion of the plant used. For example, extract from the whole plant is antioxidant, moisturizing, keratolytic, and skin conditioning. Meanwhile, extract obtained just from the fruit is antioxidant and skin conditioning but not necessarily moisturizing or helpful in removing dead surface-skin cells. The fruit itself has astringent properties, and the seed oil is both emollient and can mask odor. Sour cherry's constituents include pectin, fruit acids, sugars, flavonoids, vitamins A, B and C, polyphenols, mineral salts, and trace elements such as selenium.

southernwood extract *(Artemisia abrotanum)*—botanical sources cite it as having moisturizing, antiseptic and toning properties. The extract is obtained from the whole plant.

soy amno acids—*see* amino acid.

soy bean oil (soybean oil)—often used as a smoothing ingredient. It has a high content of phosphatides such as lecithin, sterols, and vitamins (A, E, and K). It is used in numerous forms, including hydrogenated, maleated, and unsaponified. Considered by some sources to be somewhat comedogenic, soy bean oil is not irritating.

soy bean oil (unsaponified)—possibly has a similar action to true biological precursors. It has a small molecular structure and is thought to act more as a hormone-like cellular messenger once it reaches the epidermal keratinocytes and, particularly, the dermal fibroblast. It is said to stimulate the synthesis of collagen, elastin, proteoglycans, and structural glycoproteins. *See also* isoflavones.

S

soy bean glycerides (hydrogenated)—can be used by a cosmetic formulator for emollient, emulsifying, and surfactant purposes.

soy bean protein—has good anti-irritant properties.

soy germ oil—*see* soy bean oil.

soy oil—*see* soy bean oil.

soy lecithin—a mild refattening agent that can be effectively used in facial cleansers formulated for dry skin.

soy phytosterols—anti-inflammatory and conditioning. These sterols are derived from the soy plant. *See also* plant sterols.

soy sterol—an emulsifier, emollient, and emulsion stabilizer. Soy sterol is considered a noncomedogenic raw material.

spearmint oil (Mentha viridis)—a cooling, aromatic stimulant described as having cleansing and decongesting properties. Indicated for acne and oily skin. Its fragrance and therapeutic activity is similar to that of peppermint but fresher and less harsh. *See also* mint oil.

spermaceti—a waxy substance used in the manufacture of cosmetics to thicken the products and give them shine. Originally obtained from whales as a source of fish oil, it is now synthetic. Spermaceti is nontoxic and nonirritating.

sphingolipids—ceramide precursors with unique moisturizing properties. They appear to work with the cellular system in providing a restorative effect on a damaged or disturbed corneum layer. Sphingolipids may also exhibit cell-regulating functions. Found naturally occurring in both animals and plants, it is difficult to isolate naturally occurring sphingolipids in an efficient and economical manner given their size and quantities available in an organism. The synthesized version does not exhibit exactly the same properties as the natural one, but is generally considered emollient and useful for protecting the skin against external harm (such as environmental pollutants), while also maintaining skin condition. The use of sphingolipids in cosmetics is limited by availability and price. Sphingolipid liposomes are called sphingosomes.

sphinogoceryl—forms a protective film that strengthens the skin's ability to protect against toxins and increases the skin's moisture-retention abilities. It can also improve skin texture.

sphingomyelin—can be used as an amphiphilic liposome component in the manufacture of the liposome capsule.

sphingomyelinase—a fluid that can enhance the skin's moisture-retention properties.

spinach (Spinacia oleracea)—generally considered beneficial for promoting and maintaining the skin in good condition, spinach contains antioxidant flavonoids (spinacetin and patuletin) and can also be used as a natural colorant. Other constituents include carotenoids, histamines, oxalic acid, lutein, vitamins A, C, E and H, thiamine, niacin, and a variety of minerals.

Spiraea extract—*see* meadowsweet.

spirulina amino acids—an amino acid complex with high moisturizing capabilities derived from *Spirulina platensis*.

spirulina extract—said to have a hydrating effect on the skin's surface layers. Botanical claims also maintain that certain spirulina proteins contribute to the stimulation of the fibroblast and to tissue regeneration.

spruce oil (Picea excelsa)—like sandalwood, rosemary, and jasmine oils, spruce oil has been observed to stimulate fibroblast growth. While the relevance of this observation has not been scientifically established, it has been noticed that stimulation of fibroblast activity could result in an increase in epidermal cell turnover. Spruce oil is produced by distillation of spruce branches.

squalane (squalene)—an excellent moisturizer and lubricant, it softens and smoothes the skin while also replenishing skin lipids. Its compatibility with skin lipids can be attributed to the fact that human sebum is made up of 25 percent squalane. Squalane is obtained by hydrogenation of shark liver oil or other natural oils. Components found in fish oils may reduce skin irritation and allergic responses. It can also be obtained from plant sources.

squalane and squalene and glycolipids and phytosterols and tocopharol—a light emollient that contains natural lipids also found in the skin. This is a natural plant cell oil extract, not a mixture as the name suggests.

squalene—like squalane, squalene replenishes skin lipids while softening and smoothing. It helps maintain the skin in good condition. When used in hair care products, it serves as a hair-conditioning and antistatic agent.

starch gum—*see* dextrin.

stearalkonium hectorite—*see* hectorite.

stearamide DEA (stearic acid diethanolamide)—a thickener and a wax emulsifier used in soaps, creams, and lotions.

S

stearamidopropyl dimethylamine—a surfactant and conditioner for facial cleansers, hand cleansers, and baby products. It is very mild to the skin and eyes.

stearate—*see* sodium stearate.

stearate SE—*see* sodium stearate.

steareth-2, -7, -10, -20, -21—these are emulsifiers for water-in-oil formulations, adding stability, and preventing the separation of the two phases. They are the polyoxyethylene ether of fatty alcohol. -10 is used particularly in creams and lotions of high stability though some sources indicate it has a comedogenicity and mild irritancy potential. -21 may also be used as a surfactant with very minor irritation potential to the skin and eyes.

stearic acid—an emulsifier and thickening agent found in many vegetable fats. Stearic acid is the main ingredient used in making bar soaps and lubricants. It occurs naturally in butter acids, tallow, cascarilla bark, and in other animal fats and oils. Stearic acid may cause allergic reactions in people with sensitive skin and is considered somewhat comedogenic. *See also* essential fatty acid entry in Chapter 4.

stearic acid diethanolamide—*see* stearamide DEA.

stearoxy dimethicone—an emollient and skin-conditioning agent. *See also* dimethicone.

stearyl alcohol—used in cosmetic formulations for emulsions and antifoaming and lubricating action. Stearyl alcohol is also a viscosity agent and builder. It is a saturated alcohol of high purity.

stearyl acrylate—generally found in combination with other chemicals, it acts as a film former to help maintain moisture in the skin.

stearyl heptanoate—a nongreasy emollient that produces a highly water-repellent film. Stearyl heptanoate is a natural preen gland wax.

sterols—steroid alcohols that can be used as lubricants in a variety of cosmetic preparations. Such alcohols contain the common steroid nucleus. Sterols are widely distributed in plants and animals, both in the free form and esterified to fatty acids. Cholesterol is a most important sterol and is often used in cosmetic creams. Ergosterol is an important plant sterol.

stinging nettle extract—traditionally used for mild acne conditions. *See also* nettle extract.

***stonecrop** (Sempervivum tectorum)*—also known as houseleek; hens and chicks. Anti-inflammatory and astringent, studies indicate antioxidant properties, as well. Its constituents include carbohydrates, isocitric acid, citric acid, malic acid, free amino acids (asparagine), caffeic acid, and flavonoids. *See also* citric acid, malic acid, flavonoids.

***strawberry extract** (Fragaria vesca)*—astringent. The fruit, in addition to malic and citric acids, sugar, mucilage, pectin, woody fiber, and water, also contains ascorbic acid, thereby supporting early claims of bleaching properties. Extract from the fruit was recommended for use on sunburned areas to soothe the skin. Both the leaves and the fruit were in early pharmacopoeias; however, there is no scientific evidence of benefit or harm.

sucrose (table sugar)—an emollient, mild emulsifier, and humectant. It can be used in place of glycerin.

sucrose cocoate—soothing and anti-irritant. It is also an emulsifying agent.

sucrose cocoate sorbitan stearate—a sucrose-based emulsifier.

sucrose polybehenate—an emollient and emulsifier, this is a film-forming agent that forms semi-occlusive films. It can also be used as a surfactant, and to help keep the skin looking in good condition. It exhibits good wear and wash-off resistance. Considered a natural ingredient, it is used in skin care creams and lotions.

sucrose polycottonseedate—a skin conditioner, emollient, and emulsifying agent.

sucrose polysoyate—an emollient and emulsifier.

sucrose stearate—an emollient and emulsifying agent used primarily in makeup preparations. Sucrose stearate enables the formulation of clear gel microemulsion systems with a reduced physiological effect on the skin and eyes.

sucrose trisearate—incorporated into a cosmetic for softening and smoothing, it is also an emulsifier and helps maintain the skin in good condition.

sulfated castor oil—a surfactant used as a cleansing agent.

sulfur—a mild antiseptic used in acne creams and lotions. Stimulates healing when used on skin rashes. May cause skin irritation. *See also* sulfur (colloidal).

sulfur (colloidal)—reduces oil-gland activity and dissolves the skin's surface layer of dry, dead cells. This ingredient is commonly used in acne soaps and lotions, and is a major component in many acne preparations. It can cause allergic skin reactions.

sulisobenzone—the drug name for benzophenone-4, a sunscreen chemical. *See* benzopheone-4.

sumac extract (Rhus glabra) (sumach)—astringent, antiseptic, and tonic properties are attributed to this botanical. It also helps control oil gland secretion. Depending on the variety of sumac employed, extracts for skin problems are either made from the bark or the leaves. They may also be used for eczema and skin diseases. There are several varieties of sumac, some of which are poisonous. Those that are poisonous cause swelling, inflammation, and pain, ending in ulceration at the touch.

sumach—*see* sumac extract.

sunflower oil (Helianthus annuus)—commonly used as a carrier oil, it softens and smooths the skin. Sunflower oil has a high linoleic acid and other essential fatty acid content. In addition, it contains lecithin, carotenoids, and waxes. This oil is considered a noncomedogenic raw material.

sunflower seed oil—expressed from sunflower seeds. *See also* sunflower oil.

superoxide dismutase (SOD)—an enzyme that can serve as an inhibitor of free-radical production and a free-radical scavenger. In cells, it constitutes a natural defense system against activated oxygen species. SOD converts superoxide radicals into hydrogen peroxide, which are then changed into molecular oxygen and water.

superoxide dismutase (polyoxyalkylene-modified)—used in cosmetic preparations to prevent drying and aging of the skin without causing irritation. *See also* superoxide dismutase.

sweet almond oil—an emollient with soothing properties. *See also* almond oil.

sweet clover extract—*see* clover extract.

sweet lime oil—*see* lime oil.

sweet marjoram oil (Origanum majorana)—the volatile oil distilled from the leaves of *Origanum majorana*. It is used by formulators for its refreshing action, as well as for its perfuming and odor masking action. *See also* marjoram.

sweet orange extract—*see* orange extract.

synthetic spermaceti—*see* cetyl palmitate; spermaceti.

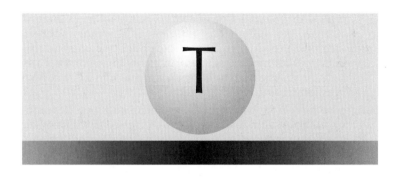

table salt—*see* sodium chloride.

table sugar—*see* sucrose.

talc—adds softness and sliding ability to a cosmetic formulation. Talc is used as a bulking and opacifying agent, and as an absorbent in makeup preparations. This is an inert powder, generally made from finely ground magnesium silicate, a mineral.

tallow—considered an occlusive skin-conditioning agent. Tallow is used primarily in the manufacture of soaps. It is the fat derived from the fatty tissue of sheep or cattle and is considered comedogenic.

tallow glycerides—a surfactant used as an emulsifying agent. Incorporated more often into makeup than skin care preparations. A mixture of triglycerides derived from tallow. *See also* tallow.

tamanu oil (Calophyllum inophyllum)—emollient, it is attributed with antioxidant, antimicrobial, anti-inflammatory, anti-scarring, healing, and astringent properties. It is also a natural UV absorber. Its composition includes neutral lipids, glycolipids, and phospholipids. Tamanu oil can be found in products used to protect the skin against sun exposure (sun and post-sun creams), antiaging and regenerating creams, acne preparations, and products for dry and very dry skin, The oil is obtained from the seeds of this evergreen tree.

tamarind (Tamarindus indica)—astringent and antiseptic. Researchers have isolated xyloglucan from extracts of the plant's seeds. Xyloglucan has demonstrated strong immunostimulating properties. It may have some antioxidant

287

capabilities, as well. Constituents of this plant include citric, tartaric, and malic acids; potassium, bitartrate; polysaccharides; proteins; and lipids. Scientists recommend this botanical for protecting the skin against environmentally induced damage, stimulating skin repair, and for skin with low immunodefenses.

tangerine oil (Citrus reticulata)—has botanical properties similar to those of orange, though with greater antispasmodic and sedative properties. Its fragrance, reminiscent of bergamot, is sweeter than that of orange. *See also* orange oil.

tapioca flour (Manihot utilissima or Jatropha manihot)—used as a thickener. This is a starch derived from cassava.

tarragon (Artemisia dracunculus)—said to have tonic and stimulating properties. Its primary active is estragol, a phenol also known as methyl chavicol. Other constituents include cymene and phellandrene.

tartaric acid—the second largest AHA in size (glycolic acid being the smallest AHA and citric acid the largest). It is not frequently used in cosmetic or antiaging preparations as formulators find it difficult to work with, and it can be somewhat irritating. *See also* alpha hydroxyacid.

TEA (triethanolamine)—an emulsifier and pH adjuster.

TEA-carbomer—used to create a gel formulation and to control viscosity.

TEA-dodecyl benzene sulfonate—a surfactant often mixed with other surfactants as a cleansing agent.

TEA-isostearate—classified as a soap. This ingredient is a surfactant used as a cleansing and emulsifying agent.

TEA-lactate—a surfactant.

TEA-lauryl sulfate—a surfactant used as a cleansing agent with a moderate level of skin irritancy.

TEA-oleamide PEG-2 sulfosuccinate—a surfactant with a very low level of skin irritancy.

TEA-oleate—a mild emulsifier and surfactant.

TEA-salicylate—a chemical UVB absorber. This is one of the 21 FDA-approved sunscreen chemicals with an approved usage level of 5 to 12 percent. TEA-salicylate is a water-soluble chemical with limited UV absorption capability. Formulators also may use it as a preservative.

TEA-stearate—a surfactant considered to be a powerful oil-in-water (hydrophilic) emulsifying and cleansing agent.

TEA-stearate is also a moisture absorber used in formulating emulsions. It may be irritating to the skin.

tea extract—studies indicate antioxidant, bacteriostatic, and an antiallergenic action. Green tea extract in particular has been noted to be rich in potent antioxidants called catechins. Tea extract has been effectively used in eye treatment products to reduce puffiness.

tea tree oil (*Melaleuca alternifolia***) (Australian tea tree oil)**—considered a natural preservative with antiseptic, germicidal, and expectorant properties. Its antimicrobial activity toward a wide array of bacteria allows it to promote healing. It is becoming recognized as a topical remedy for yeast, fungus, and skin disorders and infections. Tea tree oil exhibits positive benefits against seborrhea, psoriasis (reduces scaling and redness), eczema (stops itching and reduces redness), and dermatitis. It has been used by Australian Aborigines to treat cuts, wounds, and skin infections, and by European explorers as an herbal tea. This oil's ability to dissolve pus without causing visible or apparent damage to the skin's surface was noted by doctors when using it to clean the surface of infected wounds. It is also ideal for aromatherapy, given its low toxicity. Although effectively used on almost any skin type, except sensitive or couperose skins, it is particularly beneficial to acne, problem, and/or congested skins. Tea tree oil is obtained from distilling the tree's leaves to produce a pale yellow to colorless oil that has a camphor-like scent similar to eucalyptus. Studies indicate it to be nontoxic with negligible to no irritancy.

tepescohuite—*see mimosa tenuiflora.*

terephthalylidene dicamphor sulfonic acid—an FDA-approved sunscreen chemical with UV-filtering and absorbing capacities. It has an approved usage level of up to 10 percent in the European Union.

Terminalia cerise extract—a botanical with properties said to include firming, restructuring, and cellular stimulation. In addition, it is claimed to improve tissue drainage and, therefore, reduce puffiness. In traditional medicine, it was used for its antibacterial properties. It can be found in various types of skin care preparations such as those for anti-aging, sensitive skin, after-sun care, cellulite control, and stretch-mark prevention.

4-tertbutyl 4'-methoxydibenzoylmethane—*see* butylmethoxydibenzoylmethane.

tetradibutyl pentaerithrityl hydroxyhydrocinnamate—a stabilizer that can protect products from discoloration due to exposure to light, particularly UV.

tetrahexyldecyl ascorbate—an antioxidant that inhibits lipid peroxidation (thereby protecting skin lipids from free-radical damage), it is also used for improving and maintaining the skin's overall condition. Manufacturers also cite an ability to lessen UV damage and stimulate collagen. Studies indicate that tetrahexyldecyl ascorbate may promote a more even skin tone by inhibiting pigment production and by providing skin-lightening and brightening characteristics to a formulation. This is an oil-soluble, stable ester of vitamin C. Considered less irritating than ascorbic acid.

tetrahydroxypropyl ethylenediamine—used as a solvent and preservative. A component of the bacteria-killing substance in sugar cane. It is very alkaline and may be irritating to the skin and mucous membranes. It might also cause skin sensitization.

tetrasodium EDTA—used as a preservative and also as a sequestering and chelating agent in cosmetic solutions.

tetterwort extract (Sanguinaria canadensis) (bloodroot)—herbal lore cites external application as helpful in treatment of eczema and other skin problems. It is used for its refreshing, tonic, and cleansing action. The rootstock is the part that is used.

Theobroma grandiflorum seed butter—see cupuassu butter.

theophylline—tonic and skin conditioning. Its cosmetic activity is not clearly or definitively established. It is most often found in anticellulite products. Theophylline is in the same family of biochemicals as caffeine. Naturally occurring in tea.

thiamine HCL (vitamin B₁)—used as an emollient. *See also* vitamin B.

thioctic acid—also known as alpha lipoic acid. An antioxidant. *See* alpha lipoic acid.

thuja extract—credited with healing and anti-irritant properties. It is potentially effective against pigmentation. The oil is obtained by the distillation of small branches and twigs of yellow or white cedar. *See also* cedarwood oil.

thyme extract (Thymus sp.)—its botanical properties have been listed as antiseptic, tonic, antibacterial, deodorizing, fungicidal, and circulation stimulating. Certain fractions may have collagenase inhibitor abilities. Thyme extract might also have insect-repellent properties. Its active principle is thymic acid, which has disinfectant properties similar to those of carbolic acid. Thyme extract may cause skin irritation.

thyme oil—widely used in botanical therapy since antiquity for its warming, stimulating, and cleansing properties, it is also considered a powerful antiseptic and tonic. Thyme oil serves as a natural preservative with antibacterial activity against a wide spectrum of bacterial classes. The genus *Thymus* produces a variety of species, subspecies, and chemotypes, many with completely different chemical compositions. This includes citriodora thyme, lemon thyme, and red thyme. Lemon thyme is also described as healing and soothing for its use in skin care, while red thyme may cause skin irritation at high concentrations. The oil is obtained from the herb's branches and flowers.

tilia (linden)—botanical properties are described as antiseptic, soothing, and emollient. *See also* linden extract.

TiO₂—*see* titanium dioxide.

tissue respiratory factor (TRF) (live yeast cell derivative)—described by manufacturers as a powerful anti-inflammatory and moisturizing agent that can promote wound-healing. TRF is found to deliver its moisturizing, skin-soothing benefits more effectively than the traditional cosmetic raw materials. It also works with the skin to help improve the skin's appearance and overall health. It is obtained by stimulating living cells into producing protective substances. TRF can be described as a glyconucleopeptide and has been safely used for more than 40 years.

tissulan—a tissue extract with a high amino acid content. Claimed to improve the skin's surface and structure. *See also* amino acid.

titanium dioxide (TiO₂)—a nonchemical SPF contributor. Titanium dioxide is one of the 21 FDA-approved sunscreen chemicals with an approved usage level of 2 to 25 percent. When applied, titanium dioxide remains on the skin's surface, scattering UV light. It is often used in conjunction with other sunscreen chemicals to boost the product's SPF value, thus reducing the risk of irritation or allergies attributed to excessive usage of chemical sunscreens. Its incorporation into sunscreen formulations, makeup bases, and daytime moisturizers depends on the particular size of titanium dioxide employed. The smaller the particle size, the more unobtrusive TiO$_2$'s application. Large particles, on the other hand, leave a whitish wash or look on the skin. Some companies list "micro" or "ultra" as a reference to the size of the titanium dioxide particle. According to some sources, titanium dioxide could be the ideal UVA/UVB protection component given its chemical, cosmetic, and physical characteristics. Titanium dioxide is also used to provide a white color to cosmetic preparations.

titanium dioxide (micro)—*see* titanium dioxide.

titanium dioxide (ultra)—*see* titanium dioxide.

T

tocopherol (vitamin E)—an antioxidant obtained by vacuum distillation of edible vegetable oils. *See also* vitamin E.

tocopherol acetate—an antioxidant that helps prevent unsaturated oils and sebum from becoming rancid. It is considered a noncomedogenic raw material. *See also* vitamin E.

tocopherol ester—considered an effective free-radical scavenger.

tocopherol linoleate—a moisturizer. *See also* tocopherol.

tocopherol nicotinate—used as an antioxidant and a skin-conditioning agent.

tocophersolan—an antioxidant, this is a water-soluble form of vitamin E.

tocopheryl linoleate—used as an antioxidant and a skin-conditioning agent.

tocopheryl phosphate—added to a cosmetic formulation for cleansing, emulsifying, and surfactant activity.

tocopheryl sorbate—most likely used as an antioxidant. This is a modified form of tocopherol. *See also* vitamin E; vitamin E acetate.

tocotrienols—an antioxidant with UV absorption and skin-conditioning activity. This is a form of vitamin E, and studies indicate that it might be more potent than tocopherol. It could be incorporated into antioxidant and antiaging products. Naturally occurring in oils derived from rice bran, barley, wheat, oat, and palm; the highest levels are contained in palm oil.

tomato (*Solanum lycopersicum***)**—therapeutic skin care properties depend on the part of the plant that is used. For example, the extract made from the whole plant is astringent, while the fruit itself is considered a humectant and emollient. Tomato water has an ability to mask odor. Sources also cite antioxidant activity. The common property to all tomato derivatives in cosmetics is skin conditioning. Tomato's constituents include beta-carotene, carotenoids (lycopene), histamine, fructose, glucose, vitamins A, C, and E, mineral salts, and trace elements.

tomato oil—oil derived from the fruit can help improve and maintain a good skin condition in terms of texture, tone, and look. Oil from the seed softens and smoothes the skin, in addition to being conditioning. Some sources cite it as particularly appropriate for combination skin.

tonka bean (Dipteryx odorata) (tonquin bean)—aromatic and tonic, it was traditionally used as a fixative in perfume manufacturing. Its primary constituent is coumaric acid. The seed is the part that is used.

tormentil extract (Potentilla tormentilla)—considered one of the safest and most powerful herbal astringents. It also has mildly antiseptic and anti-inflammatory properties. Used in Old England for sores, wounds, bruises, and infections. Important constituents of tormentil extract include tannin, phytosterols, flavonoids, chinovic acid, tormentoside, and pseudosaponine. The extract is obtained from the plant's root.

trace elements (micronutrients; oligoelements)—different elements, usually inorganic, are considered essential to plant and animal nutrition in trace concentrations. The value of their topical application through cosmetic preparations is not clear, although some sources indicate a potential moisturization value.

trace element complex—*see* trace elements.

tragacanth gum—an effective emulsifying agent, binder, film former, and viscosity controller, it is also used as a stabilizing ingredient in lotions. Tragacanth gum is derived from the resin of the *Astragalus gummifer* shrub.

transglutaminase—an enzyme said to activate the skin's physiological functions.

treemoss extract (Evernia furfuracea)—a botanical ingredient that helps mask odor in a product.

trehalose—a humectant and moisturizer, it helps bind water in the skin and increase the skin's moisture content. A naturally occurring plant sugar.

tretinoin—*see* retinoic acid.

tribehenin—also known as glyceryl tribehenate. An emollient and skin conditioner.

tricaprylin—a skin-conditioning agent. *See also* caprylic/capric triglyceride.

tricaprylyl citrate—an emollient and skin conditioner.

Trichilia emetica seed butter (natal mahogany)—it is considered skin nourishing and revitalizing, with moisturizing and antiaging activity. It is an emollient and keeps the skin soft and supple.

triclosan—a preservative considered to have a low sensitizing potential in leave-on preparations.

tricontanyl PVP—a film-forming, waterproofing, and wearproofing agent. It is oil soluble and easily formulated into sunscreens, skin care creams, lotions, and general cosmetic products. Tricontanyl PVP is a very versatile ingredient. When used in sunscreens, it facilitates the formulation of high SPFs without the need to significantly increase the use of sunscreen chemicals. The result is products with higher SPF, less or lower irritancy, and greater cost effectiveness. Tricontanyl PVP is also used as a pigment dispersant in color cosmetics, and is particularly useful when titanium dioxide is used to increase SPF values. Studies indicate little to no photoallergy or toxicity.

tridecyl stearate—a skin-conditioning agent and an emollient.

tridecyl trimelliatate—an occlusive skin-conditioning agent.

triethanolamine—*see* TEA.

triethanolamine oleate—*see* TEA oleate.

triethanolamine salicylate—*see* TEA salicylate.

triethanolamine stearate—*see* TEA stearate.

triethylene glycol—a solvent prepared from ethylene oxide and ethylene glycol.

triglycerides—consistency regulators for creams, lotions, and makeup. Facilitates skin blending and imparts good flow properties to products. These are the chief constituents of fats and oils. Fatty acids such as caprylic, capric, and lauric react with glycerin to produce triglyceride oils. These oils, such as those of almond, safflower, and cocoa butter, are utilized in cosmetics for enhanced lubricity and emolliency of a product. There are a variety of triglycerides, including caprylic/capric, lauric, myristic, palmitic, and stearic.

triisostearin—*see* glyceryl tri-isostearate.

triisostearyl citrate—an occlusive skin-conditioning agent. This is the triester of isostearyl alcohol and citric acid.

triisostearyl trilinoleate—a skin-conditioning and viscosity-controlling agent with occlusive properties.

trilinolein—an emollient, it replenishes the lipids present in the stratum corneum, thereby improving skin look, feel and texture. Depending on a formulator's requirements, it can also be used as a solvent and to control a formula's viscosity.

trimethyl siloxy silicate—in combination with dimethicone, it works as a waterproofing material for sunscreen preparations. It also reduces skin whitening and greasiness commonly associated with high SPF sunscreen formulations.

trisodium ascorbyl palmitate phosphate—an antioxidant and antiwrinkle ingredient, this is a vitamin C derivative with good penetration capacities. According to manufacturers, it helps promote collagen synthesis.

trisodium EDTA—a preservative. *See also* tetrasodium EDTA.

trisodium HEDTA (trisodium hydroxy EDTA)—a preservative. *See also* tetrasodium EDTA.

trisodium hydroxy EDTA—*see* trisodium HEDTA.

tristearin—an emollient.

trolamine—*see* triethanolamine.

tropocollagen—sometimes known as soluble collagen. It has excellent moisture-binding properties and forms a moisture-retentive film on the skin. Formulations using tropocollagen instead of regular collagen are reported to provide a smoother, silkier afterfeel on the skin. The fibroblast produces tropocollagen, which is polymerized into collagen. Tropocollagen is obtained from animal connective tissues. *See also* collagen.

tropoelastin (soluble elastin)—the soluble precursor to elastin, it plays a role in elastin production. Apparently it can compensate for the loss of (and aging of) the skin's own elastin. Reported to be more effective when applied on the skin than regular elastin. *See also* elastin.

tryptophan—one of the 21 amino acids comprising a protein. Tryptophan is a component of the skin's natural moisturizing factors. *See also* amino acid.

turmeric (Curcuma longa)—healing, tonic, mildly stimulating, anti-inflammatory, and has blood-purifying properties. This common spice (used frequently in curry) and coloring agent is used in traditional medicine for a variety of curative purposes, including the treatment of eczema, skin infections, ulcers, burns, and rashes. It may have skin-softening properties and could be beneficial in products for acne.

T

tyramine—clinical studies indicate skin-lightening capacities. Tyramine is a tyrosine derivative.

l-tyrosine—an amino acid. Experiments conducted with *l*-tyrosine in the form of water-soluble derivatives proved that it penetrates the epidermis to the basal layer where the melanocytes are located. Used in suntan accelerators and in skin-bronzing cosmetics to accelerate the tanning process.

tyrosine—an amino acid. Cutaneous applications may produce an extra reserve of tyrosine in the skin, assisting or "activating" melanin synthesis. This in turn should increase and prolong the effect of the tanning process. Tyrosine's effect is improved if the product contains vitamin B (riboflavin) plus an additional compound referred to chemically as ATP (adenosine triphosphate). *See also l*-tyrosine.

T

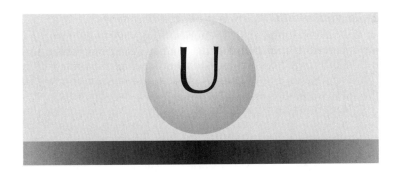

ubiquinone—also known as coenzyme Q10. A powerful antioxidant that is naturally found in the cells. It acts as a free radical neutraliser.

ucuuba oil—also known as *Virola sebifera nut oil.* Emollient, humectant, skin conditioning, and antiseptic. This nut oil is said to be rich in myristic acid. It is used generally in soaps, cleansers, massage lotions, and hair products. *See also* myristic acid.

Ulmus davidiana root extract—an extract derived from the root of the Japanese elm, it is considered anti-inflammatory and moisturizing, with an ability to help improve skin barrier functions. Manufacturers indicate for use in antiaging and acne care products.

ultramarine blue—a color additive. Ultramarines can also be green, pink, red, or violet, and are synthetic pigments composed of complex sodium aluminum sulfosilicated with the proportions of each element varying in each color. It was originally obtained naturally from ground lapis but is now produced synthetically. Used primarily in eye shadows, mascaras, and face powders. *See also* color entry in Chapter 4.

ulve extract—*see* seaweed extract.

ulve seaweed—*see* seaweed extract.

Uncaria tomentosa extract—also known as cat's claw. It is credited with anti-inflammatory, antioxidant, antibacterial, and immunostimulant properties. Among its constituents are alkaloids and tannins. The plant is a woody vine, native to the tropical rainforests of Central and South America.

undecylenoyl PEG 5 paraben—a preservative.

urea—incorporated into cosmetics for a variety of purposes, including moisturizing, desquamating, antimicrobial, and buffering. Urea is regarded as a "true" moisturizer rather than a humectant since it attracts and retains moisture in the corneum layer. It facilitates the natural exfoliation of keratinocytes given its ability to dissolve intercellular cement in the corneum layer. Through its antimicrobial properties that inhibit the growth of micro-organisms in a product, urea's incorporation into a formulation can also be as part of a larger preservative system. This ingredient's buffering action is attributed to its ability to regulate the hydrolipid mantle. In addition, urea is found to enhance the penetration and absorption of other active ingredients, relieve itchiness, and help leave the skin feeling soft and supple. Anti-inflammatory, antiseptic, and deodorizing actions allow it to protect the skin's surface against negative changes and help maintain healthy skin. Studies show that urea does not induce photoallergy, phototoxicity, or sensitization. The safest concentration of use in skin care preparations is between 2 percent and 8 percent. High concentrations of urea seem to be unstable when incorporated into skin care preparations and can also be irritating. Acidic urea solutions can produce burning or stinging sensations.

ursolic acid—helps maintain the look and feel of the skin, and acts as a perfume and to mask odor. Therapeutic benefits in skin care include anti-inflammatory activity. Ursolic acid has demonstrated antimicrobial, antibacterial and antifungal action, as well.

UV absorber 3—a UV absorber. *See* octocrylene.

UVA screen (oil soluble)—a method of indicating that a given product contains sunscreen against UVA without revealing which or of what type. Refer to sunscreen entry in Chapter 4.

UVB screen (oil soluble)—a method of indicating that a given product contains sunscreen against UVB without revealing which or of what type. Refer to sunscreen entry in Chapter 4.

U

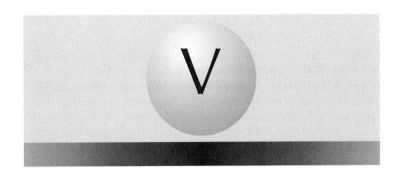

valerian oil *(Valeriana officinalis)*—therapeutic activities include calming, soothing and antispasmodic. It is also incorporated into cosmetic formulations for perfuming, and odor-masking action. Valerian was held in such esteem as a remedy during medieval times that it was called "All Heal." Its composition is complex, with constituents including alkaloids (catinine and valerine), gamma-aminobutyric acid (GABA), volatile oils (particularly valerenic acid to which valerian's sedative properties are attributed), formate, flavones such as hesperidin, and terpenes (for example l-camphene, l-limonene, and l-pinene). The oil is present in the dried root in quantities of 0.5 to 2 percent depending on the plant variety and place of growth. It is obtained by steam distillation. It is reported that when used frequently and in large quantities, valerian oil will produce headaches.

valeric acid—obtained from valerian extract. *See also* valerian oil.

valine—an amino acid used as a skin-conditioning and odor-masking agent. It is more commonly used in hair care preparations than in skin care.

vanilla fruit extract—vanilla fruit is commonly known as vanilla bean. This extract has skin soothing, conditioning, protecting, and smoothing properties.

vanilla fruit oil *(Vanilla planifolia)*—emollient and skin conditioning, it is obtained from the cured, full-grown, unripe fruit of vanilla. It may cause a skin reaction in overly sensitive skin.

vanilla resinoid—part of a natural preservative mixture that also includes linalool, ex-*bois de rose*, *bois de rose*, lemongrass,

V

cedarwood oil, neroli bigarde petals oil, and other such exotic components.

Vaseline fluid—*see* petrolatum.

veegum—*see* magnesium aluminum silicate.

vegetable glyceride (hydrogenated)—an emollient and emulsifying agent obtained from vegetable oil. It is also used as a stabilizer, a viscosity controller, and to facilitate the spreading of a product. The oil source in this case is not identifiable.

vegetable oil—a carrier and an occlusive skin-conditioning agent which may also be incorporated for skin-softening purposes. Such a listing may refer to a variety of oils alone or in combination, including peanut, corn, sesame, olive, and cottonseed. As the extract type of oil is not specified when listed in this fashion, it is difficult to determine the ingredient value or any skin reactions that may arise from the ingredient's use. Vegetable oil is an expressed oil of vegetable origin consisting primarily of triglycerides of fatty acids.

vegetable starch—a thickener.

verbena—*see* vervain oil.

veronica extract (Veronica officinalis)—credited with anti-inflammatory, healing, purifying, tonic, and soothing properties. Some say it promotes healthy tissue growth and a refinement of the pores. There are many species of veronica, with about 20 having been medicinally employed. Regardless of the species, the extract is generally obtained from the plant's flowers, leaves, and stems.

vervain oil (Verbena officinalis) (verbena)—has been credited with astringent and antispasmodic properties. It is a perennial bearing many small, pale lilac flowers.

vetiver oil (Vetiveria zizanioides) (khus-khus)—considered stimulant and tonic, and used in perfumery as well as in cosmetics. The oil, which has an aromatic to harsh woodsy odor, is produced from the roots of a fragrant grass.

violet extract (Viola sp)—traditionally used for soothing and anti-itching skin treatments, and as an antiseptic in skin creams and burn preparations. Violet extract also has cleansing properties. Its important constituents include saponins, antiseptic glycosides (viola quercitin), violine, an alkaloid, salicylic acid, and dye-matter for a blue color. The extract has a slightly sweet, floral scent. While the violet

V

family comprises over 200 species, it is the sweet-scented violet that appears to be most appropriate for botanical use. Violet extract may produce a skin rash in those allergic to this particular plant.

vipers bugloss oil *(Echium plantagineum)*—one fraction of this botanical lipid includes stearidonic acid, a fatty acid with known anti-inflammatory properties. Manufacturer studies indicate that it may reduce the skin's inflammatory response to UV rays. It is useful in sunscreens and sun care products, as well as in antiaging products and anti-inflammatory preparations. Found within the same family as black cohosh and bugbane. *See also* black cohosh extract.

vitamin A—can act as a keratinization regulator, helping to improve the skin's texture, firmness, and smoothness. Vitamin A esters, once in the skin, convert to retinoic acid and provide antiaging benefits. Vitamin A is believed to be essential for the generation and function of skin cells. Continued vitamin A deficiency shows a degeneration of dermal tissue, and the skin becomes thick and dry. Surface application of vitamin A helps prevent skin dryness and scaliness, keeping the skin healthy, clear, and infection resistant. Its skin regeneration properties appear enhanced when combined with vitamin E. Vitamin A is a major constituent of such oils as cod liver and shark, and many fish and vegetable oils. *See also* retinol; retinoic acid; retinyl palmitate.

vitamin A palmitate—known as a skin "normalizer." It acts as an antikeratinizing agent, helping the skin stay soft and plump, and improving its water-barrier properties. It is also an antioxidant. Because of its impact on the skin's water-barrier properties, it is useful against dryness, heat, and pollution. It is also suggested for use in sunscreens. Clinical studies with vitamin A palmitate indicate a significant change in skin composition, with increases in collagen, DNA, skin thickness, and elasticity. Vitamin A palmitate's stability is superior to retinol.

V

vitamin B—the literature tends to indicate that B vitamins cannot pass through the layers of the skin and, therefore, are of no value in the skin surface. Current experiments demonstrate, however, that vitamin B_2 acts as a chemical reaction accelerator, enhancing the performance of tyrosine derivatives in suntan-accelerating preparations. *See also* biotin for B_7; panthenol for B_5; pyridoxine tripalmitate for B_6; riboflavin for B_2; thiamine HCL for vitamin B_1.

vitamin C—a well-known antioxidant. Its effect on free-radical formation when topically applied to the skin by means of a cream has not been clearly established. The effectiveness of topical applications has been questioned due to vitamin C's instability (it reacts with water and degrades). Some forms are said to have better stability in water systems. Synthetic analogues such as magnesium ascorbyl phosphate are among those considered more effective, as they tend to be more stable. When evaluating its ability to fight free-radical damage in light of its synergistic effect with vitamin E, vitamin C shines. As vitamin E reacts with a free radical, it, in turn, is damaged by the free radical it is fighting. Vitamin C comes in to repair the free-radical damage in vitamin E, allowing E to continue with its free-radical scavenging duties. Past research has indicated that high concentrations of topically ap-plied vitamin C are photoprotective, and apparently the vitamin preparation used in these studies resisted soap and water, washing, or rubbing for three days. More current research has indicated that vitamin C does add protection against UVB damage when combined with UVB sunscreen chemicals. This would lead one to conclude that in combi-nation with conventional sunscreen agents, vitamin C may allow for longer-lasting, broader sun protection. Again, the synergism between vitamins C and E can yield even better results, as apparently a combination of both provides very good protection from UVB damage. However, vitamin C appears to be significantly better than E at protecting against UVA damage. A further conclusion is that the combination of vitamins C, E, and sunscreen offers greater protection that the sum of the protection offered by any of the three ingredi-ents acting alone. Vitamin C also acts as a collagen biosyn-thesis regulator. It is known to control intercellular colloidal substances such as collagen, and when formulated into the proper vehicles, can have a skin-lightening effect. It is said to be able to help the body fortify against infectious condi-tions by strengthening the immune system. There is some evidence (although debated) that vitamin C can pass through the layers of the skin and promote healing of tissue damaged by burns or injury. It is found, therefore, in burn ointments and creams used for abrasions. Vitamin C is also popular in antiaging products. Current studies indicate possible anti-inflammatory properties as well. *See also* ascorbic acid.

vitamin C ester—said to promote a visible renewal of the skin's appearance, resulting in skin that looks brighter, firmer,

V

and healthier. This is a general category, however, and the listing does not indicate the form of the ester incorporated into the product. For example, the ester could be either ascorbyl palmitate or magnesium ascorbyl phosphate, where the first has both antioxidant and odor-masking properties, while the second is used for antioxidant activity but does not provide an odor-masking function.

vitamin D—acts as a keratinization regulator, helping to improve skin feel and firmness with repeated use. This vitamin is absorbed through the skin's outer layers. Studies are indicating that vitamin D is an important factor in epidermal cell turnover. It is generally found in combination with vitamin A, as such a mixture appears to help epithelial growth and promote good skin pigmentation. Like vitamin A, vitamin D is a major constituent of many fish and vegetable oils.

vitamin E (D-alpha-tocopherol; DL-alpha-tocopherol; tocopherol)—considered the most important oil-soluble antioxidant and free-radical scavenger. Studies indicate that vitamin E performs these functions when applied topically. It is also a photoprotectant, and it helps protect the cellular membrane from free-radical damage. In addition, vitamin E serves a preservative function due to its ability to protect against oxidation. This benefits not only the skin, but also the product in terms of longevity. As a moisturizer, vitamin E is well-absorbed through the skin, demonstrating a strong affinity with small blood vessels and an ability to enhance blood circulation in the skin. It is also considered to improve the skin's water-binding ability. In addition, vitamin E emulsions have been found to reduce transepidermal water loss, thereby improving the appearance of rough, dry, and damaged skin. This vitamin is also believed to help maintain the connective tissue. There is evidence that vitamin E is effective in preventing irritation due to sun exposure: studies show that vitamin E topically applied prior to UV irradiation is protective against epidermal cell damage caused by inflammation. This indicates possible anti-inflammatory properties. Lipid peroxidation in tissues may be one cause of skin aging. Vitamin E, however, appears to counteract decreased functioning of the sebaceous glands and reduce excessive skin pigmentation, which is found to increase almost linearly with age. It is available also as a tocopherol-polypeptide complex that delivers the vitamin in a water-dispersable form. In this way, when incorporated into cosmetic formulations, it does not need other compounds to

V

---

assist in its solubilization. Useful in antiaging creams and lotions, and in UV protective products, tocopherol is a naturally occurring vitamin E found in a variety of cereal germ oils including wheat germ oil. It can also be produced synthetically.

vitamin E acetate (tocopherol acetate)—an antioxidant with skin-moisturizing activity. Given its free-radical scavenging properties, it is useful in UV protective products. Vitamin E acetate is commonly used to replace vitamin E because it is more stable and is converted to vitamin E by the body. *See also* vitamin E.

vitamin E linoleate—a synthetic version of vitamin E. *See also* tocopheryl linoleate; vitamin E.

vitamin F—used in the treatment and care of dry skin. This is the group name for a family of essential fatty acids comprised of arachidonic, linoleic, and alpha-linoleic acids. *See also* arachidonic acid; linoleic acid.

vitamin H—*see* biotin.

vitamin K—helps promote blood clotting and has been used medically to reduce the possibility of bruising after surgery. It is being incorporated into cosmetic preparations, particularly those used for treating dark circles. It could also be used in acne products, and there are studies underway on its efficacy for the treatment of spider veins.

vitamin P—considered a vascular protector and an anti-inflammatory agent, vitamin P is said to promote capillary health and increase resistance to collagen destruction. Vitamin P is a bioflavonoid that can work in conjunction with vitamin C, helping prevent oxidation of the latter. Vitamin P is found in such food sources as apricots, broccoli, citrus fruit pulp, grapes, prunes, and spinach. *See also* bioflavonoid.

VP/eicosene copolymer—can be used for a variety of purposes, including binding, film forming, and to control viscosity.

volcanic sand—mildly abrasive it is used in exfoliating products.

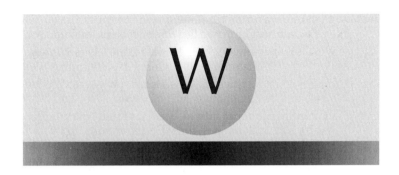

W

walnut extract (Juglans sp.)—traditionally used topically for soothing and anti-itching, as well as against sunburns and other superficial burns. It can be used in cases of acne and skin diseases because of its fungistatic, antiseptic, and astringent properties. Extract is obtained either from the walnut leaf, which is said to be astringent and cleansing, or from the shell, which is considered astringent and emollient with some masking activity. Tannin is a primary constituent of walnut extract.

walnut leaves (Juglans regia)—incorporated into a cosmetic product for astringent, cleansing, scrubbing, skin conditioning, or soothing purposes. They can also be used as bulking agents and to mask odor. Constituents include tannin, flavonoids, vitamin C, and a volatile oil. Studies indicate a potential ability to impact oxidative stress, thereby functioning as an antioxidant.

walnut meal—a mild abrasive. *See also* walnut shell powder.

walnut oil—hydrating, toning, anti-inflammatory, nourishing, and emollient. Walnut oil can help maintain skin suppleness. Its constituents include vitamin E, oleic acid, linolenic acid, and a high percentage of linoleic acid (some sources cite up to 60 percent). Its application includes use in moisturizers, eye creams, and body oils.

W

walnut shell meal—an abrasive. *See also* walnut shell powder.

walnut shell powder—used as an abrasive and bulking agent in cleansers, scrubs, soaps, and masks. It is the powder ground from the shell of English walnuts.

water—listed also as catalyzed, deionized, demineralized, distilled, pure spring, and purified water. Water is an important skin component and is essential for its proper functioning. It is the most common ingredient used in cosmetic formulations and, therefore, is generally listed first on product labels. Water is usually processed to eliminate hardness and minerals, and to avoid product contamination.

water lily extract *(Nymphaea alba)*—soothing. It appears to reduce the temperature and decrease the pain of sun-exposed skin. It is most likely to be incorporated into sensitive skin and post-sun cosmetics. An extract can be obtained from the plant's flower and its root. *See also* lily extract.

watercress extract *(Nasturtium officinale)*—used in folklore for cleansing external ulcers and in night creams for freckles, spots, and acne. An extract derived from both the plant's flower and leaves is credited with helping reduce sebum production. Watercress extract is utilized as a moisture regulator and skin activator for sunburn (and bath) preparations. Important constituents of watercress include minerals, flavonoids, and vitamins. This is a hardy perennial found in abundance near springs and open running watercourses.

wax (self-emulsifying)—can be obtained from insects, animals, and plants such as roses, and each has its own set of characteristics. Beeswax, for example, is glossy and hard but changes to a plastic texture when warm. Wax esters such as lanolin or spermaceti are less greasy, harder, and more brittle than fats. Waxes are generally nontoxic to the skin but, depending on their source, may cause allergic reactions in some sensitive people.

wheat bran extract—considered a moisturizer due to its carbohydrate/sugar components. This is the extract from the broken coat material of wheat grains.

wheat germ extract—used in cosmetics because of its high vitamin E content. This extract is obtained from the wheat kernel embryo separated in milling. *See also* vitamin E.

wheat germ glycerides—softens the skin and has good penetration ability. Commonly used in moisturizers in concentrations of 0.1 to 5 percent. Wheat germ glycerides contain polyunsaturated fats, key for healthy skin. This mixture of mono-, di-, and triglycerides is produced by the transesterification of wheat germ oil. Although some sources indicate it as having an irritancy potential, safety tests show it to be nonsensitizing and nonirritating to the skin. It is considered by some to be somewhat comedogenic.

W

wheat germ oil—an emollient, it helps improve the feel and texture of the skin. The therapeutic benefits associated with wheat germ oil include antioxidant and free-radical scavenging properties, given its vitamin E content, as well as regenerating activity. Additional constituents include vitamins A, B, and D and lecithin. It is cited as appropriate for use in antiaging products, as well as for dry skin, sunburned skin, eczema, and on stretch marks. The oil is obtained by the expression or extraction of wheat germ.

wheat germ oil (unsaponifiable)—acts as a hormone-like cellular messenger. Studies indicate that this activity results in a stimulation of the fibroblast to produce collagen, elastin, proteoglycans, and structural glycoproteins.

wheat protein—has elastic and binding properties, helps reduce the irritating effect of surfactants, and apparently, demonstrates excellent emulsifying action. Given its film-forming abilities on the skin's surface, it also moisturizes and conditions the skin, increasing skin firmness by helping minimize transepidermal water loss. Some forms of wheat protein are said to be able to penetrate down into the wrinkles, forming a film that contracts on drying, causing the flattening out of the skin and a reduction in surface roughness. Wheat protein has an unusually low irritation potential.

wheat protein (soluble)—*see* wheat protein.

wheat starch—used as a demulcent and emollient and in face powders. Wheat starch swells when water is added. It is obtained from wheat.

whey protein—*see* milk protein.

white clover—*see* melilot.

white dead-nettle—*see* white nettle.

white lily bulb extract (Lilium candidum) (Madonna lily)—has antiseptic and soothing properties. The roots contain tannin, gallic acid, mucilage, starch, gum, resin, sugar, ammonia, tartaric acid, and fecula. This is a perennial aquatic herb that grows to the surface of the water from a thick horizontal rootstock.

W

white nettle (Lamium album) (White dead-nettle)—considered astringent, it also is used to mask odor. It is obtained from the plant's flowers or leaves. *See also* nettle.

white sweet lupine extract—*see* lupine extract.

white willow extract (Salix alba)—deodorant with tonic and astringent properties. It is used effectively in products for acne and eczema. The extract is obtained from the bark of this large tree which contains tannin as a chief constituent and a small quantity of salicin. See also willow extract.

wild alum *(Geranium maculatum)*—astringent and deodorant. It is cited as good for oily skin.

wild basil *(Ocimum gratissimum)*—primarily used as a fragrance component in a cosmetic formulation, the essential oil has demonstrated antibacterial and antifungal properties as well.

wild marjoram—*see* wild Spanish marjoram.

wild pansy extract—*see* pansy extract.

wild Spanish marjoram (wild marjoram)—described as having antiseptic and anti-inflammatory botanical properties. *See also* marjoram.

wild thyme extract *(Thymus serpyllum)*—an emollient, tonic, and antiseptic extract traditionally used to clean wounds after washing. Believed not to be as effective as the common variety of thyme. It contains 30 to 70 percent phenols, including thymol and carvacrol. When distilled, some 225 pounds of dried material yield 150 grams of essence. Wild thyme is a perennial herb.

wild yam extract *(Dioscorea villosa)*—helps maintain the skin looking healthy, supple, and in good condition. Given its phtyoestrogen content, sources cited it for use in antiaging and antiwrinkle skin care preparations. The root is the part that is used.

willow extract *(Salix sp.)*—described as antiseptic and skin clearing. The roots and leaves have demulcent, tonic, and astringent properties. Apparently, it is very mild, hence its incorporation in lotions and creams for infants. Willow bark extract provides a natural source of salicylic acid, beneficial for its exfoliating activity.

winterbloom infusion—*see* witch hazel extract.

W

witch hazel distillate—an aqueous solution obtained by distillation of *Hamamelis virginiana* twigs. *See also* witch hazel extract.

witch hazel extract *(Hamamelis virginiana)* **(hamamelis; winterbloom)**—traditionally used in the topical treatment of burns, sunburns, skin irritation, insect bites, and bruises. It is credited with anti-inflammatory, astringent, and wound-healing properties. It is often used for its anti-itching, softening, and emollient properties. In addition, anti-free radical activity is now associated with witch hazel, thereby helping counter the damaging effects of UVA, while acting as an absorber of both UVA and UVB. Ideal applications for witch hazel are in sun preparations, after-sun preparations, and creams that strive to regenerate overstrained skin. It can be formulated effectively into gels as an antiseptic preparation for treating impure, greasy skin. Some sources cite a recommended dosage of 2 to 5 percent for use in formulations. Obtained from the leaves and bark of the plant.

wood alcohol—*see* alcohol.

wood sage—*see* germander extract.

wool wax alcohols—*see* lanolin alcohol.

wormwood *(Artemisia absinthium)*—attributed actions include perfuming, antimicrobial, and skin conditioning. Given its azulene content, it might also be used for some natural coloring. Among its other constituents are a complex bitter (absinthin), succinic acid, thujyl alcohol, thujyl acetate, thujone, phellandrene, candinene, tannin, and vitamins B and C.

woundwort extract *(Stachys sylvatica and Stachys palustris)*—in herbal medicine, it is considered antiseptic, astringent, and tonic. The extract, obtained from the leaves, has been credited with an ability to stop bleeding and to heal wounds.

W

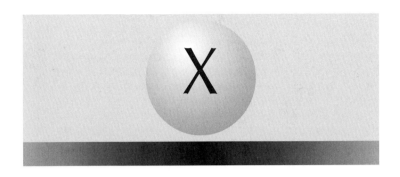

xanthan gum (corn starch gum)—serves as a texturizer, carrier agent, and gelling agent in cosmetic preparations. It also stabilizes and thickens formulations. This is the gum produced through a fermentation of carbohydrate and *Anthomonas camestris.*

xanthophylls—a family of biochemicals that are oxygenated derivatives of caratenoids. They can be used as colorants (red to yellow) and for apparent antioxidant and anti–free radical properties. Some studies now indicate UV protection capacities, as well. Astaxanthin, lutein, and zeaxanthin are examples of xanthophylls. Both lutein and zeaxanthan appear to limit UV-induced skin damage. *See also* astaxanthin.

xylitol—a humectant and skin conditioning agent. It acts as a humidifier, drawing moisture from the air for skin absorption. Some manufacturers also cite a soothing and antimicrobial action. Xylitol is a naturally occurring sugar in birch bark and a range of fibrous fruits and vegetables, including corn.

xyloglucan—a fraction of tamarind extract. *See* tamarind.

X

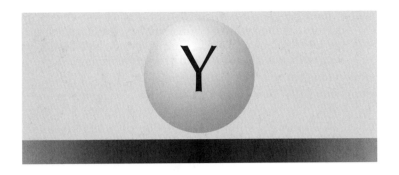

yarrow extract *(Achillea millefolium)* ***(Achillea extract; milfoil)***—general effects attributed to yarrow include anti-inflammatory and antispasmodic. It is famous in folkloric medicine for stopping the bleeding of wounds and nosebleeds. Studies indicate an antibiotic effect and an ability to reduce the blood's clotting time. Yarrow extract is also described as having astringent, antiseptic, anti-inflammatory, healing, and calming properties. Considered good in the care of oily and acne skins. Yarrow's important constituents include flavonoids, amino acids, sugars, and phytosterols. It grows everywhere: in grass, meadows, pastures, and by the roadside. Since it creeps by its roots and multiplies by its seeds, yarrow becomes a troublesome weed in gardens. The whole plant is used in making the extract.

yeast—has a rubefactant effect on the skin, making it good for pale, yellow skins. It is used in face masks designed to give the skin a ruddy color. Yeast is a fungus whose usual and dominant growth form is unicelluar. It can be irritating to dry or sensitive skins. *See also* malt.

yeast extract—manufacturers claim it is able to revitalize the skin with moisture, fight dryness, and give the skin a radiant appearance. In addition, it is claimed that yeast extract has the ability to minimize the dryness and pain associated with sunburned and wind-chapped skin; restore the comfort of soft, elastic, and healthy skin; reduce facial lines; and improve dry skin. Its constituents include enzymes, vitamins, sugars, and mineral substances.

Y

yellow toadflax (Linaria vulgaris)—also known as wild snap-dragon. Credited with anti-inflammatory, astringent, cleansing, and draining properties. Constituents include flavonoids such as linarin, glycosides, and a variety of organic acids.

ylang-ylang extract—*see* ylang-ylang oil.

ylang-ylang oil (Cananga odorata and Unona odorantissimum)—used in folklore as a scenting agent and for insect bites. Ylang-ylang is found to be relaxing and an excellent anti-stress agent. In addition, it is credited with antiseptic, softening, smoothing, rejuvenating, calming, soothing, and antispasmodic properties. It is good for inflamed and/or irritated skin and for controlling acne. Ylang-ylang oil is said to help balance the skin and work to reduce oiliness. Along with its therapeutic effects, ylang-ylang is also believed to be effective in its tension-relieving properties, since a variety of skin disorders such as acne and eczema can be aggravated by stress. Some sources cite that it takes roughly 100 pounds of blossoms to produce about two pounds of essential oil. This oil is produced by means of steam distillation into a fragrant, yellowish oil of varying grades.

ylang-ylang water—*see* ylang-ylang oil.

yomogi extract—a botanical said to have moisturizing and soothing properties.

yucca (Yucca sp.)—the various species of yucca are used in cosmetic formulations for masking odor and protecting the skin against aggressive factors (extreme climates, for example). An extract made from the leaves, stems, and roots of the *schidigera* variety is also attributed with cleaning and surfactant action. Some studies indicate anti-inflammatory and antioxidant/free-radical scavenging activity. Yucca's constituents include phytoestrogen and a high level of saponins. Generally, the root or the stalk is the part that is used. However, the flower can also be used and is said to have antifungal properties.

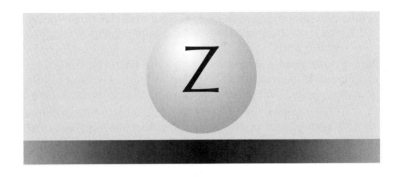

zinc—described as an oligoelement, trace element, or micro-nutrient. Zinc is believed to accelerate wound-healing and offer protection against UV radiation. It appears to favor the sulfur uptake in sulfurated amino acids and facilitates the incorporation into the skin of the cystine amino acid. It also has a synergistic effect with vitamins A and E. Zinc is a structural component or, at the very least, a part of more than 70 metal enzymes, and promotes collagen synthesis in the dermis and keratinization of the corneum layer. Zinc is useful for acne treatments since it lowers sebaceous secretion, and is also used in the treatment of psoriasis.

zinc aspartate—a skin-conditioning agent. Zinc aspartate is the zinc salt of aspartic acid.

zinc gluconate—helps maintain the skin in good condition and is a deodorant. Zinc gluconate could also be effectively used in antiacne products. *See also* zinc.

zinc oxide—has been used to protect, soothe, and heal the skin. Zinc oxide provides an excellent barrier to the sun and other irritants. It is somewhat astringent, antiseptic, and antibacterial. When used in sunscreen preparations, it provides both UVA and UVB protection, and can contribute to and/or increase SPF. At the appropriate particle size, zinc oxide is transparent in the visible light spectrum but opaque in the UVC ranges, thereby avoiding a whitening effect when incorporated into sunscreen preparations. Zinc oxide is included on the FDA's list of approved sunscreen chemicals. It demonstrates an impressive synergistic effect when combined with organic sunscreens. Zinc oxide is also used when a white color is desired for a product. It is obtained from zinc ore, a commonly found mineral, and is relatively nonallergenic.

zinc pyrithione—a preservative against bacteria, fungi, and yeast. It is unstable in light and in the presence of oxidizing agents. Zinc pyrithione is useful in gels, creams, heavy lotions, and talcum powder.

zinc stearate—used in cosmetic formulations to increase adhesive properties. It is also used as a coloring agent. This is a mixture of the zinc salts of stearic and palmitic acids.

zinc sulfate—a cosmetic astringent and biocide produced through the reaction of sulfuric acid with zinc. It is irritating to the skin and mucous membranes, and may cause an allergic reaction.

Zingiber cassumunar—also known as plai. The extract is obtained from the plant's leaves and flowers and can help improve a product's smell, as well as helping improve skin feel. The root may be used either in extract, oil, or powder forms to mask odor, maintain skin condition, and serve as a humectant. The essential oil has exhibited antifungal and antimicrobial capacities.

PART III

Appendix: Botanical Latin Names

Botanical Latin Names

Acacia senegal—acacia
Achillea millefolium—milfoil, yarrow
Aesculus hippocastanum—horse chestnut
Agrimonia eupatoria—agrimony
Alchemilla vulgaris—alchemilla, lady's mantle
Aleurites moluccana—kukui nut oil
Allium satiuum—garlic
Aloe vera—aloe vera
Alternifolia—see *Melaleuca alternifolia*
Althaea officinalis—althea
Andira araoba—goa
Anemone sp.—anemone
Angelica sp.—angelica
Anthemis nobilis—Roman chamomile
Arboresenes artemesia—southernwood
Arctium lappa—burdock
Arctostaphylos uva-urusi—bearberry
Areca catechu—areca nut palm, betel nut palm
Armoracia lapathifolia—horseradish
Arnica montana—arnica
Artemisia absinthium—wormwood

Artemisia dracunculus—tarragon
Avena sativa—oat

Bellis perennis—daisy
Berberis vulgaris—barberry
Beta vulgaris—beet
Betula sp.—birch
Bixa orellana—annatto
Borago officinalis—borage
Boswellia thurifera—frankincense

Calamintha officinalis—calamint
Calendula officinalis—calendula
Calophyllum inophyllum—tamanu
Camellia sinensis L.—green tea
Cananga odorata—ylang-ylang
Capsella bursa pastoris—shepherd's purse
Capsicum annuum—pepper
Carduus marianus—milk thistle
Carica papaya—papaya
Caroba balsam—carob
Carthamus tinctorius—safflower
Carum carvi—caraway
Caryophyllus aromaticus—clove
Cassia angustifolia—senna
Castanea sativa—chestnut
Centaurea cyanus—cornflower
Centella asiatica—gotu kola
Certraria islandica—Iceland moss
Chondrus crispus—carrageen, Irish moss
Chrysanthemum parthenium—feverfew

Cimicifuga racemosa—black cohosh
Cinchona ledgeriana—cinchona
Cinnamomum camphora—camphor
Cinnamomum zeylanicum—cinnamon
Citrus acida—lime
Citrus aurantifolia—lime
Citrus aurantium—bitter orange, Italian orange
Citrus bergamia—bergamot
Citrus limonum—lemon extract
Citrus paradisi—grapefruit
Citrus reticulata—tangarine
Citrus sinensis—sweet orange
Cochlearia officinalis—scurvy grass
Cola acuminata—kola tree
Coleus barbatus—coleus
Commiphora meccanensis—balm of Gilead
Commiphora myrrha—myrrh
Commiphora opobalsamum—balm of Gilead
Coriandrum sativum—coriander
Crataegus oxyacantha—hawthorn
Cucumis sativus—cucumber
Cupressus sp.—cypress
Curcubita pepo—pumpkin
Curcuma longa—turmeric
Cymbopogon citratus—lemongrass
Cymbopogon martini—palmarosa
Cymbopogon nardus—citronella
Cynara scolymus—artichoke

Daucus carota—carrot
Dioscorea villosa—wild yam
Dipteryx odorata—tonka bean
Dryopteris sp.—fern

Echinacea angustifolia—echinacea
Echium plantagineum—vipers bugloss oil
Elettaria cardamomum—cardamom
Equisetum arvense—horsetail
Eucalyptus globulus—eucalyptus
Eugenia caryophyllus—clove
Euphrasia officinalis—eyebright
Euterpe oleracea—açai
Evernia furfuracea—treemoss
Evernia prunastri—oakmoss

Fagus sylvatica—beech
Filipendula ulmaria—meadowsweet
Foeniculum vulgare—fennel
Fragaria vesca—strawberry
Fucus vesiculosus—fucus seaweed
Fumaria officinalis—fumitory

Galium aparine—cleavers
Gentiana sp.—gentian
Geranium maculatum—crane's bill
Geum urbanum—avens
Ginkgo biloba—ginkgo
Glycyrrhiza glabra—licorice
Gnaphalium polycephalum—everlasting
Guaiacum officinale—guaiac

Hamamelis virginiana—witch hazel
Harpagophytum procumbens—devil's claw
Hedera helix—ivy
Helianthus annuus—sunflower
Hibiscus sp.—hibiscus
Hordeum vulgare—barley
Humulus lupulus—hops
Hydrastis canadensis—goldenseal
Hydrocotyl asiatica—gotu kola
Hypericum perforatum—St. John's wort
Hyssopus officinalis—hyssop

Inula helenium—elecampane
Iris sp.—iris

Jacaranda procera—carob
Jasminum officinale—jasmine
Jatropha manihot—tapioca
Juglans sp.—walnut
Juniperus communis—juniper

Lactuca virosa—lettuce
Laminaria digitata—seaweed
Lamium album—white nettle, blind nettle
Lamnanthes alba—meadowfoam
Laurus nobilis—laurel

Lavandula officinalis—lavender
Lawsonia inermis—henna
Lentinus edodes—shiitake mushroom
Levisticum officinale—lovage
Lilium candidum—white lily
Linaria vulgaris—common toadflax; yellow toadflax
Lonicera fragrantissima—honeysuckle
Lycium barbarum—boxthorn, goji berry, matrimony vine, wolfberry
Lycopodium clavatum—club moss

Macademia integrifolia—macadamia nut tree
Malva sylvestris—mallow
Manihot utilissima—tapioca
Matricaria chamomilla—German chamomile
Medicago sativa—alfalfa
Melaleuca alternifolia—tea tree
Melaleuca leucadendron—cajeput
Melilotus officinalis—melilot
Melissa officinalis—balm mint
Mentha sp.—mint
Mentha piperita—peppermint
Mentha viridis—spearmint
Monarda didyma—bergamot
Morus sp.—mulberry
Myrica cerifera—bayberry
Myristica fragrans—nutmeg
Myrospermum toluiferum—balsam of tolu
Myroxylon pereirae—balsam of Peru

Narcissus poeticus—narcuissus
Nasturtium officinale—watercress
Nymphaea alba—water lily

Ocimum basilicum—basil
Ocimum gratissimum —wild basil
Oenothera biennis—evening primrose
Olea europaea—olive
Ononis arvensis—restharrow
Ononis spinosa—restharrow
Orchis sp.—orchid
Origanum majorana—sweet marjoram
Origanum vulgare—marjoram
Oryza sativa—rice

Paeonia officinalis—peony
Panax sp.—ginseng
Papaver sp.—poppy
Papaver rhoeas—red poppy
Passiflora incarnata—passion flower
Pelargonium sp.—geranium
Petroselinum sativum—parsley
Phaseolus aureus—mung bean
Phaseolus vulgaris—bean
Phoradendron flavescens—American mistletoe
Picea excelsa—spruce
Picraena excelsa—quassia
Pimpinella anisum—anise
Pinus sp.—pine

Plantago sp.—plantain
Pogostemon patchouli—patchouli
Potentilla anserina—cinquefoil
Potentilla tormentilla—tormentil
Primula officinalis—primula
Prunus amygdalus amara—bitter almond
Prunus amygdalus dulcis—sweet almond
Prunus cerasus—sour cherry
Prunus persica—peach
Psoralea coryfolia—potato
Pyrola elliptica—shinleaf
Pyrus cydonia—quince
Pyrus malus—apple

Quercus sp.—oak

Rhamnus purshiana—casacara sagrada
Rheum palmatum—rhubarb
Rhus glabra—sumac
Ribes nigrum—black currant
Ribes rubrum—red currant
Ricinus communis—castor oil plant
Rosa sp.—rose
Rosa moscatta—musk rose
Rosmarinus officinalis—rosemary
Rubus idaeus—raspberry
Rubus villosus—blackberry
Rumex acetosa—sorrel
Ruscus aculeatus—butchersbroom

Salix sp.—willow
Salvia officinalis—sage
Salvia sclarea—clary sage
Sambucus sp.—elder
Sanguinaria canadensis—bloodroot, tetterwort
Santalum album—sandalwood
Saponaria officinalis—soapwort
Sassafras albidum—sassafras
Satureia hortensis—savory
Scrophularia nodosa—figwort
Sempervivum tectorum—hens and chicks; houseleek; stonecrop
Silybum marianum—lady's thistle
Simmondsia chinensis—jojoba
Smilax officinalis—sarsasparilla
Solanum lycopersicum—tomato
Solidago sp.—goldenrod
Sorbus aucuparia—mountain ash; rowan
Spinacia oleracea—spinach
Spireae ulmaria—meadowsweet
Stachys officinalis—betony
Stachys palustris—woundwort, marsh
Stachys syluatica—woundwort, hedge
Symphytum officinale—comfrey
Syzygium aromaticum—clove

Tamarindus indica—tamarind
Taraxacum officinale—dandelion
Taraktogenos kurzii—chaulmoogra
Teucrium scorodonia—germander
Thuja occidentalis—cedar
Thymus sp.—thyme

Thymus serpyllum—wild thyme
Tilia sp.—linden
Trifolium sp.—clover
Trigonella foenumgraecum—fenugreek
Tropaeolum majus—nasturtium
Turnera aphrodisiaca—damiana
Tussilago farfara—coltsfoot

Ulmus sp.—elm
Ulmus fulva—slippery elm
Unona odorantissimum—ylang-ylang
Urtica dioica—nettle

Valeriana officinalis—valerian
Vanilla planifolia—vanilla
Verbena officinalis—vervain
Veronica officinalis—veronica
Vetiveria zizanioides—vetiver, khus-khus
Viola sp.—violet
Viola tricolor—pansy
Virola sebifera—ucuuba
Viscum album—European mistletoe

Zingiber officinale—ginger